Technology and Mental Disorders: A Clinician's Guide to Improving Mental Health

Technology and Mental Disorders: A Clinician's Guide to Improving Mental Health

Editor: John Dalvi

AMERICAN
MEDICAL PUBLISHERS
www.americanmedicalpublishers.com

AMERICAN
MEDICAL PUBLISHERS
www.americanmedicalpublishers.com

Cataloging-in-Publication Data

Technology and mental disorders : a clinician's guide to improving mental health / edited by John Dalvi.
p. cm.
Includes bibliographical references and index.
ISBN 979-8-88740-488-2
1. Psychotherapy--Technological innovations. 2. Psychotherapy--Data processing.
3. Psychology, Pathological. 4. Mental illness. 5. Mental health. 6. Information storage and retrieval systems--Mental health. I. Dalvi, John.
RC489.D35 T43 2023
616.891 402 85--dc23

American Medical Publishers,
41 Flatbush Avenue,
1st Floor, New York,
NY 11217, USA

ISBN 979-8-88740-488-2 (Hardback)

Contents

Preface

Mental illness or mental health disorders refer to a group of mental health conditions that affect the mood, thinking, and behavior. There are several types of mental health disorders including depression, anxiety disorders, schizophrenia, eating disorders, and addictive behaviors. Mental illnesses can be caused by a variety of environmental and genetic factors such as inherited traits, brain chemistry, and environmental exposure to stressors and toxins before birth. Some common signs and symptoms of mental disorders are feeling sad, confused thinking, lower concentration, excessive fears or worries, extreme feelings of guilt, extreme mood changes of highs and lows, withdrawal from friends and activities, etc. Psychiatrists diagnose mental disorders through medical history, lab tests, and psychological evaluation. The treatment of mental disorders varies according to the type of disorder. Some of the commonly used classes of prescription psychiatric medications include antidepressants, anti-anxiety disorders, and mood-stabilizing medications. Lately, technological advancements such as AI-assisted therapy, virtual reality, digital pills, and digital symptom tracking are being increasingly used in the treatment of mental disorders. This book is a comprehensive guide to improving mental health. It aims to shed light on the relationship between mental disorders and technology. This book is a vital tool for all researching and studying this field.

The researches compiled throughout the book are authentic and of high quality, combining several disciplines and from very diverse regions from around the world. Drawing on the contributions of many researchers from diverse countries, the book's objective is to provide the readers with the latest achievements in the area of research. This book will surely be a source of knowledge to all interested and researching the field.

In the end, I would like to express my deep sense of gratitude to all the authors for meeting the set deadlines in completing and submitting their research chapters. I would also like to thank the publisher for the support offered to us throughout the course of the book. Finally, I extend my sincere thanks to my family for being a constant source of inspiration and encouragement.

Editor

Telemonitoring in Chronic Pain Management Using Smartphone Apps: A Randomized Controlled Trial Comparing Usual Assessment Against App-Based Monitoring with and without Clinical Alarms

Carlos Suso-Ribera [1,*], Diana Castilla [2,3], Irene Zaragozá [3], Ángela Mesas [4], Anna Server [4], Javier Medel [4] and Azucena García-Palacios [1,3]

1 Department of Basic and Clinical Psychology and Psychobiology, Universitat Jaume I, 12071 Castellón, Spain; azucena@uji.es
2 Department of Personality, Assessment, and Psychological Treatments, Universidad de Valencia, 46010 Valencia, Spain; diana.castilla@uv.es
3 Ciber Fisiopatologia Obesidad y Nutricion (CB06/03 Instituto Salud Carlos III) (Ciber Physiopathology Obesity and Nutrition, CB06/03 Instituto Salud Carlos III Health Institute), 28029 Madrid, Spain; irenezaragoza@gmail.com
4 Pain Clinic, Vall d'Hebron Hospital, 08035 Barcelona, Spain; amesas@vhebron.net (Á.M.); aserver@vhebron.net (A.S.); fjmedel@vhebron.net (J.M.)
* Correspondence: susor@uji.es

Abstract: Background. The usefulness of mHealth in helping to target face-to-face interventions for chronic pain more effectively remains unclear. In the present study, we aim to test whether the Pain Monitor mobile phone application (app) is well accepted by clinicians, and can help improve existent medical treatments for patients with chronic musculoskeletal pain. Regarding this last goal, we compared three treatment conditions, namely usual treatment, usual treatment with an app without alarms and usual treatment with an app with alarms. All treatments lasted one month. The three treatments were compared for all outcomes, i.e., pain severity and interference, fatigue, depressed mood, anxiety and anger. Methods. In this randomized controlled trial, the usual monitoring method (i.e., onsite; $n = 44$) was compared with daily ecological momentary assessment using the Pain Monitor app—both with ($n = 43$) and without alarms ($n = 45$). Alarms were sent to the clinicians in the presence of pre-established undesired clinical events and could be used to make treatment adjustments throughout the one-month study. Results. With the exception of anger, clinically significant changes (CSC; 30% improvement) were greater in the app + alarm condition across outcomes (e.g., 43.6% of patients experienced a CSC in depressed mood in the app + alarm condition, which occurred in less than 29% of patients in the other groups). The clinicians were willing to use the app, especially the version with alarms. Conclusions. The use of apps may have some benefits in individual health care, especially when using alarms to tailor treatments.

Keywords: chronic pain; smartphone app; telemonitoring; ecological momentary assessment; randomized controlled trial

---

1. Introduction

Chronic Pain: A Major Public Health Challenge

Chronic pain is a multidimensional, distressing experience that can occur with or without tissue damage and persists over extended periods of time (at least three months) [1]. This disease is a public health problem worldwide [2]. Specifically, it is currently estimated that chronic pain affects between 20% and 30% of the adult population worldwide [3–8] and up to 70% of adults older than 65 years [9]. As a consequence, chronic pain has become the most expensive disease in the world [10] and accounts for up to 2% of the annual European gross domestic product [11]. Additionally, with the age distribution shifting towards the elderly [12], the economic burden of this disease is likely to increase in the coming years.

In this scenario, various efforts have been made to improve chronic pain treatments in recent decades. However, existing reviews only provide modest support for the most popular chronic pain treatments, including medical interventions, physical therapy, psychological treatment—or a combination of these [13–15]. Several factors, such as patient characteristics, unexplored genetic or biomechanical mechanism factors or the experience of therapists, could help explain the modest effectiveness of existing treatments for chronic pain. However, some authors have suggested that inadequate monitoring of patient progress and response to treatment is likely to be, at least in part, responsible for the limited impact of current therapies for chronic pain [16,17].

Due to its chronic nature, management of chronic pain often requires prolonged and regular contact with the health care system [18]. In this sense, it is important to note that a move towards self-management will be needed, rather than relying on the care of health professionals [19]. However, in doing so, monitoring could still remain a challenge because limited resources and existing waiting lists in public health settings limit the quality of patient monitoring in chronic pain settings [20,21]. For example, pain treatment follow-up is still predominantly discrete during on-site appointments. This is problematic because pain-related variables, such as pain intensity, mood, and fatigue can vary across and within days [22,23], even in patients with chronic pain such as osteoarthritis [24], rheumatic diseases [25], multiple sclerosis [23] and fibromyalgia [26].

The aforementioned variability of symptoms in patients with chronic pain means that a single measure may not be representative of the entire experience. Furthermore, retrospective pain assessment leads to recall bias and reduces accuracy [27]. This could be minimized with paper diaries. However, research has shown that the use of paper diaries is problematic due to participant noncompliance (missing data and back-filling) and errors associated with manual data entry [28,29]. Additionally, neither episodic on-site assessment nor paper diaries permit timely communication and response to undesired events experienced by the patient during the course of treatment [20].

Another problem related to the current model of care in chronic pain refers to decision-making in the face of unwanted events. Specifically, the current approach to care requires patients to judge when an undesired event is problematic and what is the preferred action to take in the face of that event [30–32]. This approach is problematic, as some patients may tolerate serious or even urgent problems (e.g., tachycardia, severe drowsiness, or persistent vomiting, diarrhea or urine retention) for too long, while others may seek care for symptoms that are less urgent or not problematic (e.g., very mild or short-term). For patients with chronic pain, an added problem is that patients combine appointments with their general practitioner, emergency services and specialized pain clinics for the treatment of their pain and related symptoms [33]. This practice is likely to be problematic, as the alternation of different specialized and nonspecialized services could lead to unpredictable treatment plans in response to unwanted events.

Telemonitoring with episodic phone calls, which is becoming an increasingly common practice, also only partially solves the aforementioned problems. First, because undesired events (e.g., side medication effects or decreased treatment effectiveness) can occur at different treatment stages [34], which means that control calls will often occur before or long after unwanted events occur. Additionally, because such phone calls require the active participation of a healthcare professional, which makes this procedure resource-consuming and ineffective [18].

Taking all the previous into account, it has been argued that our societies will not be able to sustain the current model of care for this condition [20,21,35,36], especially due to the aging of the population and the dramatic increase in the prevalence of this disease in the elderly [9]. Indeed, this appears to be true now more than ever as a result of the COVID-19 crisis, imposed restrictions on circulation and saturation of health systems [37]. Our team has already achieved some important goals in the design, development and implementation of a new tool, namely a smartphone app called Pain Monitor, which facilitates regular assessment of patient outcomes using mobile technology and minimal healthcare professional involvement in assessment. The app, which has been developed by a multidisciplinary team including physicians, nurses, psychologists and engineers following guidelines on pain research and eHealth [38–41], was found to have valid content (i.e., comparable to well-established paper-and-pencil measures) and high patient acceptability (i.e., response rates greater than 70% for daily responses over a period of one month) [42]. While important milestones have been achieved, the utility of the app in terms of increased treatment effectiveness (e.g., further reduction in pain severity and associated symptoms) remains unclear.

In fact, although it has been argued that mobile technology (mHealth)—especially the use of smartphone apps—facilitates this paradigm shift towards telemonitoring in chronic pain care, reviews on this topic have evidenced that randomized controlled trials (RCT) evaluating the usefulness of these tools are lacking in the chronic pain literature [39,41,43–45]. Therefore, the current investigation constitutes an important step forward into the literature on this important public health condition. In particular, the goal of the present study is to test whether incorporating the Pain Monitor app into routine medical treatment results in better pain-related outcomes in patients with chronic musculoskeletal pain. As a secondary objective, we want to investigate the opinion of healthcare professionals on the app (the patients' opinion was already evaluated in the validation study [42]), which is key for future implementation [46].

This RCT had three conditions, i.e., usual treatment (TAU) with the usual assessment method (episodic, combined on-site and by phone call), TAU with app-based assessment without clinical alarms and TAU with app-based assessment with clinical alarms. Eligible patients were adults with chronic musculoskeletal pain, the most common chronic pain condition, which included pain in the bones, muscles, nerves, ligaments or tendons [47]. As recommended in the guidelines, we focus not only on the effectiveness of mHealth in pain severity levels [38]. In particular, outcomes also include interference of pain on functioning, fatigue and mood (depression, anxiety and anger).

The study goal is to compare the response to one month of usual pain treatment for patients in the three monitoring conditions, namely usual episodic monitoring, monitoring with an app without clinical alarms and monitoring with an app with clinical alarms. All patients received the usual treatment for their pain, so differences in outcomes (pain severity and interference, fatigue and mood) across outcomes were expected to occur as a consequence of the assigned monitoring condition. Another goal was to investigate the opinions about the app of health professionals involved in the study (e.g., in charge of disseminating the study, helping download the app and proposing the treatment).

We expected that the use of the app with alarms that were sent to the healthcare professional in the presence of unwanted clinical events would allow a quick detection of patient suffering (see the alarms in Appendix A), including severe pain levels, side medication effects, high interference of pain on functioning and psychological distress, as well as a quick reaction to these events. As a consequence of the above, we anticipated that patients in the app + alarm condition (telemonitoring) would report a greater reduction in pain severity, pain interference, fatigue, depressed mood, anxiety and anger. Additionally, we expected that patients in this condition would also experience unwanted clinical events (e.g., poor treatment response or undesired clinical events associated with treatment onset) for a shorter time compared to treatment as usual or treatment as usual with the app, but without alarms. In relation to the professionals' opinion on the app, we expected that the professionals would experience some burden as they help patients to download the app and respond to alarms. However, we also anticipated that they would perceive the app to be useful and would be willing to use it in the future, preferably the version with alarms.

2. Materials and Methods

The study protocol—including a description of the planned procedures and analyses—was published before starting the recruitment [18]. However, we summarize the main study characteristics, as well as any deviations from the original plan, in the next lines.

The study started in late 2017 and ended in late 2018. All procedures were approved by the ethical review board of the Vall d'Hebron Hospital in Barcelona on 25th, June 2017 and registered on clinicaltrials.gov on 25th, July 2017 (NCT03247725).

2.1. Design

This is a superiority RCT with three conditions: (1) treatment as usual (TAU); (2) TAU + daily assessment using the Pain Monitor app (TAU + app); or (3) TAU + daily assessment using the Pain Monitor app with alarms (TAU + app + alarm). Because we want to ensure that telemonitoring and not the daily response to pain-related items in the app is responsible for patient benefits, we allocated patients using the app into two conditions: telemonitoring (i.e., use of the app with alarms to the physician in the presence of unwanted events detected by the app) and daily app use without alarms. Patients were randomly assigned to the study condition before agreeing to participate. Randomization was performed by an independent researcher with an online randomization tool. There was no allocation ratio. The patients' treating physicians performed the enrollment and assignment to previously randomized conditions. Patients were assigned to conditions based on a random allocation sequence. If they refused to participate because of the assigned condition, the TAU was offered, but they were excluded from the study.

Patients and treating physicians were not blinded to allocation. In the case of patients, this was done for ethical and safety reasons, especially for those using the app without alarms, as they needed to know that the app would not report any adverse event to the physicians. Regarding the medical staff, blinding was not possible because the clinicians had to know that they would receive alarms from a subset of patients, and they had to check their electronic clinical records to decide whether a change in the treatment was required after receiving an alarm. Most assessments were completed by patients, who, as noted earlier, were not blind to their assigned condition for ethical and safety reasons. The only evaluation that was conducted by health professionals, i.e., the follow-up assessment in the TAU group, was as well not blinded. There are several reasons to explain why assessment was not blinded in this case either. For example, calling the patient required accessing to patient personal data, which is restricted to health professionals. Additionally, the TAU condition aimed at recreating the usual practice at the pain clinic, which implies that a health professional is in charge of patient episodic monitoring between appointments. All the physicians at the pain clinic participated in the study, so calls could not be performed by a clinical external to the study and blinded to the patients' condition.

2.2. Participants

The study was advertised by physicians at the pain unit of the Vall d'Hebron Hospital, a tertiary care hospital in Barcelona. The study was presented to all consecutive patients with chronic pain that met the inclusion criteria. Eligibility included being over 18 years of age, not presenting any psychological disorders or problems with language that would make participation difficult, having a mobile phone with Android operating system, accepting the assigned condition and signing the informed consent form. There were no exclusion criterion in terms of previous or existing treatment for pain at study onset or treatment changes during the study, so that the study was as naturalistic as possible, and the sample representative of patients treated at the clinic. In relation to the limitation to Android operating systems, note that by the time the study was conducted the app was only available for Android for economic reasons, as this is the operating system used by more than 90% of phones in Spain [48].

Sample size was calculated a priori with the statistical software G*Power [49] considering previous studies on complications of pain treatments [30,50]. We expected that the rapid detection of such problems using alarms would result in moderate between-group differences in primary outcomes (see below). Taking 80% power, an alpha level of 0.05 and an expected Cohen's d of 0.5, we calculated that 50 participants would be needed in each condition.

2.3. Interventions

All patients received the same intervention (TAU). This consisted of the usual medical treatment for their pain at the pain unit according to the usual practice at the pain clinic and pain guidelines [51,52]. The treatment could include medication (e.g., opioids, antidepressants or anticonvulsants), more invasive techniques (e.g., infiltration) or a combination of both. This treatment was proposed during the first appointment at the clinic (day of baseline assessment). However, if only an infiltration was proposed, because this could only be scheduled one or two weeks later, baseline assessment was postponed until the infiltration was performed. This was done to ensure that baseline assessment occurred on the day of initiation of treatment, regardless of the prescribed treatment.

The prescribed treatment (TAU) remained unchanged during the whole study duration (one month), except when an alarm was received by the clinicians (TAU + app + alarm condition only). Only in this scenario, phone calls were made by the physicians to explore whether a treatment change was required. Alarms were notified to the clinicians on the following working day after their occurrence. These were expected to be responded to on the same day or the next two days, depending on the severity of the alarm.

The duration of the study was set to one month since treatment onset because the clinicians considered that this is a critical period in which most problems with the treatment occur (e.g., poor effect on outcomes or side effects).

2.4. Pain Monitor App

Pain Monitor is a mobile phone app developed for Android, in which patients are asked to respond twice daily during 30 days (morning and evening, at flexible times from 10 am to 12 am and from 7 pm to 9 pm). A reminder is sent to the participant at 10 am and 7 pm and again 90 min later if a response had not been provided. The app incorporates different algorithms which allow sending clinical alarms to professionals (consult Appendix A to see a summary of the parameters that these algorithms follow). The alarms included in this study were established by the medical staff in a joined decision based in clinical experience and research data. The assessment protocol used in the app was validated in a previous study which allowed a reduction of items which can be more effectively used in ecological momentary assessments [42].

In accordance with recommendations from RCT guidelines in pain settings [38], outcomes included pain severity and side effects of the medication (primary outcomes), as well as fatigue, pain interference and mood states, namely depression, anxiety and anger (secondary outcomes). All these items used a 11-point numerical rating scale where 0 indicated the less severe symptomatology (e.g., no pain or sadness) and 10 reflected the most severe levels of symptoms (e.g., most intense pain or sadness). Pain interference on functioning was composed of 4 items, namely interference of pain on sleep, work/housework, leisure and social interactions. Similar to the brief pain inventory [53], an overall interference score was computed as a mean of these items to obtain a measure of overall interference of pain on functioning. For all items, with the exception of pain interference, patients were asked to report on their current status (i.e., current pain severity, fatigue and mood). For interference of pain on functioning, patients were asked to report the experienced interference during the night (interference of pain on sleep) or during the day (interference on work/housework, leisure and social interactions).

In past research, single items for each of these constructs were validated to be used in the Pain Monitor app [42]. To do so, a single item for each construct was correlated with well-established measures of pain severity, pain interference, fatigue and mood. Specifically, pain severity and interference items were validated against the brief pain inventory [53], while fatigue and mood items were validated against the Profile of Mood States [54], the hospital anxiety and depression scale for depression and anxiety [55] and the Beck depression inventory-II for depression [56]. The correlations were found to be significant and moderate in strength. The validated app items can be found in the current study protocol, which can be accessed for free [18]. For the present study purposes, only a subset of the full protocol was used. See items used in the RCT in Appendix B.

The list of adverse symptoms included the most frequent side effects of treatments for pain [52,57,58]. Note that the item that evaluated these physical symptoms did not explicitly refer to side medication effects. This was done to avoid inducing the idea that, if experienced, symptoms were due to the proposed treatment. Thus, the item stated "Please, indicate which of the following symptoms you experienced today (select only those that you do not normally experience)." Note that, even if patients experienced unusual symptoms after treatment onset, these cannot be only attributed to pain treatment, as they could be a consequence of many other factors (e.g., an infection, stress, hormonal changes, etc.).

Daily symptoms were only tracked in the TAU + app and TAU + app + alarm conditions, because these were assessed with the app. Tacking daily symptoms in the TAU group would have required daily calls, which was not feasible and would largely imply a deviation from usual practice at the clinic.

All conditions (TAU, TAU + app and the TAU + app + alarm) completed the aforementioned measures (i.e., single items on pain severity, side effects of the medication, fatigue, pain interference and mood) at baseline (the same day treatment was proposed) and the end of the study (30 days after). However, patients in the TAU + app and the TAU + app + alarm conditions also responded to the protocol twice daily. This was done to control for the effect of daily measuring (TAU + app) and to generate the alarms (TAU + app + alarm). The protocol was automatically prompted in the morning and in the evening to reduce the reliance on the patient's memory.

Patients in the TAU condition completed the protocol as usual, i.e., with paper and pencil at baseline and by phone at the end of study (30 days later). This second measurement was not done face-to-face because patients are usually scheduled no earlier than 4–5 months after the previous appointment. In the TAU follow-up assessment, one of the pain clinic physicians, AM, made the phone calls to the participants. If patients were unavailable, they were called daily for up to three consecutive days. If no response was obtained, this was considered a missing value. The other two groups (TAU + app and TAU + app + alarms) were assessed with the Pain Monitor app at all times. The comparability of the paper-and-pencil and app assessments was not conducted here because the validity of the current assessment protocol across measurement modalities was already performed in past research [42].

The participating clinicians helped patients download the app during the initial appointment and provided support during this first use (completion of baseline evaluation). Patients also received the contact information from the lead researcher, CSR, in case technical problems occurred with the app.

In addition to patient measurement, we explored the professionals' experience with the app. Consistent with the technology acceptance model [59], we evaluated perceived utility ("To what extent do you believe the app is useful for pain management?"), acceptability ("To what extent did you experience burden due to the alarms generated by the app?") and intention to use ("To what extent would you like to use the app with alarms in the future?"). All physicians participating in the study and working at the pain clinic (n = 6) were invited to participate in this survey at the end of the study. All questionnaires were anonymized.

2.5. Data Analysis

First, a descriptive analysis of the sample (i.e., age, sex, marital status, job status, educational level, pain localization and pain duration), including the study flow chart, was conducted. This included an analysis of means and standard deviations for age and percentages for the remaining variables.

Next, we investigated whether randomization resulted in comparable groups in terms of study outcomes (multivariate analysis of variance, MANOVA).

Originally, we planned to explore between and within changes in all study outcomes using a repeated measures MANOVA. However, during the review process it was noted that nonparametric statistics should be used due to the ordinal nature of the measures used (11-point numerical rating scales) [60]. Therefore, we calculated a Kruskal–Wallis H test to compare the change in outcomes under three conditions, as a well as a Friedman test to investigate baseline-to-follow-up changes for each condition. Both analyses were complementary, since the Kruskal–Wallis test provides evidence on between-group differences and the Friedman test reports on within-group evolution. In the Kruskal–Wallis test, the dependent variables were change scores (e.g., end of study pain severity—baseline pain severity) because the test cannot be computed with repeated measures. In Friedman's test, analyses were computed separately for each condition because between-group changes cannot be investigated. Due to multiple comparisons, a more restrictive alpha level of 0.01 was set for the analyses.

Again different from that which was planned, we added an analysis of clinically meaningful improvements at the individual level due to insufficient power and loss in sample size (see the results section). This analysis is recommended in guidelines for pain trials and a reduction in 30% of severity of symptoms is argued to be a useful benchmark, representing at least moderate clinically significant changes (CSC) for the individuals [61,62]. Therefore, a CSC in an outcome for a given individual occurred if follow-up scores (e.g., one month after treatment, i.e., end of study) improved when compared to baseline scores by at least 30% of baseline score. For example, a baseline pain level of 5 and a follow-up pain level of 3 would represent a positive CSC reduction (the follow-up pain level is smaller than $5 - 5 \times 0.3 = 3.5$). Note that this 30% benchmark is only a recommended value based on past research with different outcomes and response scales, including 11-point numeric rating scales as the ones used in the present study [62]. However, change scores have ranged from 30% to 60% across investigations depending on the outcomes and the measures used [61], so the generalizability of our findings should be taken with caution.

As a final step, an analysis of variance (ANOVA) was computed to compare the number of side effects experienced by patients in the app + alarm and patients in the app without alarm conditions. This was followed by an analysis of frequencies of the types of alarms received and the clinicians' opinion about the app. As planned, interim analyses were not conducted because no harm was expected from adding the app to TAU [18].

2.6. *Trial Registration and Ethics*

Trial registration code in ClinicalTrials.gov is NCT03247725. The ethics committee of the Vall d'Hebron Hospital approved the present study and its procedures (code PR(ATR)381/2015).

3. Results

The study flowchart is shown in Figure 1. The initial recruitment plan included 150 chronic pain patients (at least 50 were needed per condition). Because we anticipated some attrition due to the longitudinal nature of the study and the occurrence of technological problems, we recruited 165 patients which were randomly assigned to conditions prior to recruitment. This resulted in 56 patients in the TAU condition, 56 in the TAU + app condition and 53 in the TAU + app + alarms condition. Finally, data were obtained from 44 patients in the TAU condition, 45 patients in the TAU + app condition and 43 patients in the TAU + app + alarm condition, which corresponds to 78.6%, 80.4% and 81.1% of the initial sample, respectively. In the TAU condition, attrition was mainly due to the fact that patients failed to respond to follow-up assessment phone calls (for each patient, up to six phone calls were made over three consecutive days to obtain the follow-up assessment). In the two app conditions, attrition was mainly a result of problems with the phone (e.g., lack of memory or buying a new smartphone during the study due to a failure or malfunction of the old one).

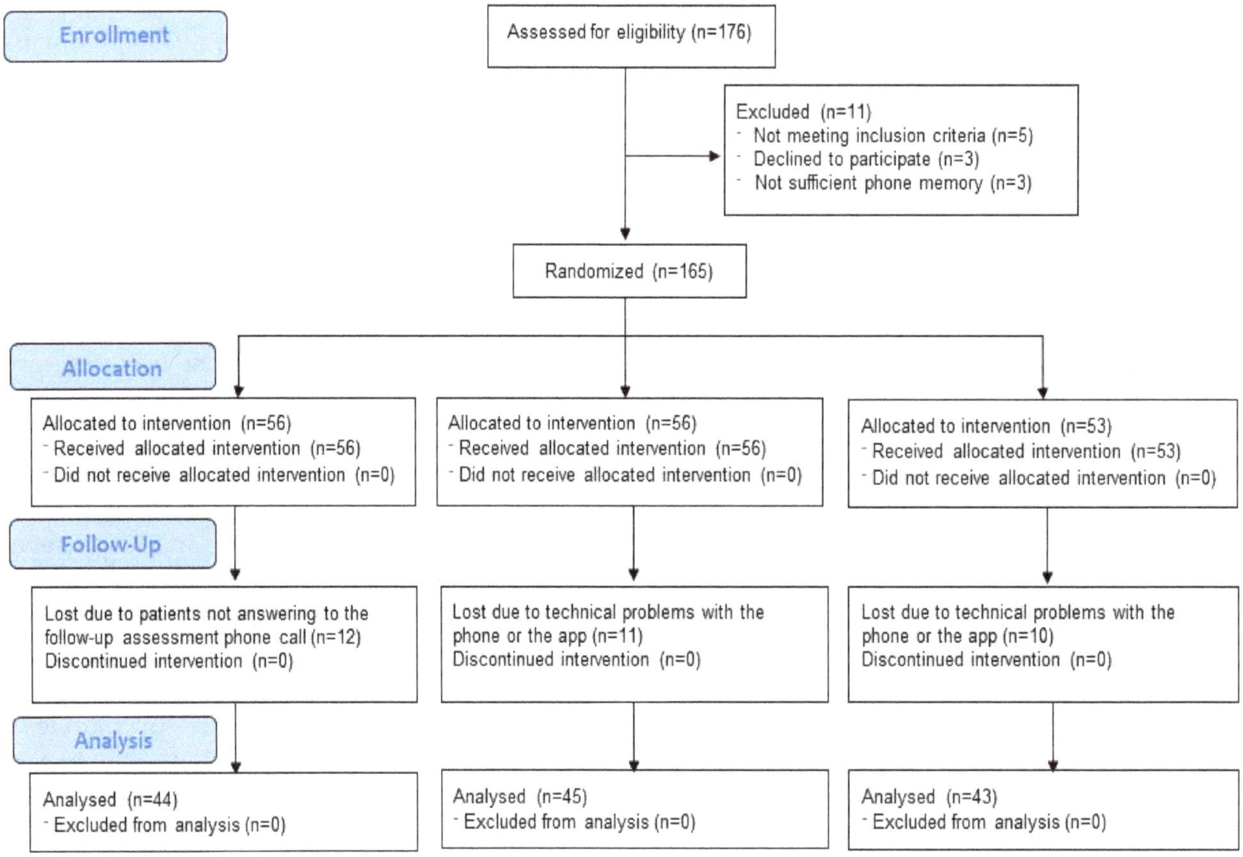

Figure 1. Study flowchart.

Overall, the response to the prompted daily questions in app was good (on average, patients responded to 77.0% of daily evaluations) and comparable to past research [42]. Note that an alarm was set to indicate when a patient was not responding to the app items (e.g., over two consecutive missing days), so that the principal investigator, CSR, could call patients and explore reasons for missing data (e.g., technical problems or lack of time or motivation).

3.1. Sample Characteristics

Patients had a mean age of 52.1 years (range = 23–82, SD = 11.2) and the majority were women (73.8%). Most of the participants were married or in a relationship (73.2%). One third of the patients were working at the time of assessment (34.4%). The rest of the participants were on temporary sick leave (20.6%), had compensation for permanent disability (19.1%) or were retired (11.5%), unemployed (7.6%) or homemakers (6.9%). Regarding educational level, 33.1% had only completed primary education, 32.3% had completed secondary studies, and 34.6% had completed tertiary education (technical or university studies).

Patients had musculoskeletal pain, most frequently pain in the low back or in the neck. Patients had been experiencing pain for between 6 months and 1 year (9.9%), 1–5 years (37.2%), 5–10 years (24.0%) or over 10 years (28.9%).

3.2. Baseline Differences in Study Variables

A MANOVA was conducted to investigate whether the randomization had effectively resulted in comparable patient profiles at baseline. The results supported the success of randomization. Specifically, baseline pain severity ($F = 1.65$, $p = 0.196$), pain interference ($F = 1.58$, $p = 0.211$), fatigue ($F = 0.42$, $p = 0.656$), sadness ($F = 0.22$, $p = 0.806$), anxiety ($F = 1.01$, $p = 0.368$) and anger ($F = 0.42$, $p = 0.656$) were comparable across conditions. The same occurred with sociodemographic characteristics, namely age ($F = 2.33$, $p = 0.101$), gender ($\chi^2 = 1.86$, $p = 0.395$), marital status ($\chi^2 = 7.9$, $p = 0.660$), educational level ($\chi^2 = 4.72$, $p = 0.318$), job status ($\chi^2 = 7.59$, $p = 0.669$) and pain duration ($\chi^2 = 3.16$, $p = 0.789$).

3.3. Changes in Pain Severity, Pain Interference, Fatigue and Mood across Treatment Conditions

As explained in the data analysis section and the beginning of the results section, two analytical approaches were followed due to sample size and reduced power. The first was the planned analysis of differences at the group level (Kruskal–Wallis and Friedman test). As indicated in Table 1, the Friedman test indicated that a treatment main effect was not observed for any outcome in the TAU and the TAU + app conditions. Only in the TAU + app + alarm condition a change (e.g., reduction) in pain interference was revealed ($Z = -3.32$, $p < 0.001$). The Kruskal–Wallis test revealed that none of the change scores differed across conditions (all $p > 0.01$).

In addition to changes at the group level, we also investigated changes at the individual level by means of an analysis of CSC (i.e., improvement of 30% or more with respect to baseline scores). The results are reported on Table 2. Again, the statistical analyses did not indicate significant differences in the proportion of clinically improved patients across conditions. However, this may again be due to insufficient sample size. Note, however, that the proportion of patients showing a CSC in outcomes was consistently higher in the TAU + app + alarm condition, with the only exception of anger, where the numbers were similar in the previous and the TAU condition. For example, 33.3% of patients in the TAU + app + alarm condition experienced a CSC reduction in pain severity after one month of treatment, while only half of this proportion improved in the other two conditions (15.4 in TAU and 16.7 in TAU + app). Similarly, a CSC in sadness was obtained by 43.6% of patients in the TAU + app + alarm condition and less than 30% of patients in the other two groups. Comparable results were revealed for pain interference, fatigue and anxiety, always in favor of the TAU + app + alarm condition.

Table 1. Group-level changes in study outcomes across conditions.

	TAU			TAU + App			TAU + App + Alarm			Kruskal–Wallis Test
Outcomes	Baseline Mean (SD)	Follow-Up Mean (SD)	Friedman Z	Baseline Mean (SD)	Follow-Up Mean (SD)	Friedman Z	Baseline Mean (SD)	Follow-Up Mean (SD)	Friedman Z	Chi-Squared
Pain severity	6.28 (0.34)	5.90 (0.37)	−1.25	5.56 (0.33)	5.50 (0.36)	−0.22	5.58 (0.34)	5.14 (0.37)	−1.22	1.60
Pain interference	5.81 (0.37)	5.42 (0.38)	−0.83	4.94 (0.37)	4.75 (0.38)	−0.30	5.13 (0.37)	4.28 (0.38)	−3.32 **	4.61
Fatigue	6.41 (0.37)	5.85 (0.39)	−1.94	4.94 (0.36)	4.65 (0.37)	−1.07	5.44 (0.37)	5.14 (0.39)	−2.05	1.19
Sadness	4.26 (0.43)	4.13 (0.42)	−0.25	3.94 (0.41)	3.69 (0.40)	−0.78	4.11 (0.43)	3.47 (0.42)	−1.76	1.79
Anxiety	3.89 (0.48)	5.03 (0.45)	−2.07	3.20 (0.45)	3.50 (0.42)	−0.63	3.70 (0.47)	3.35 (0.44)	−0.75	6.55
Anger	2.73 (0.43)	3.60 (0.46)	−1.29	2.57 (0.42)	3.29 (0.45)	−1.65	2.51 (0.43)	2.60 (0.46)	−0.19	0.55

TAU—treatment as usual. ** $p < 0.001$.

Table 2. Percentage of participants showing a clinically significant improvement in study outcomes across conditions.

Outcomes	TAU	TAU + App	TAU + App + Alarm	χ^2	p
Pain severity	15.4	16.7	33.3	4.65	0.098
Pain interference	17.5	20.0	38.5	5.27	0.072
Fatigue	17.9	14.3	25.6	1.74	0.419
Sadness	26.3	28.6	43.6	3.13	0.209
Anxiety	16.2	21.4	30.8	2.36	0.308
Anger	25.0	14.3	23.7	1.70	0.427

TAU—treatment as usual.

3.4. *Differences in Frequency of Experienced Physical Symptoms*

As noted earlier, the daily frequency of undesired and unusual physical symptoms was evaluated with the app only, so these were not assessed in the TAU condition for reasons of feasibility and fidelity to usual practice. The ANOVA results indicated that the average daily number of unwanted symptoms was slightly, but not significantly higher (F = 1.49, $p = 0.226$) in the group without alarms (mean = 1.47, SD = 0.64) compared to the group with alarms (mean = 1.33, 0.38).

In total, 51 alarms were received in the TAU + app + alarm condition. The most frequent were related to recurrent headache ($n = 11$), gait instability ($n = 10$), interference of pain on sleep ($n = 5$), urine retention ($n = 4$), very severe pain levels that do not improve with treatment ($n = 3$) and sleepiness ($n = 3$). These data were collected by the app daily based on patient self-reports. In total, 93% of alarms were considered sufficiently relevant to call the patient and further investigate whether an action (e.g., a change in the medication) was required.

3.5. *Professionals' Experience with the App*

As indicated in Table 3, the pain clinic physicians ($n = 6$) generally perceived that the app was useful for pain management (e.g., increased treatment safety and effectiveness) and for their own comfort as health care providers. Importantly, they were keener on using the app version with alarms than the version without alarms.

Table 3. Physician opinions about the mHealth solution.

To What Extent the App ...	Completely Disagree	Slightly Disagree	Neither Agree Nor Disagree	Slightly Agree	Completely Agree
Was useful for pain management	0	0	0	3	3
Increases treatment safety	0	0	0	4	2
Increases treatment effectiveness	0	0	1	5	0
Gives me comfort	0	1	1	3	1
Is useful for me as a professional	0	0	0	4	2
Can be useful for patients	0	0	0	2	4
With alarms is something I want To use in the future	0	0	0	4	2
Without alarms is something I want to use in the future	0	2	1	2	1
Alarms impact daily job burden	0	4	1	0	1
Has an impact on burden (help patient downloading the app)	2	2	1	1	0

We also investigated burden. On average, the physicians perceived that helping the patient download the app and guiding them during the first use required 13 min (7–20 min range, median = 15 min) and responding to all daily alarms (e.g., looking at the patient's medical record and calling them) required 28 min in total (10–45-min range; median = 27.5 min). As reported in Table 3, the burden was generally perceived as low or average.

4. Discussion

The present study aimed to compare the effectiveness of three monitoring approaches in patients with chronic pain, namely usual episodic monitoring, monitoring with an app without clinical alarms and monitoring with an app with clinical alarms. For one month, all patients received the usual treatment for their pain, but different effects on outcomes (pain severity and interference, fatigue, depression, anxiety and anger) were expected to emerge across monitoring conditions. Another goal was to investigate the opinion of health professionals about the app.

In relation to the first goal and contrary to our expectations, monitoring with the app and alarms did not have a significantly greater impact on outcomes compared to the usual monitoring method or the app without alarms condition, both at the group and individual level. However, consistent with our hypotheses there was only a reduction in pain interference in the group of patients using the app with clinical alarms for telemonitoring. In addition, the analyses at the individual level showed that the proportion of patients reporting a clinically meaningful reduction (i.e., over 30%) in almost all outcomes, namely pain severity, pain interference, fatigue, depression and anxiety, was higher in patients who were monitored using the app with alarms. Regarding the second objective, the healthcare professionals involved generally perceived that the app was useful for pain management in the sense that it improved treatment safety and effectiveness. They also believed that it increased their sense of comfort as healthcare providers. Importantly, they were more satisfied with the version of the app that included alarms. Regarding the burden of using the app, they reported that helping patients download the app and respond to alarms required some extra time, but they found this burden to be low or moderate.

For several years, it has been argued that eHealth and particularly mHealth will inevitably change our health systems in general [63] and pain management in particular [45]. To date, the focus of existing eHealth and mHealth solutions in pain settings has been mostly placed on self-administered treatments, mostly of psychological or alternatively of physical therapy nature [64–66]. While developing alternatives to face-to-face multidimensional treatments for chronic pain is indeed important, most patients still advocate individual, face-to-face treatments [67] and the first-line intervention for patients with chronic pain, namely medical treatment, will probably continue to require some patient-professional face-to-face interaction. Thus, the development of tools that improve face-to-face interventions and allow for a rapid adaptation of treatments as a function of patient evolution during treatment, as in measurement-based care [68], should be a major focus of research in chronic pain settings. This study may provide some novel insights about the potential utility, as well as the implementation challenges of this new approach to monitoring. In fact, to the best of our knowledge, this is the first randomized controlled trial that explored the utility of telemonitoring adults with chronic pain between onsite appointments using a smartphone app.

One of the findings regarding the implementation of mHealth in chronic pain management was that this system was well accepted by the pain physicians involved, which is critical for implementation purposes [69]. Importantly, they preferred the app version that included alarms, even when these generated some burden. While these results are encouraging, a lesson learned based on this perceived burden is that, if mHealth telemonitoring is to be implemented in the future, it may be advisable to allocate some time for clinicians to assist patients with the first app use, as well as to check daily alarms and call patients to make treatment adjustments. This will be especially relevant if a similar technology is to be implemented in routine care for all patients (note that, on average, it took around 30 min for each alarm, considering the time to check the electronic medical record, call the patient and make adjustments to the treatment if necessary). This time, however, clinicians found it beneficial—as indicated by reports showing overall low burden and high perceived usefulness of alarms. Additionally, these costs in terms of time spent dealing with alarms must be weighed against the potential costs of not receiving such alarms (e.g., patients attending the emergency services or taking ineffective medications). While acknowledging the previous positive findings in terms of clinician's acceptability and the potential benefits of using alarms, it is important to note that conclusions about the actual sustainability and cost-effectiveness of this new approach to monitoring at a large scale should be taken with caution.

In relation to the utility of this new approach to monitoring, one of the main study goals was to explore whether the inclusion of telemonitoring (app with alarms) would lead to improved outcomes thanks to a rapid detection of poor treatment response, chronic low mood or high interference of pain on functioning. One problem was sample loss. Thus, even though a visual inspection of mean-level differences across conditions suggested somewhat larger improvements in the app + alarm condition in pain interference, sadness and anxiety, these results should not be overemphasized. Even the fact that pain interference only significantly improved in the app + alarm condition should be interpreted with caution due to sample size loss during the study. An interesting and more promising finding, however, was the fact that the percentage of patients reporting a clinically meaningful improvement in almost all outcomes, i.e., pain severity, pain interference, fatigue, sadness and anxiety was always higher in the app + alarm condition. This is important because, different from the analysis of changes at the group mean level, CSC is explored at the individual level. As noted in past research, while "managers and trialists may be happy for treatments to work on average, patients expect their doctors to do better than that" [70]. At the individual level, our results support the idea that the use of the app with alarms may indeed result in more patients benefiting from medical treatment. For example, while 15.4% and 16.7% of patients in the TAU and TAU + app conditions showed a clinically significant reduction in pain severity, twice the number of patients in the TAU + app + alarm condition (33.3%) showed such reductions.

An important finding in the present study was that the use of the app with alarms as adjunct to medical treatments for pain may as well provide some benefits on the functioning and mental well-being of individuals, again when explored at the individual level. Chronic pain is a very disabling and mentally distressing experience. Not surprisingly, musculoskeletal diseases, which were the type of conditions included in the present study, have become the leading cause of sick leave in Europe and account for approximately half of work-related illnesses [12] and the prevalence of anxiety and mood disorders in patients with chronic pain is two-to-three times higher than in the general population [71]. While the impact of pain on the physical functioning status and mental well-being of individuals is patent, the first-line treatments for the disease, namely medical interventions, have shown to exert a modest effect on daily functioning and, especially, on the mental health status of individuals, even when pain is effectively reduced [72–74]. Therefore, the finding that the use of the app with alarms resulted in a larger number of patients reporting improved pain interference with functioning, fatigue and mental well-being, is encouraging. Note for example, that depression and anxiety levels were meaningfully reduced in 43.6% and 30.8% of patients in the app + alarm condition, while reductions in depression and anxiety in the other two conditions occurred in less than 29% and 22% of patients, respectively. Again, note that these results refer to the percentage of patients with clinically significant improvements. By contrast, the analyses at the group level indicated that the effect of the condition was insufficient to reveal group differences with the recruited sample, even when pain interference only significantly improved in the app + alarm condition.

In addition to exploring the effectiveness of usual medical treatment in several conditions, this study aimed to investigate whether physical symptoms rarely experienced by the patient before treatment onset were minimized in the app + alarm condition compared to the group using the app without alarms. Of course, one thing to keep in mind is that there is no guarantee that these physical symptoms are actually due to the recently proposed pain treatment. By mentioning that patients should only report symptoms that they do not usually experience, we expected to reduce possible misinterpretation of symptoms. However, it is also possible for patients to experience unusual symptoms for reasons other than the onset of a new pain treatment (e.g., an infection, hormonal changes or a stressful daily event, to name some examples). This limitation is difficult to address, so the results regarding the number of daily symptoms should be taken with caution. While acknowledging the previous, an important finding was that algorithms can be effectively created so that the determination of when an event becomes alarming (e.g., experiencing nausea or dizziness for a given number of days) no longer depends solely on the interpretation of the patient. Of course, reporting of symptoms rather than signs requires patient self-report. However, the contribution of the present study is that an algorithm can be used to effectively send an alarm to professionals, so that action can be taken. Note that these alarms could be generated because of the ecological momentary assessment with the app, which current and past research has revealed to be feasible in terms of patient response rates [42].

As a final remark, which may be important for implementation purposes, the study revealed that patient follow-up using phone calls was difficult and technical and phone-related problems are likely to occur when implementing mHealth. In relation the former, calling patients in the TAU condition for follow-up assessment was very time consuming and largely ineffective. Specifically, if often took several calls to get in contact with the participants and these were not always available to complete the survey at the time of the call. This occurred despite the fact that patients were informed that a follow-up call would be made one month after the baseline assessment. This supports the need for more flexible and patient-dependent assessment tools, such as smartphone apps. In this sense, patient daily self-monitoring eliminated the need for physician active monitoring, so only when the app algorithm detected an undesired event, this was notified to the physician and only then a phone call was made. In relation to technical problems, such as app malfunctioning or problems with the patients' phone, such as crashing or low battery or memory, these did occur in the study and resulted in almost 20% of loss in sample size. Recent research into telemonitoring in chronic pain states that these technical problems are something we will probably have to accept [37]. One lesson we learned, however, is that the inclusion of an alarm that sends a notification when patient responses are missing for a number of days (e.g., two in the present study) may be a good strategy to minimize technical problems. This strategy was implemented in the present investigation and it helped us identify some technical problems (e.g., patients that changed their phone or patients that were not receiving the push notifications). These problems would have probably remained undetected otherwise. Similar to past research [75], a technical team will probably be needed to address such technical problems if technological solutions are to be implemented in routine care. In addition to using alarms, another option to minimize missing data are to create a plan to maintain the app after the initial development is completed, which may help reduce technical problems associated with operating system updates [76].

To the best of our knowledge, this is the first study to use an alarm-based telemonitoring system in a randomized controlled trial in chronic pain settings. Some study limitations, including loss of sample due to technical or phone-related problems or the reduced power in the analyses have been already discussed. However, in relation to sample size it is important to mention that the anticipation of a 10% drop-out was clearly insufficient. At least 25% should have been expected based on our results. We expect that this will help researchers when calculating the required sample size for similar future studies. It is also important to acknowledge additional shortcomings, such as the reliance on subjective outcomes only (e.g., the inclusion of wearable devices could have provided more objective data on physical functioning) and the focus on musculoskeletal pain only, which prevents us from generalizing the findings to specific populations or to all chronic pain populations. In relation to wearable devices, however, it is important to note that their inclusion in routine practice may be less ecological than the use of smartphones since the latter are much more frequently utilized by the population. Another shortcoming that should be acknowledged is that the required sample size was obtained based on an uncorrected alpha level of 0.05. Corrections such as Bonferroni–Holm [77] should be considered in future similar investigations conducting multiple comparisons as this may significantly impact on sample size requirements. For instance, by correcting the alpha level to 0.01 due to multiple comparisons in the present study, the sample size needed would have increased from 150 to 222. Furthermore, in relation to sample size, it is important to note that the patient's ability to use the technology was not evaluated in the present investigation because excellent usability findings had already been reported in the original validation study [42]. Therefore, it is difficult to know to what extent technical ability impacted on study completion and, ultimately, on the final sample size. Additionally, as mentioned earlier during the text, the selection of a 30% cutoff to determine the benchmark for a clinically significant change may also have influenced the results. It is possible that more restrictive benchmarks would have resulted in different percentages of change across conditions and, therefore, to different conclusions. The inclusion of a midpoint response, as in the "Neither agree nor disagree" option in the healthcare professionals' questionnaire, may have also been problematic. In this sense, even though the use of a midpoint response may be useful when participants are ambivalent or neutral, they may also be used when participants have no opinion or when they want to provide a response that is socially desirable [78]. In addition, the use of midpoint responses negatively impacts score reliability [79]. In the present study, the prevalence of midpoint responses was 8.3%, which appears to be an acceptable level of uncertainty according to past research [80]. However, future research should consider whether the inclusion of such midpoint response options is crucial for the study's needs and should preferably include a very clear midpoint response or a response scale without midpoints [78]. Finally, because no analysis of costs was made, it is difficult to know to what extent the implementation of mHealth was cost-effective. This should be addressed in future hybrid designs.

5. Conclusions

The present study may contribute to the field of mHealth in chronic pain in a number of ways. First, the study showed that mobile apps can be effectively implemented for patient monitoring. In this sense, the Pain Monitor app allowed us to collect a large number of data associated with pain and treatment in an automated way. This information has never before been collected with this level accuracy (i.e., daily assessment as opposed to the traditional retrospective assessment). This is important given the heterogeneity both in the etiology and the treatment of chronic pain, as ecological momentary assessment could help us obtain a more accurate picture of treatment response which may help guide interventions in a more effective manner [42]. Second, this RCT may serve guide future research in a more effective matter as it provided data on the impact that telemonitoring is likely to have on physical and mental health outcomes in patients with musculoskeletal chronic pain. Third, it showed that, if effective, telemonitoring is more likely to have an impact on outcomes if an alarm system that allows for a rapid response to unwanted events occurs, which suggests that daily assessment only is not likely to be sufficient to have an impact on outcomes. Finally, the lessons learned in terms of physicians' burden and technology problems and solutions may help researchers, clinicians and policy makers interested in the field of mHealth.

Author Contributions: Conceptualization, C.S.-R., D.C., I.Z., Á.M., A.S., J.M. and A.G.-P.; methodology, C.S.-R., D.C., I.Z., Á.M., A.S., J.M. and A.G.-P.; software, A.G.-P., C.S.-R., I.Z. and D.C.; validation, C.S.-R., Á.M., A.S. and J.M.; formal analysis, C.S.-R.; investigation, C.S.-R., Á.M., A.S. and J.M.; resources, C.S.-R., D.C., I.Z., Á.M., A.S., J.M. and A.G.-P.; data curation, I.Z., D.C. and C.S.-R.; writing—original draft preparation, C.S.-R.; writing—review and editing, C.S.-R., D.C., I.Z., Á.M., A.S., J.M. and A.G.-P.; visualization, C.S.-R.; supervision, A.G.-P., C.S.-R. and Á.M.; project administration, A.G.-P., C.S.-R. and Á.M.; funding acquisition, A.G.-P., D.C., I.Z. and C.S.-R. All authors have read and agreed to the published version of the manuscript.

Appendix A

Alarms Generated by the Pain Monitor App

- Morning pain > 7 during 5 consecutive days
- Evening pain > 7 during 5 consecutive days
- Morning sadness >7 during 5 consecutive days
- Evening sadness >7 during 5 consecutive days
- Morning anxiety >7 during 5 consecutive days
- Evening anxiety >7 during 5 consecutive days
- Vomiting during 2 consecutive days
- Tachycardia during 2 consecutive days
- Blurred vision during 2 consecutive days
- Headache during 2 consecutive days
- Dry mouth during 2 consecutive days
- Constipation during 5 consecutive days
- Drowsiness during 5 consecutive days

- Nausea during 3 consecutive days
- Itching during 3 consecutive days
- Diarrhea during 2 consecutive days
- Fever during 2 consecutive days
- Facial redness during 2 consecutive days
- Urine retention during 2 consecutive days
- Unsteady walking during 3 consecutive days
- Excessive sweating during 7 consecutive days
- Dizziness during 3 consecutive days
- Do not take the medication and there is no intention to take it
- Number of rescue medication > 3
- Sleep interference > 7
- Missing data = 2 consecutive days

Appendix B

Items in the Pain Monitor App Used in the Randomized Controlled Trial

Appendix B.1

Sociodemographic Items (Assessed Once, the First Day of App Use):

1. Please indicate your date of birth (DD/MM/YYYY)
2. What type of user are you?
    a. I am a person with chronic pain
    b. I do not have chronic pain, but I want to see the app
3. Please indicate your gender:
    a. Male
    b. Female
4. Please indicate your type of pain. You may select more than one option:
    a. Fibromyalgia
    b. Low back pain
    c. Cervical pain
    d. Rheumatoid arthritis
    e. Osteoarthritis; Headache
    f. Neuropathic pain
    g. Cancer pain
    h. None of the above.
5. If you selected "None of the above" please indicate your type of pain. Otherwise, leave this question blank. Press OK to continue.
6. Please indicate the location where your pain is more intense:
    a. Head
    b. Shoulder
    c. Neck
    d. High back
    e. Lower back

f. Arm
g. Elbow
h. Wrist
i. Hand
j. Abdomen
k. Chest
l. Buttock
m. Hip
n. Leg
o. Knee
p. Foot
q. Whole body
r. Somewhere not listed

7. Who is currently treating your pain? You may select more than one option:

a. General practitioner
b. Rheumatologist
c. Orthopedic specialist
d. Rehabilitation physician
e. Psychiatrist
f. Pain Unit
g. Neurosurgeon
h. Neurologist
i. Oncologist
j. Another professional.

8. When did your current pain start?

a. Less than one year ago
b. Between 1 and 5 years ago
c. Between 5 and 10 years ago
d. More than 10 years ago

9. What is your current treatment for pain? You may select more than one option:

a. Physiotherapy
b. Pharmacotherapy
c. Infiltrations
d. Psychological treatment
e. Natural / alternative treatments
f. My pain is not being treated

10. Did you start a new treatment for pain in the last month?

a. Yes
b. No

11. Please select the treatment/s you started in the last month. You may select more than one option:

a. Physiotherapy
b. Pharmacotherapy
c. Infiltrations

d. Psychological treatment
e. Natural / alternative treatments
f. I have not started a new treatment

12. What is your marital status?

a. Single
b. Married
c. In a relationship
d. Divorced
e. Separated
f. Widowed

13. What is your job status?

a. Active worker
b. Sick leave
c. Permanent disability
d. Unemployed
e. Homemaker
f. Retired
g. Student

14. What is the highest level of education you have completed?

a. No studies
b. Less than high school
c. High school graduate
d. Technical training
e. University degree

15. Do you currently have a diagnosis of depression by a physician or a psychologist?

a. Yes
b. No

16. Do you currently have a diagnosis of anxiety by a physician or a psychologist?

a. Yes
b. No

Appendix B.2

Outcomes (Assessed Twice per Day)

1. Please indicate the intensity of your CURRENT PAIN: 0 No pain ———10 Extreme pain
2. Please indicate the intensity of your CURRENT FATIGUE: 0 No fatigue ———10 Extreme fatigue
3. Please indicate the intensity of your CURRENT SADNESS: 0 No sadness ——— 10 Extremely sad
4. Please indicate the intensity of your CURRENT ANXIETY: 0 No anxiety ——- 10 Extremely anxious
5. Please indicate the intensity of your CURRENT ANGER: 0 No anger ——- 10 Extremely angry

Appendix B.3

Items Used for Generating Alarms Only (Assessed Once Daily, in the Evening Except for Pain Interference on Sleep Which Was Evaluated in the Morning Assessment)

1. Did your PAIN interfere with the quality of your SLEEP LAST NIGHT? 0 No interference —— 10 Maximum interference
2. Did your PAIN interfere with your SOCIAL INTERACTIONS TODAY? 0 No interference —— 10 Maximum interference
3. Did your PAIN interfere with the quality of your LEISURE ACTIVITIES TODAY? 0 No interference —— 10 Maximum interference
4. Did your PAIN interfere with your USUAL WORK or HOUSEWORK TODAY? 0 No interference —— 10 Maximum interference
5. Did you experience any of these symptoms TODAY? You may select more than one option. Only select symptoms that were not present before pain treatment onset:

   a. Nausea
   b. Vomiting
   c. Tachycardia
   d. Constipation
   e. Drowsiness / sedation
   f. Blurred vision
   g. Dry mouth
   h. Headache
   i. None of the above

6. Did you experience any of these symptoms TODAY? You may select more than one option. Only select symptoms that were not present before pain treatment onset:

   a. Dizziness
   b. Itching
   c. Diarrhea
   d. Gait instability
   e. Excessive sweating
   f. Fever
   g. Urine retention
   h. Facial redness
   i. A different symptom
   j. None of the above

7. Did you take your prescribed medication TODAY?

   a. Yes
   b. No, but I will do it later
   c. No and I do not plan to take it
   d. I have not been prescribed a pain medication

8. How many times did you take a rescue medication TODAY?

   a. 0
   b. 1
   c. 2
   d. 3
   e. 4
   f. 5
   g. 6

h. 7
i. 8
j. 9
k. 10
l. More than 10

References

1. de C. Williams, A.C.; Craig, K.D. Updating the definition of pain. *Pain* **2016**, *157*, 2420–2423. [CrossRef] [PubMed]
2. Bevan, S.; Quadrello, T.; Mcgee, R.; Mahdon, M.; Vavrovsky, A.; Barham, L. *Fit for Work Pain-European Report*; The Work Fundation: London, UK, 2009.
3. Breivik, H.; Collett, B.; Ventafridda, V.; Cohen, R.; Gallacher, D. Survey of chronic pain in Europe: Prevalence, impact on daily life, and treatment. *Eur. J. Pain* **2006**, *10*, 287–333. [CrossRef] [PubMed]
4. Johannes, C.B.; Le, T.K.; Zhou, X.; Johnston, J.A.; Dworkin, R.H. The prevalence of chronic pain in United States adults: Results of an Internet-based survey. *J. Pain* **2010**, *11*, 1230–1239. [CrossRef] [PubMed]
5. Wong, W.S.; Fielding, R. Prevalence and characteristics of chronic pain in the general population of Hong Kong. *J. Pain* **2011**, *12*, 236–245. [CrossRef] [PubMed]
6. Fayaz, A.; Croft, P.; Langford, R.M.; Donaldson, L.J.; Jones, G.T. Prevalence of chronic pain in the UK: A systematic review and meta-analysis of population studies. *BMJ Open* **2016**, *6*, e010364. [CrossRef] [PubMed]
7. Azevedo, L.F.; Costa-Pereira, A.; Mendonça, L.; Dias, C.C.; Castro-Lopes, J.M. Epidemiology of chronic pain: A population-based nationwide study on its prevalence, characteristics and associated disability in Portugal. *J. Pain* **2012**, *13*, 773–783. [CrossRef] [PubMed]
8. Reid, K.J.; Harker, J.; Bala, M.M.; Truyers, C.; Kellen, E.; Bekkering, G.E.; Kleijnen, J. Epidemiology of chronic non-cancer pain in Europe: Narrative review of prevalence, pain treatments and pain impact. *Curr. Med. Res. Opin.* **2011**, *27*, 449–462. [CrossRef] [PubMed]
9. Miró, J.; Paredes, S.; Rull, M.; Queral, R.; Miralles, R.; Nieto, R.; Huguet, A.; Baos, J. Pain in older adults: A prevalence study in the Mediterranean region of Catalonia. *Eur. J. Pain* **2007**, *11*, 83–92. [CrossRef] [PubMed]
10. Gaskin, D.J.; Richard, P. The economic costs of pain in the United States. *J. Pain* **2012**, *13*, 715–724. [CrossRef]
11. Bevan, S. Economic impact of musculoskeletal disorders (MSDs) on work in Europe. *Best Pract. Res. Clin. Rheumatol.* **2015**, *29*, 356–373. [CrossRef]
12. Bevan, S.; Quadrello, T.; Mcgee, R.; Mahdon, M.; Vavrovsky, A.; Barham, L. Fit for Work? Musculoskeletal Disorders in the European Workforce. Available online: http://www.bollettinoadapt.it/old/files/document/3704FOUNDATION_19_10.pdf (accessed on 15 February 2018).
13. Geneen, L.J.; Moore, R.A.; Clarke, C.; Martin, D.; Colvin, L.A.; Smith, B.H. Physical activity and exercise for chronic pain in adults: An overview of Cochrane Reviews. *Cochrane Database Syst. Rev.* **2017**, *1*, CD011279. [CrossRef] [PubMed]
14. Gatchel, R.; McGeary, D.; McGeary, C.; Lippe, B. Interdisciplinary chronic pain management: Past, present, and future. *Am. Psychol.* **2014**, *69*, 119–130. [CrossRef] [PubMed]
15. Hughes, L.S.; Clark, J.; Colclough, J.A.; Dale, E.; McMillan, D. Acceptance and commitment therapy (ACT) for chronic pain: A systematic review and meta-analyses. *Clin. J. Pain* **2017**, *33*, 552–568. [CrossRef] [PubMed]
16. Salaffi, F.; Sarzi-Puttini, P.; Atzeni, F. How to measure chronic pain: New concepts. *Best Pract. Res. Clin. Rheumatol.* **2015**, *29*, 164–186. [CrossRef] [PubMed]
17. Dansie, E.J.; Turk, D.C. Assessment of patients with chronic pain. *Br. J. Anaesth.* **2013**, *111*, 19–25. [CrossRef] [PubMed]
18. Suso-Ribera, C.; Mesas, Á.; Medel, J.; Server, A.; Márquez, E.; Castilla, D.; Zaragozá, I.; García-Palacios, A. Improving pain treatment with a smartphone app: Study protocol for a randomized controlled trial. *Trials* **2018**, *19*, 145. [CrossRef]
19. Mann, E.G.; LeFort, S.; VanDenKerkhof, E.G. Self-management interventions for chronic pain. *Pain Manag.* **2013**, *3*, 211–222. [CrossRef]

20. OECD; EU. *Health at a Glance: Europe 2016—State of Health in the EU Cycle*; OECD Publishing: Paris, France, 2016; ISBN 9789264265585.
21. Busse, R.; Blümel, M.; Scheller-Kreinsen, D.; Zentner, A. *Tackling Chronic Disease in Europe: Strategies, Interventions and Challenges*; WHO: Copenhagen, Denmark, 2010; Volume 20.
22. Kikuchi, H.; Yoshiuchi, K.; Miyasaka, N.; Ohashi, K.; Yamamoto, Y.; Kumano, H.; Kuboki, T.; Akabayashi, A. Reliability of recalled self-report on headache intensity: Investigation using ecological momentary assessment technique. *Cephalalgia* **2006**, *26*, 1335–1343. [CrossRef]
23. Kratz, A.L.; Murphy, S.L.; Braley, T.J. Ecological Momentary Assessment of Pain, Fatigue, Depressive, and Cognitive Symptoms Reveals Significant Daily Variability in Multiple Sclerosis. *Arch. Phys. Med. Rehabil.* **2017**, *98*, 2142–2150. [CrossRef]
24. Allen, K.D.; Coffman, C.J.; Golightly, Y.M.; Stechuchak, K.M.; Keefe, F.J. Daily pain variations among patients with hand, hip, and knee osteoarthritis. *Osteoarthr. Cartil.* **2009**, *17*, 1275–1282. [CrossRef]
25. Schneider, S.; Junghaenel, D.U.; Keefe, F.J.; Schwartz, J.E.; Stone, A.A.; Broderick, J.E. Individual differences in the day-to-day variability of pain, fatigue, and well-being in patients with rheumatic disease: Associations with psychological variables. *Pain* **2012**, *153*, 813–822. [CrossRef] [PubMed]
26. Bartley, E.J.; Robinson, M.E.; Staud, R. Pain and fatigue variability patterns distinguish subgroups of Fibromyalgia patients. *J. Pain* **2018**, *19*, 372–381. [CrossRef] [PubMed]
27. García-Palacios, A.; Herrero, R.; Belmonte, M.A.; Castilla, D.; Guixeres, J.; Molinari, G.; Banos, R.M.; Baños, R.M.; Botella, C.; Garcia-Palacios, A.; et al. Ecological momentary assessment for chronic pain in fibromyalgia using a smartphone: A randomized crossover study. *Eur. J. Pain* **2014**, *18*, 862–872. [CrossRef]
28. Kirchner, T.R.; Shiffman, S. Ecological Momentary Assessment. In *Wiley-Blackwell Handb. Addict. Psychopharmacology*; MacKillop, J., de Wit, H., Eds.; John Wiley & Sons: Hoboken, NJ, USA, 2013; pp. 541–565. [CrossRef]
29. Smyth, J.M.; Stone, A.A. Ecological momentary assessment research in behavioral medicine. *J. Happiness Stud.* **2003**, *4*, 35–52. [CrossRef]
30. Deyo, R.A.; Mirza, S.K.; Turner, J.A.; Martin, B.I. Overtreating chronic back pain: Time to back off? *J. Am. Board Fam. Med.* **2009**, *22*, 62–68. [CrossRef]
31. Dargan, P.J.; Simm, R.; Murray, C. New approaches towards chronic pain: Patient experiences of a solution-focused pain management programme. *Br. J. Pain* **2014**, *8*, 34–42. [CrossRef] [PubMed]
32. Fashler, S.R.; Cooper, L.K.; Oosenbrug, E.D.; Burns, L.C.; Razavi, S.; Goldberg, L.; Katz, J. Systematic review of multidisciplinary chronic pain treatment facilities. *Pain Res. Manag.* **2016**, *2016*, 5960987. [CrossRef]
33. Hong, J.; Reed, C.; Novick, D.; Happich, M. Costs associated with treatment of chronic low back pain: An analysis of the UK general practice research database. *Spine (Phila. Pa. 1976)* **2013**, *38*, 75–82. [CrossRef]
34. Breivik, H.; Borchgrevink, P.C.; Allen, S.M.; Rosseland, L.A.; Romundstad, L.; Breivik Hals, E.K.; Kvarstein, G.; Stubhaug, A. Assessment of pain. *Br. J. Anaesth.* **2008**, *101*, 17–24. [CrossRef]
35. World Health Organization. *Innovative Care for Chronic Conditions*; WHO: Geneva, Switzerland, 2002.
36. Christensen, H.; Hickie, I.B. Using e-health applications to deliver new mental health services. *Med. J. Aust.* **2010**, *192*, 53–56. [CrossRef]
37. Eccleston, C.; Blyth, F.M.; Dear, B.F.; Fisher, E.A.; Keefe, F.J.; Lynch, M.E.; Palermo, T.M.; Reid, M.C.; de C. Williams, A.C. Managing patients with chronic pain during the COVID-19 outbreak. *Pain* **2020**, *161*, 889–893. [CrossRef] [PubMed]
38. Dworkin, R.H.; Turk, D.C.; Farrar, J.T.; Haythornthwaite, J.A.; Jensen, M.P.; Katz, N.P.; Kerns, R.D.; Stucki, G.; Allen, R.R.; Bellamy, N.; et al. Core outcome measures for chronic pain clinical trials: IMMPACT recommendations. *Pain* **2005**, *113*, 9–19. [CrossRef] [PubMed]
39. Rosser, B.A.; Eccleston, C. Smartphone applications for pain management. *J. Telemed. Telecare* **2011**, *17*, 308–312. [CrossRef] [PubMed]
40. Kaiser, U.; Kopkow, C.; Deckert, S.; Neustadt, K.; Jacobi, L.; Cameron, P.; De Angelis, V.; Apfelbacher, C.; Arnold, B.; Birch, J.; et al. Developing a core outcome-domain set to assessing effectiveness of interdisciplinary multimodal pain therapy. *Pain* **2017**, *1*, 673–683. [CrossRef] [PubMed]
41. Portelli, P.; Eldred, C. A quality review of smartphone applications for the management of pain. *Br. J. Pain* **2016**, *10*, 135–140. [CrossRef]

42. Suso-Ribera, C.; Castilla, D.; Zaragozá, I.; Ribera-Canudas, M.V.; Botella, C.; García-Palacios, A. Validity, reliability, feasibility, and usefulness of Pain Monitor. A multidimensional smartphone app for daily monitoring of adults with heterogeneous chronic pain. *Clin. J. Pain* **2018**, *34*, 900–908. [CrossRef]
43. Alexander, J.; Joshi, G. Smartphone applications for chronic pain management: A critical appraisal. *J. Pain Res.* **2016**, *9*, 731–734. [CrossRef]
44. Wallace, L.S.; Dhingra, L.K. A systematic review of smartphone applications for chronic pain available for download in the United States. *J. Opioid Manag.* **2014**, *10*, 63–68. [CrossRef]
45. Sundararaman, L.V.; Edwards, R.R.; Ross, E.L.; Jamison, R.N. Integration of Mobile Health Technology in the Treatment of Chronic Pain. *Reg. Anesth. Pain Med.* **2017**, *42*, 488–498. [CrossRef]
46. Lemey, C.; Larsen, M.E.; Devylder, J.; Courtet, P.; Billot, R.; Lenca, P.; Walter, M.; Baca-García, E.; Berrouiguet, S. Clinicians' concerns about mobile ecological momentary assessment tools designed for emerging psychiatric problems: Prospective acceptability assessment of the memind app. *J. Med. Internet Res.* **2019**, *21*, e10111. [CrossRef]
47. Araya Quintanilla, F.; Cuyul Vásquez, I.A. Influence of psychosocial factors on the experience of musculoskeletal pain: A literature review. *Rev. Soc. Española Dolor* **2018**, *26*, 44–51. [CrossRef]
48. Ericsson Mobility Report. 2016. Available online: https://www.ericsson.com/en/mobility-report/reports (accessed on 8 September 2020).
49. Faul, F.; Erdfelder, E.; Lang, A.-G.; Buchner, A. G*Power 3: A flexible statistical power analysis program for the social, behavioral, and biomedical sciences. *Behav. Res. Methods* **2007**, *39*, 175–191. [CrossRef] [PubMed]
50. Furlan, A.D.; Sandoval, J.A.; Mailis-gagnon, A.; Tunks, E. Opioids for chronic noncancer pain: A meta-analysis of effectiveness and side effects. *Can. Med. Assoc. J.* **2006**, *174*, 1589–1594. [CrossRef] [PubMed]
51. Turk, D.C.; Wilson, H.D.; Cahana, A. Treatment of chronic non-cancer pain. *Lancet* **2011**, *377*, 2226–2235. [CrossRef]
52. Attal, N.; Cruccu, G.; Baron, R.; Haanpää, M.; Hansson, P.; Jensen, T.S.; Nurmikko, T. EFNS guidelines on the pharmacological treatment of neuropathic pain: 2010 revision. *Eur. J. Neurol.* **2010**, *17*, 1113-e88. [CrossRef]
53. Cleeland, C.S.; Ryan, K.M. Pain assessment: Global use of the brief pain inventory. *Ann. Acad. Med. Singapore* **1994**, *23*, 129–138. [PubMed]
54. McNair, D.; Lorr, M.; Droppleman, L. *Profile of Mood States*; Educational and Industrial Testing Service: San Diego, CA, USA, 1971.
55. Zigmond, A.S.; Snaith, R.P. The hospital anxiety and depression scale. *Acta Psychiatr. Scand.* **1983**, *67*, 361–370. [CrossRef]
56. Beck, A.; Ward, C.H.; Mendelson, M.; Mock, J.; Erbauch, J. An inventory for measuring depression. *Arch. Gen. Psychiatry* **1961**, *4*, 561. [CrossRef]
57. Trescot, A.; Glaser, S.E.; Hansen, H.; Benyamin, R.; Patel, S.; Manchikanti, L. Effectiveness of opioids in the treatment of chronic non-cancer pain. *Pain Physician* **2008**, *11*, 181–200.
58. Varrassi, G.; Müller-Schwefe, G.; Pergolizzi, J.; Orónska, A.; Morlion, B.; Mavrocordatos, P.; Margarit, C.; Mangas, C.; Jaksch, W.; Huygen, F.; et al. Pharmacological treatment of chronic pain—The need for CHANGE. *Curr. Med. Res. Opin.* **2010**, *26*, 1231–1245. [CrossRef]
59. Davis, F.D.; Bagozzi, R.P.; Warshaw, P.R. User Acceptance of computer technology: A comparison of two theoretical models. *Manag. Sci.* **1989**, *35*, 982–1003. [CrossRef]
60. Kersten, P.; White, P.J.; Tennant, A. Is the pain visual analogue scale linear and responsive to change? An exploration using rasch analysis. *PLoS ONE* **2014**, *9*, e99485. [CrossRef] [PubMed]
61. Scott, W.; Wideman, T.H.; Sullivan, M.J.L. Clinically meaningful scores on pain catastrophizing before and after multidisciplinary rehabilitation: A prospective study of individuals with subacute pain after whiplash injury. *Clin. J. Pain* **2014**, *30*, 183–190. [CrossRef] [PubMed]
62. Ostelo, R.W.J.G.; Deyo, R.A.; Stratford, P.; Waddell, G.; Croft, P.; Von Korff, M.; Bouter, L.M.; de Vet, H.C. Interpreting change scores for pain and functional status in low back pain. *Spine (Phila. Pa. 1976).* **2008**, *33*, 90–94. [CrossRef]
63. Borrelli, B.; Ritterband, L.M. Special issue on ehealth and mhealth: Challenges and future directions for assessment, treatment, and dissemination. *Health Psychol.* **2015**, *34*, 1205–1208. [CrossRef]
64. Thurnheer, S.E.; Gravestock, I.; Pichierri, G.; Steurer, J.; Burgstaller, J.M. Benefits of mobile apps in pain management: Systematic review. *JMIR mHealth uHealth* **2018**, *6*, e11231. [CrossRef]

65. Martorella, G.; Boitor, M.; Berube, M.; Fredericks, S.; Le May, S.; Gélinas, C. Tailored web-based interventions for pain: Systematic review and meta-analysis. *J. Med. Internet Res.* **2017**, *19*, e385. [CrossRef]
66. Mehta, S.; Peynenburg, V.A.; Hadjistavropoulos, H.D. Internet-delivered cognitive behaviour therapy for chronic health conditions: A systematic review and meta-analysis. *J. Behav. Med.* **2019**, *42*, 169–187. [CrossRef]
67. Osma, J.; Suso-Ribera, C.; Martínez-Borba, V.; Barrera, A.Z. Content and format preferences of a depression prevention program: A study in perinatal women. *An. Psicol.* **2020**, *36*, 56–63. [CrossRef]
68. Gual-montolio, P.; Martínez-borba, V.; Bretón-lópez, J.M.; Osma, J. How Are Information and Communication Technologies Supporting Routine Outcome Monitoring and Measurement-Based Care in Psychotherapy? A Systematic Review. *Int. J. Environ. Res. Public Health* **2020**, *17*, 3170. [CrossRef]
69. Peters, D.H.; Tran, N.T.; Adam, T. Implementation research in health: A practical guide. Alliance for Health Policy and Systems Research, World Health Organization: Geneva, Switzerland, 2013; p. 69. ISBN 978-92-4-150621-2.
70. Evans, J.G. Evidence-based and evidence-biased medicine. *Age Ageing* **1995**, *24*, 461–463. [CrossRef] [PubMed]
71. Pereira, F.G.; França, M.H.; de Paiva, M.C.A.; Andrade, L.H.; Viana, M.C. Prevalence and clinical profile of chronic pain and its association with mental disorders. *Rev. Saude Publica* **2017**, *51*, 96. [CrossRef] [PubMed]
72. da C. Menezes Costa, L.; Mahera, C.G.; McAuleya, J.H.; Hancock, M.J.; Smeets, R.J.E.M. Self-efficacy is more important than fear of movement in mediating the relationship between pain and disability in chronic low back pain. *Eur. J. Pain* **2011**, *15*, 213–219. [CrossRef]
73. Sullivan, M.J.L.; Adams, H.; Horan, S.; Maher, D.; Boland, D.; Gross, R. The role of perceived injustice in the experience of chronic pain and disability: Scale development and validation. *J. Occup. Rehabil.* **2008**, *18*, 249–261. [CrossRef]
74. Suso-Ribera, C.; Jornet-Gibert, M.; Ribera-Canudas, M.V.; McCracken, L.M.; Maydeu-Olivares, A.; Gallardo-Pujol, D.; Maydeu-Olivares, A.; Gallardo-Pujol, D. A reduction in pain intensity is more strongly associated with improved physical functioning in frustration tolerant individuals. *J. Clin. Psychol. Med. Settings* **2016**, *23*, 192–206. [CrossRef]
75. Lubans, D.R.; Smith, J.J.; Skinner, G.; Morgan, P.J. Development and implementation of a smartphone application to promote physical activity and reduce screen-time in adolescent boys. *Front. Public Health* **2014**, *2*, 1–11. [CrossRef]
76. Price, M.; Yuen, E.K.; Goetter, E.M.; Herbert, J.D.; Forman, E.M.; Acierno, R.; Ruggiero, K.J. mHealth: A mechanism to deliver more accessible, more effective mental health care. *Clin. Psychol. Psychother.* **2014**, *21*, 427–436. [CrossRef]
77. Holm, S. A simple sequential rejective method procedure. *Scand. J. Stat.* **1979**, *6*, 65–70.
78. Nadler, J.T.; Weston, R.; Voyles, E.C. Stuck in the middle: The use and interpretation of mid-points in items on questionnaires. *J. Gen. Psychol.* **2015**, *142*, 71–89. [CrossRef]
79. Weems, G.H.; Onwuegbuzie, A.J. The impact of midpoint responses and reverse coding on survey data. *Meas. Eval. Couns. Dev.* **2001**, *34*, 166–176. [CrossRef]
80. Garland, R. The mid-point on a rating scale: Is it desirable. *Mark. Bull.* **1991**, 2, 66–70.

2

Manipulating the Perceived Shape and Color of a Virtual Limb Can Modulate Pain Responses

Marta Matamala-Gomez [1,2,3,*], Birgit Nierula [1,2,4], Tony Donegan [1], Mel Slater [2] and Maria V. Sanchez-Vives [1,2,5,6]

1. Institut d'Investigacions Biomèdiques August Pi i Sunyer (IDIBAPS), 08036 Barcelona, Spain; bnierula@gmail.com (B.N.); tonydonegan@gmail.com (T.D.); msanche3@clinic.cat (M.V.S.-V.)
2. Event-Lab, Department of Clinical Psychology and Psychobiology, Universitat de Barcelona, 08035 Barcelona, Spain; melslater@gmail.com
3. Dipartamento di Scienze Umane per la Formazione 'Ricardo Massa', Università degli studi Milano-Bicocca, 20126 Milan, Italy
4. Max Planck Institute for Human Cognitive and Brain Sciences, 04103 Leipzig, Germany
5. Departament de Cognició, Desenvolupament i Psicologia de l'Educació, Facultat de Psicologia, Universitat de Barcelona, 08035 Barcelona, Spain
6. Institució Catalana de Recerca i Estudis Avançats (ICREA), 08010 Barcelona, Spain

* Correspondence: marta.matamala10@gmail.com

Abstract: Changes in body representation may affect pain perception. The effect of a distorted body image, such as the telescoping effect in amputee patients, on pain perception, is unclear. This study aimed to investigate whether distorting an embodied virtual arm in virtual reality (simulating the telescoping effect in amputees) modulated pain perception and anticipatory responses to pain in healthy participants. Twenty-seven right-handed participants were immersed in virtual reality and the virtual arm was shown with three different levels of distortion with a virtual threatening stimulus either approaching or contacting the virtual hand. We evaluated pain/discomfort ratings, ownership, and skin conductance responses (SCRs) after each condition. Viewing a distorted virtual arm enhances the SCR to a threatening event with respect to viewing a normal control arm, but when viewing a reddened-distorted virtual arm, SCR was comparatively reduced in response to the threat. There was a positive relationship between the level of ownership over the distorted and reddened-distorted virtual arms with the level of pain/discomfort, but not in the normal control arm. Contact with the threatening stimulus significantly enhances SCR and pain/discomfort, while reduced SCR and pain/discomfort were seen in the simulated-contact condition. These results provide further evidence of a bi-directional link between body image and pain perception.

Keywords: virtual reality; pain perception; telescoped effect; amputee patients

---

1. Introduction

Immersive virtual reality (VR) technology has been repeatedly demonstrated to be an effective tool for modulating pain threshold perception in healthy subjects [1,2], and pain ratings in patients with chronic pain [3,4]. This is because multisensory signals, which can be integrated and manipulated in VR environments, influence our perception of pain, in part because nociceptive stimuli activate a wide network of cortical and subcortical areas in the brain, commonly known as the "pain matrix," that are also implicated in the processing of sensory information [5].

Using VR, one can feel immersed (feeling inside of and being able to interact with the virtual world), and present (the subjective illusion of "being there," when placed in the immersed virtual environment despite the knowledge that you are not there) [6] in a multisensory environment that is under the full control of the experimenter [7]. Furthermore, it is possible to induce, through VR, the illusion of owning a virtual body; this refers to the subjective illusion that a body or body part is one's own, which again is facilitated by multisensory feedback such as synchronous visual and tactile stimulation, when the virtual and the real bodies are co-located at the same position [8]. The sense of ownership over a virtual body, or "embodiment," is highly flexible regarding the visual aspect of the body, and it is possible to embody bodies that are quite different from those in real life [9,10]. The virtual body can therefore be designed with the morphological characteristics that the experimenter determines [11]. This allows the exploration of how the visual aspect of the body modulates pain perception. For example, Martini et al. [2] investigated the influence of skin color on pain perception when participants were embodied in a virtual body. They found that participants experienced pain threshold reduction when the virtual arm was represented in red compared to a "normal" or blue color. In addition, another study by the same group showed that virtual arm transparency decreases the pain threshold [12]. It is also possible to alter pain perception and anticipatory responses to pain in healthy subjects by modulating the morphological characteristics of the limb, such as showing a subject's limb becoming smaller or bigger [13]. Moreover, we can reduce pain perception in a patient with chronic pain whose painful limb feels bigger than it really is by reducing the apparent size of their painful limb [14]. This top-down modulation of pain through modification of visual input reveals the potential of VR illusions as a treatment for pain. Additionally, instead of virtual body illusions, other studies have used VR to provide immersive virtual environments as a distractive pain strategy [15,16].

Even though VR is a potential tool for modulating the pain threshold through virtual body illusions in healthy subjects [1,2,12,17–20], this cannot be extrapolated to how these strategies are going to work in chronic pain patients. Indeed, there are some conflicting results about how bodily illusions can reduce chronic pain in clinical populations [21,22]. In this regard, a study conducted with thirteen amputee patients showed that, while phantom pain was reduced after four weeks of mirror therapy training in five amputee patients, eight amputee patients who reported telescopic distortion of the phantom limb (telescopic distortion refers to the feeling that the proximal portion of the amputated limb is missing or has shrunk with the more distal portion floating near, attached to, or 'within' the stump [23,24]), reported a gradual increase in phantom pain perception after the same mirror therapy training [22]. This difference may be due to the different cortical representations of the limb, a phenomenon seen not only in amputees but also in patients with complex regional pain syndrome and other chronic pain conditions [25–29]. The altered representation of the painful part of the body in the brain seems to play a key role in the development and maintenance of chronic pain, and therapies that attempt to reverse these changes have been partially successful, especially in amputee patients [30]. However, few studies have investigated how distorting a representation of a body part affects the sensation of pain. The present study aims to ascertain whether the illusion of ownership over a telescopically distorted virtual arm can modulate pain perception. To study pain, without delivering painful stimuli and avoiding the problems associated with sensitization/adaptation to repeated painful stimuli, we have used a paradigm of anticipatory responses to pain. Since the responses to a threatening stimulus start before skin contact [13], we investigated both the responses to pain when a threatening stimulus touched the virtual hand of the participant and the anticipatory responses to pain as a threatening stimulus approached the virtual hand. In order to deliver an unpleasant sensation to the participants, we used a vibration stimulus attached to the palm associated and triggered by a virtual needle as a threatening stimulus. For this, the skin conductance responses (SCRs), corresponding to the activation of the autonomic nervous system [31], of healthy subjects were recorded while they were embodied in a virtual body in several conditions in which the virtual arm, which was co-located with their real arm, had a normal or a distorted representation. Moreover, as was done in previous investigations [2,32], we wanted to investigate the effects of the redness of a colored telescopically distorted virtual arm on pain both when a threatening stimulus touched the virtual hand of the participant, and the anticipatory response to pain as a threatening stimulus approached the virtual hand.

The current study is a proof-of-concept study that may help us understand the mechanisms of visual distortion of body image, such as the telescoping effect in amputees (the distal part of the phantom limb perceived as shrinking within the stump), and its effect on pain responses.

2. Methods

2.1. Participants

Thirty right-handed, healthy subjects above 18 years of age participated in this study. Three subjects were excluded from further analysis due to an extremely high *z*-score (>± 2.5) in the SCR data, which led to a final sample size of 27 right-handed subjects (8 males and 19 females; mean age ± SD = 24.7 ± 1.1; mean Edinburgh scale ± SD = 68.7 ± 1.1). The following conditions were considered as inclusion criteria for participation in the study: normal or normal-when-corrected vision, the absence of neurological disorders, no history of chronic pain or other conditions interfering with pain sensitivity, no presence of epilepsy, no medication in use that changed attention to pain or general perception for 24 h before the experiment, and no pregnant women. The experiment was carried out in the installations of the Eventlab for Neuroscience and Technology Laboratory at the University of Barcelona/IDIBAPS. All participants gave written informed consent and received monetary compensation for their participation (12 €). The study was approved by the local ethics committee (Comité Ético de Investigación Clínica de la Corporación Sanitaria Hospital Clínic de Barcelona, HCB/2017/1068) and was carried out according to the Declaration of Helsinki [33].

2.2. Study Design

In order to investigate whether observation of a telescopically distorted representation of the arm alters pain responses and anticipatory responses to pain in healthy subjects, participants completed one experimental session of 20 min. This study was a 3 × 2 within-subject experimental design. The experimental setup is shown in Figure 1A. In this study, there were two main factors. The first factor was Virtual Arm, with three different representations of the virtual arm: (1) the virtual arm represented in a normal position (Control); (2) the virtual arm represented in a distorted position, namely, a shortened virtual forearm shrinking within the arm (telescoped virtual arm) (Distorted); and (3) the virtual arm represented in a distorted position (telescoped virtual arm) and was red (Reddened-Distorted) (see Figure 1B). In all cases, the virtual arm was co-located with the real arm. The telescoped virtual arm representation was created following the graphical representation illustrating telescoping from the 5th edition of *Practical Management of Pain* [34]. In order to explore how these different representations of the virtual arm alter anticipatory responses to pain and pain responses itself, the second factor was *Threatening Stimulus Contact*, with two different types of threatening stimulus: (1) a tactile stimulus that contacted the skin (Real Contact); and (2) a stimulus that approached but did not touch the skin (Simulated Contact). For this, we used a vibrator attached to the palm of the hand of the participants to deliver visuo-tactile stimulations when the threatening stimulus (a virtual needle) contacted the palm of the virtual hand (see Figure 1C). Note that this is a tactile but non-nociceptive stimulus. The three virtual arm representations were combined with the two visually threatening stimulus contacts, resulting in six different conditions, each of which was presented three times. The order of the conditions was randomized among the subjects. Hence, each participant completed a total of 18 virtual arm and threatening stimulus exposures. After each exposure, participants had to indicate their level of sensory intensity (pain intensity) and affective magnitude (unpleasantness/discomfort), assessed using a visual analogue scale (VAS) [35] through a single request: "On a scale from 0 to 100, indicate the level of pain intensity/discomfort that you felt, please." Further, after each exposure, participants had to indicate their level of ownership over the virtual arm [12]. Each stimulus exposure lasted 53 s (Figure 1D). After completing the virtual reality experiment, participants had to complete a questionnaire to evaluate their overall virtual reality experience [36]. In order to measure the electrodermal response when the threatening stimulus eventually touched the skin, and the anticipatory physiological response to an incoming threatening stimulus, the SCR was recorded following exposure to the threatening stimulus [13,37], which in the real contact condition touched the virtual hand and in the simulated contact condition simply approached the virtual hand without contacting it.

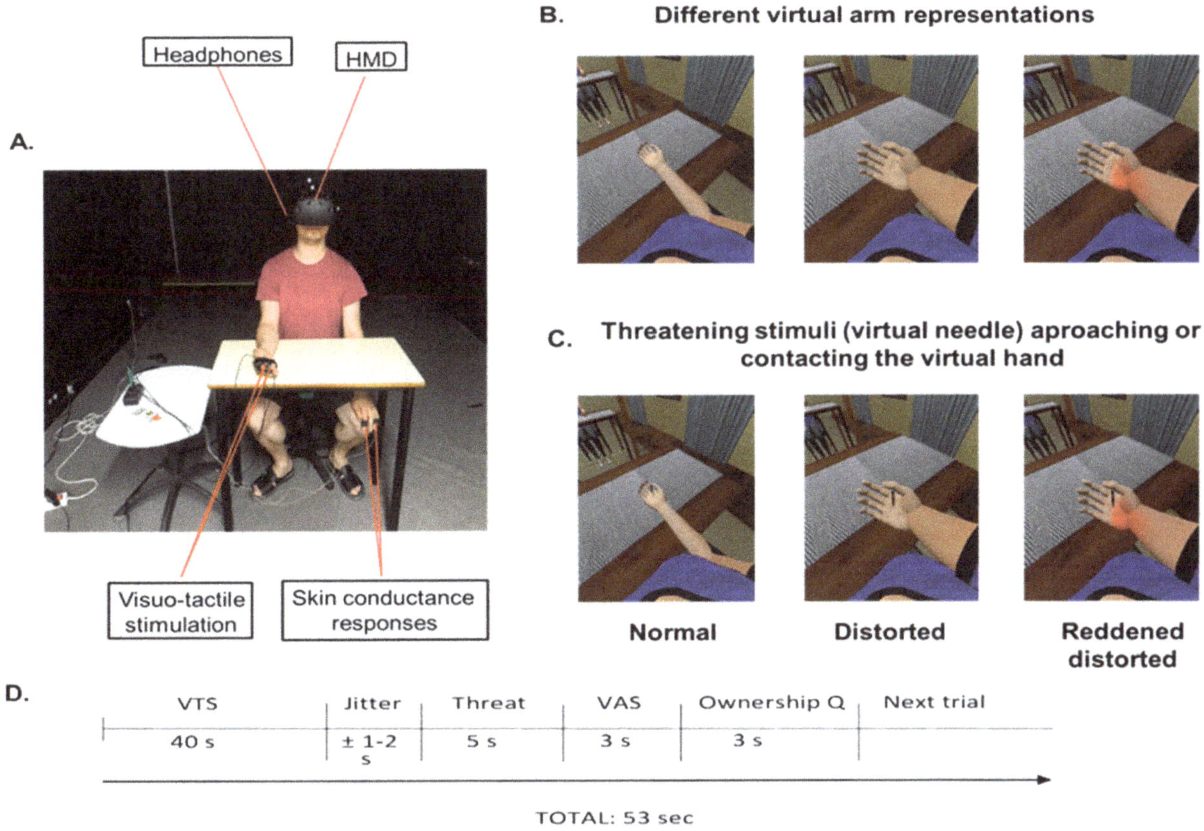

Figure 1. Experimental set-up and virtual arm and threatening stimulus conditions. (**A**) Participants wore a head-mounted display (HMD) that immersed them in a virtual environment. This allowed them to feel embodied in a virtual body, which they saw from a first-person perspective and which was co-located with their real body. Using headphones, participants heard the task instruction, "Pay attention to the right arm placed on the table, please," before each visuo-tactile stimulus phase, which lasted 45 s. During the visuo-tactile stimulation, which was used to induce ownership over the virtual arm, virtual balls tapped the virtual fingers while participants felt, simultaneously, a tactile stimulation (vibration) on their real fingers. To record skin conductance responses after each threatening stimulus, two electrodes were attached to the index and ring fingers of the participants' left hands. (**B**) Different virtual arm representations (virtual arm factor): normal representation, distorted representation (telescoped virtual arm), and reddened-distorted representation of the virtual arm. The distorted representation of the virtual forearm was shrinking within the virtual arm, as occurs with the telescoping effect in amputee patients. However, from a participant's first-person perspective it seems bigger than the normal representation. (**C**) Threatening stimulus (virtual needle) in all three levels of the virtual arm factor. (**D**) Timeline of one experimental trial. Each experimental trial lasted around 53 s and was divided into four parts: First, participants were immersed in an immersive virtual reality (VR) environment in which the virtual arm could either be distorted, reddened and distorted, or in a normal position. To induce ownership over the virtual arm, they received 45 s of synchronous visuo-tactile stimulation. Second, after a jitter of 1–2 s, the threatening event appeared (a virtual needle) for 5 s. Immediately after the threatening event, the VAS appeared on the screen of the HMD. Finally, after the VAS was taken, a question related to ownership over the virtual arm appeared. VTS, visuo-tactile stimulation VAS, visual analogue scale; Ownership Q, ownership questionnaire.

2.3. *Apparatus*

2.3.1. Head-Mounted Display

We used a head-mounted display (HMD) (Rift Development Kit 2, Oculus, Menlo Park, CA, USA) with a resolution of 960 × 1080 pixels per eye and a nominal horizontal field of view of 100° displayed at 75 Hz to show the virtual environment, which was programmed in Unity 4.5.3 (Unity Technologies, San Francisco, CA, USA). The virtual body was configured to match the gender of the participants (female or male) and was taken from the Rocketbox library (Rocketbox Studios GmbH, Hannover, Germany). The virtual environment was the same during all conditions. Headphones were used in order to allow the participants to follow the task instructions during the experimental sessions (Figure 1A).

2.3.2. Visuo-Tactile Stimulation

To increase the illusion of ownership over the virtual body, we used visuo-tactile stimulation. For this, we delivered tactile stimulation to the participants by using vibrators attached to the middle and index fingers, and to the palm of the right hand, that were controlled by Unity through an Arduino MEGA microcontroller board (Figure 1A). Each vibration had a duration of 1.0 s.

2.3.3. Skin Conductance Responses

To record skin conductance, we attached two electrodes to the index and the ring fingers of the left hands of the participants (Figure 1A). The SCR was recorded at a sampling rate of 256 Hz, using a portable biosignal acquisition device (g.MOBIlab+, g.tec), while the recording and storage of the data was handled by a Simulink model in Matlab 2012b (The MathWorks, Inc., Natick, MA, USA).

2.4. *Procedures*

2.4.1. Position of the Participants

Participants were seated on a chair with their right arm resting on the table and their left arm hidden under the table, resting on the left leg to ensure that participants only paid attention to their right arm during the experimental session. The right arm of the subject was placed within their field of view. The two vibrators attached to the dorsal distal phalanges of the right index and middle fingers were used in order to deliver visuo-tactile stimulations to induce the ownership illusion over the virtual arm. The other vibrator attached to the palm of the hand was used to deliver visuo-tactile stimulations when the threatening stimulus (the virtual needle) contacted the palm of the virtual hand. Through the HMD, participants were immersed in a virtual reality scenario in which they saw a virtual body from a first-person perspective co-located with their own real body [38]. They heard the task instructions through headphones throughout the experimental session, and their skin conductance was recorded with the two electrodes attached to their left index and ring fingers.

2.4.2. Virtual Reality Scenario

Once participants donned the HMD, the room lights were turned off to allow the participants to be fully immersed in the virtual environment. At the beginning of the experimental session, participants were instructed to look around the virtual room, to describe what they saw, and to look down at their virtual body in order to habituate to the virtual scenario and the virtual body. The right virtual arm was always placed in the field of view of the participants with the palm of the hand facing up to the celling. Once the habituation phase was over, participants were asked to focus their attention on the right virtual arm. During the entire session and before the presentation of each condition, participants listened to the following verbal instruction through the headphones: "Pay attention to the right arm that is located on the table, please." In order to induce the illusory ownership over the virtual body in each different representation of the virtual arm, each representation of the virtual arm included

40 s of visuo-tactile stimulation where participants saw a virtual ball tapping in random order their virtual right index and middle finger whilst feeling a spatiotemporal synchronous vibration on their real right index and middle finger, respectively [39]. During the experimental session, participants were exposed to six conditions in which three representations of the arm were combined with two types of stimulus contact.

2.4.3. Pain Ratings and Ownership Measures

Pain ratings and measures of the degree of ownership over the virtual arm were taken for each of the six conditions to measure the effect of visual distortion on the sensory and anticipatory aspects of pain processing. Once each virtual trial was over, the screen of the HMD turned black and a VAS appeared with a voice instruction asking the participants to judge how strong the pain feels in order to assess the intensity of pain and how discomforting the threatening stimulus was perceived, on a scale ranging from 0 (not discomfort at all/minimum pain intensity) to 100 (worst discomfort/strongest pain intensity imaginable) [13]. Participants' ratings were promptly annotated by the experimenter. After the VAS, a question related to ownership over the virtual arm in each representation appeared in the screen of the HMD, with a voice instruction asking the participant to judge their level of ownership over the virtual arm from −3 (totally disagree) to 3 (totally agree), with the following sentence: "I felt that the virtual arm was my arm" [36]. After the virtual reality exposure, the HMD and the headphones were removed and participants had to fill in a questionnaire concerning the overall virtual reality experience.

2.5. SCR Data Preprocessing

The peak-to-base response amplitude of skin conductance was used as an index of SCR [40–42]. For the assessment of SCRs, the difference between the maximum value detected in a 6 s post-stimulus time window and the baseline (3 s pre-stimulus) was computed, which is comparable with other studies in which a time frame of 1–5 s after stimulus onset was chosen [43–45]. Finally, we obtained the normalized maximum change of the SCR after each stimulus (virtual needle real contact/virtual needle simulated contact). The sample rate to extract SCR data was set to 256 Hz. The data were stored under Matlab and could be opened in the Matlab command windows with g.BSanalyze (gtec). Final SCR data were obtained by using a Matlab graphical user interface (GUI) for feature extraction of the skin conductance signal *(featextractiongui)* in Matlab2012b (The MathWorks, Inc. Natick, MA, USA). Event markers identifying each stimulus type were programmed to automatically register SCR when the stimulus—the virtual needle—contacted (real contact) or approached (simulated contact) the palm of the virtual hand.

2.6. Virtual Reality Experience Questionnaire

Once participants completed the whole VR exposure, they had to fill in a questionnaire related to their VR experience, answering the following statements from −3 (totally disagree) to +3 (totally agree) [36]:

- Q1. During the experiment there were moments in which I felt that the virtual balls were touching my real fingers.
- Q2. Although the virtual body did not seem to be physically my body, I felt that it could be my own body.
- Q3. When I saw the virtual arm distorted, I felt that my own arm was distorted as well.
- Q4. During each different representation of the virtual arm, I felt that if I moved my real arm the virtual arm would start moving too.
- Q5. During the whole experimental session, I was able to focus my attention to the right arm.

2.7. Data Handling

All statistical tests were performed in Stata 13 (StataCorp LP, College Station, TX, USA). This was a mixed-effects design, with fixed-effects virtual arm (normal, distorted, reddened-distorted) and threat contact (real contact, simulated contact), and random effects over the individual subjects. We analyzed differences in pain ratings and in SCR across conditions with a multilevel mixed-effects linear regression test (the "mixed" function in Stata). Furthermore, in order to observe differences between virtual arm conditions, we ran a pairwise comparison with the Scheffe test for multiple comparisons. Moreover, in order to observe a possible relationship between ownership and pain ratings assessed with the VAS throughout the experiment, we used Spearman's correlation test. In order to observe differences in ownership scores across conditions, we used multilevel mixed-effect ordered logistic regression test (the "meologit" function in Stata). Finally, in order to conduct mediation analyses, we used a seemingly unrelated regression test (the "sureg" function in Stata).

3. Results

3.1. Changes in Shape and Color of the Virtual Arm Modulate SCR after Threatening Stimulus Exposure

Our results show that changes in shape and color of the virtual arm modulated SCR after a threatening stimulus exposure. In this case, the SCR was taken as a proxy of pain responses, as has been established in previous work by Romano and Maravita [13]. Specifically, we observed a higher SCR when the virtual arm was distorted (telescoped virtual arm) compared with the normal virtual arm ($z = -2.93$, $p = 0.003$); we did not find a significant relationship between the shape changes of the virtual arm and SCR, but did find a significant relationship between color changes and SCR. The results show that the red color in the reddened-distorted virtual arm increase anticipatory pain responses, showing a significant difference between normal ($z = -2.93$, $p = 0.014$) and distorted ($z = -4.79$, $p < 0.0001$) virtual arm conditions. Furthermore, in relation to the dependency of the SCR on the threatening stimulus contact, our results showed a significant decrease in SCR when the threatening stimulus approached but did not contact the virtual hand (simulated contact), compared to the real contact condition ($z = -3.08$, $p = 0.002$) (Figure 2). Interestingly, the proportions between SCR in normal virtual arm, those of distorted and reddened-distorted arms, were the same both for the real contact and the simulated contact; however, the absolute values were smaller in the simulated contact. Table 1 summarizes SCR values and p-values for all of the experimental conditions.

Table 1. Values in terms of means, standard error (SE), and p-values indicating mean differences between the different experimental conditions.

	Virtual Arm			Threat Contact	
Experimental Variable	**Normal Virtual Arm (1)**	**Distorted Virtual Arm (2)**	**Reddened-Distorted Virtual Arm (3)**	**Real Contact (1)**	**Simulated Contact (2)**
Mean	8.13	10.43	4.49	9.27	6.17
SE	13.20	12.63	9.25	13.60	10.09
p-value	0.014	<0.001			<0.001
Conditions	3 vs. 1	3 vs. 2			2 vs. 1

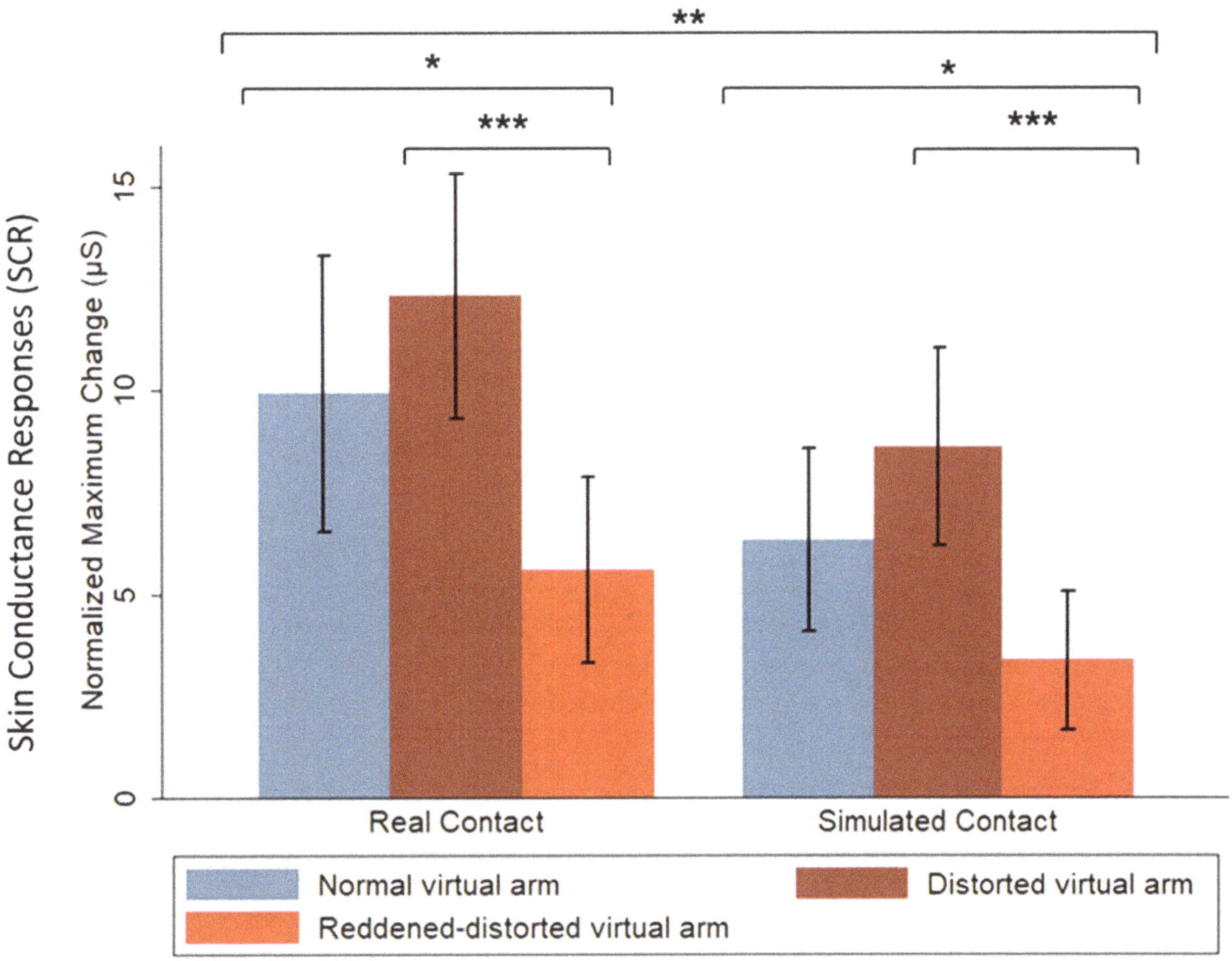

Figure 2. Skin conductance response (SCR) increased when the virtual needle contacted (real contact) the virtual hand in all three virtual arm conditions, while the reddened-distorted virtual arm showed a comparatively decreased SCR in both real and simulated contact of the threatening stimulus. Difference in SCR after the threatening stimulus contacted (real contact) or approached (simulated contact) the virtual hand in all three virtual arm conditions. Bars show mean change in SCR and error bars indicate 95% confidence interval. * $p < 0.05$, ** $p < 0.01$, *** $p < 0.001$.

3.2. Distortion of the Virtual Arm Increase Pain Ratings (VAS) after Threatening Stimulus Exposure

The data obtained in our study show a positive relationship between the level of ownership over the distorted ($r_s = 0.226$, $p < 0.01$) and reddened-distorted ($r_s = 0.225$, $p < 0.01$) virtual arms with the level of pain/discomfort assessed using the VAS. Nevertheless, this positive relationship was not found after the normal virtual arm exposure ($r_s = 0023$, $p = 0.767$) (Figure 3A–C). Thus, in the distorted virtual arm conditions, we found that the higher the level of ownership of the distorted and reddened-distorted virtual arm, the higher the pain/discomfort perception. Furthermore, in agreement with the above results in which we observed a significant difference when the threatening stimulus contacted or approached the virtual arm, again our results show a significant difference in pain/discomfort perception when the threatening stimulus contacted or approached the virtual arm. In particular, we found lower VAS scores when the threatening stimulus approached the virtual hand, but not when it contacted the virtual hand (multilevel effects mixed effects $z = -7.00$, $p < 0.001$).

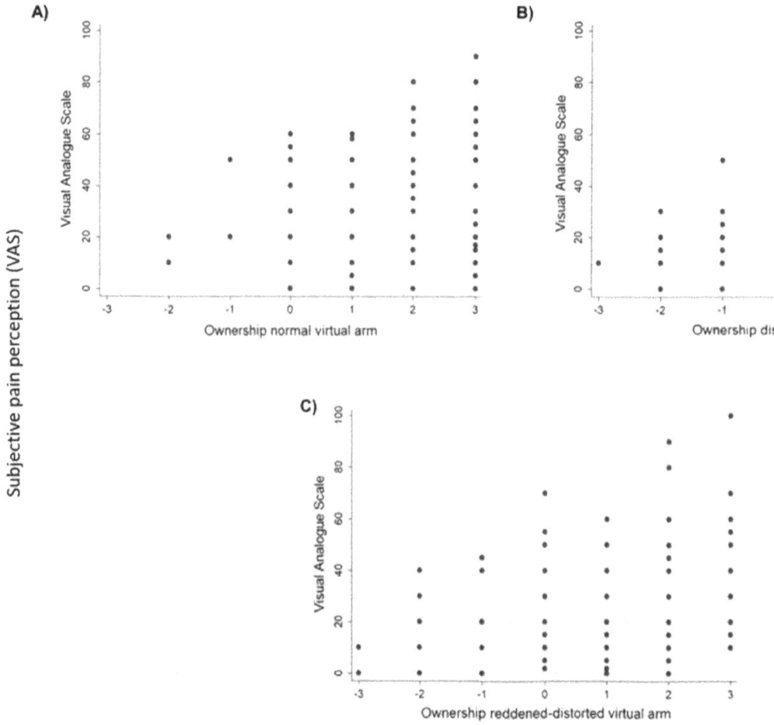

Figure 3. Pain ratings increase with the distortion of the embodied virtual arm. The relationship between pain ratings and ownership levels under the (**A**) normal virtual arm condition (no relationship); (**B**) the distorted virtual arm condition; and (**C**) the reddened-distorted virtual arm condition.

3.3. Dependency of Ownership on Shape and Color Changes of the Virtual Arm after Threatening Stimulus Exposure

The reported levels of ownership show a statistically significant difference between the different representations of the virtual arm, ownership being higher with the normal representation of the virtual arm. Indeed, we found a statistically significant difference in ownership between the normal representation of the virtual arm and both the distorted ($z = -9.16$, $p < 0.001$) and reddened-distorted virtual arm ($z = -8.92$, $p < 0.001$). In addition, contact of the threatening stimulus with the virtual hand significantly increased the level of ownership in all three virtual arm representations compared with simulated contact of the threatening stimulus ($z = -2.30$, $p = 0.021$) (Figure 4A). Table 2 summarizes ownership values and p-values for all of the experimental conditions.

Table 2. Scoring values in terms of mean, standard error (SE) and p-values for all the different experimental conditions.

Experimental Variable	Virtual Arm			Threat Contact	
	Normal Virtual Arm (1)	Distorted Virtual Arm (2)	Reddened-Distorted Virtual Arm (3)	Real Contact (1)	Simulated Contact (2)
Mean	1.89	1.03	1.05	1.42	1.38
SE	1.13	1.49	1.50	1.23	1.49
p-value		<0.001	<0.001		0.021
Condition		2 vs. 1	3 vs. 1		2 vs. 1

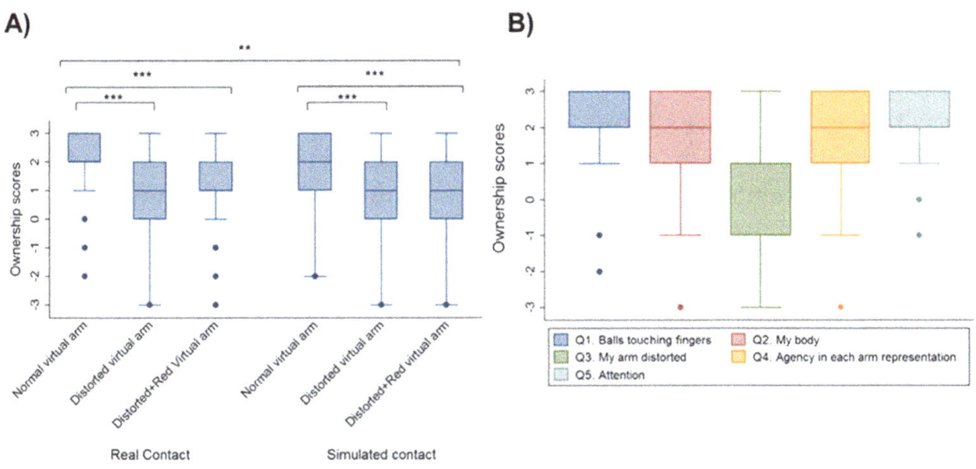

Figure 4. Ownership levels increase with the normal representation of the virtual arm. (**A**) Ownership question ratings after each virtual reality condition exposure show higher ownership scores in the normal virtual arm representation compared with the distorted and reddened-distorted conditions, in both real and simulated contact of the threatening stimulus. (**B**) Questionnaire ratings after the whole virtual reality exposure show that although participants reported high levels of agency and ownership of the virtual body, ownership scores decreased with the distorted virtual arm representation. Boxplots show medians (horizontal lines), interquartile ranges (IQR; boxes), data outside 1.5 × IQR (whiskers), and outliers (o). ** $p < 0.01$, *** $p < 0.001$.

From the results obtained in the final VR questionnaire that participants had to fill in after the VR experience, we found that participants reported high levels of ownership (Q1, Q2) and agency (Q4) of the virtual body and virtual arm. However, we also observed low scores in ownership levels with the distorted virtual arm representation (Q3). Finally, in Q5, which was related to the level of attention towards the virtual arm, participants reported high attention levels of the virtual arm throughout the whole VR exposure (Figure 4B).

We found that ownership (ownership scoring collected during the experimental sessions) mediates differences in SCR, but not subjective pain ratings (VAS), between the different virtual arm conditions. Specifically, we found a significant relationship between the independent factor virtual arm and the mediation variable ownership ($z = -5.39$, $p < 0.001$). Further, we also found a significant relationship between the SCR (dependent variable) and ownership ($z = -2.91$, $p = 0.004$), and between the SCR and the virtual arm factor ($z = -3.34$, $p = 0.001$). We calculated the mediation effect (ME) by the following calculation: ME = regression coefficient between SCR and ownership ($r_s = -1.13$) × regression coefficient between SCR and virtual arm ($r_s = -0.42$). The ME of ownership in SCR between the different virtual arm conditions is 0.472. Although we did not find a relationship between the subjective pain ratings (VAS), as a second dependent variable, and the virtual arm factor ($z = 0.90$, $p = 0.367$), we found a significant relationship between VAS and ownership ($z = 5.31$, $p < 0.001$). Nevertheless, no mediation effects of ownership can be reported in subjective pain responses ratings (VAS) between different virtual arm conditions.

4. Discussion

Through immersive virtual reality, we can induce the sense of owning a virtual arm by using a congruent multisensory correlation between the real and the virtual arm [8,46]. It is known that changes in the color and shape of a virtual arm (that is co-located with the real one) modulate pain threshold in healthy subjects (see [47] for a review). Furthermore, there is some evidence demonstrating that a distorted representation in the brain of the painful part of the body is associated with increased pain perception in chronic pain patients [48,49]. Along these lines, some studies have investigated the role of the representation of the painful part of the body in the brain, such as the telescopic effect in amputees, on pain perception [25,50]. The study by Makin and colleagues [25] highlighted the importance of the preserved representation of the amputated limb in the area of the brain where the former hand was represented [51] as a key factor involved in chronic phantom pain. In their study, the authors suggested that this preserved representation could activate phantom chronic pain through top-down (central to peripheral nervous system) mechanisms. In line with this study, Bultitude and Rafal [26] suggested that the pain in patients with complex regional pain syndrome is a consequence of a distorted representation of the affected limb in the brain. Furthermore, some patients with chronic pain report that the mental representation of their affected body part is somehow distorted in size or posture, or even absent entirely [27–29], which may be associated with a distorted cortical representation of the limb. While early investigations found that visual feedback techniques such as mirror therapy or virtual reality could reduce pain perception in amputee patients [30,52,53], it has also been shown that mirror therapy can exacerbate pain in those amputees that experience the telescopic effect [22].

Here, we conducted a proof-of-concept study in healthy subjects in order to better understand the mechanisms of pain/discomfort in amputee patients that suffer from the telescoping effect. Although the mechanisms for acute and chronic pain are different [54], and amputees and healthy individuals are likely to have significantly different cortical representation of their body [55], this study can contribute to the understanding of the effects of visual distortion of the body on pain. We observed that multisensory integration interventions using VR could be used to manipulate the shape and color of the virtual body representation in order to modulate pain perception and anticipatory responses to pain in healthy subjects. We conclude that autonomic responses (SCR) that act as proxies of pain responses are enhanced when there is a virtual threat (virtual needle) that approaches or eventually touches a virtual arm that feels a part of one's own body. This paradigm can be used in order to explore how changes in the morphological or functional characteristics of the represented virtual body can modulate pain responses while avoiding the problems derived from repetitive painful stimulation, such as sensitization and adaptation. Although existing studies have demonstrated that visual illusions in which arm size is increased or decreased can affect pain perception in both healthy and clinical populations [4,13,56], this is the first study to investigate how being embodied in a virtual body with a distorted virtual arm (simulating the telescopic effect in amputees), affects subjective (pain scores in VAS) and the related physiological responses (SCR) to a threatening event in healthy subjects.

First, regarding the virtual arm factor, we found that being embodied in a distorted virtual arm enhances SCR and pain/discomfort ratings to the threatening event compared with the normal virtual arm condition; these results are in line with later investigations [13] in which the authors found higher SCR while observing a visually magnified hand. Moreover, other studies also found that visual enlargement of the hand being viewed enhanced analgesia by increasing heat-pain thresholds, compared with the visual reduction of the viewed hand [57]. However, the opposite effect was found in clinical populations with chronic pain, in which the visual enlargement of the affected hand increased pain perception compared with the visual reduction of the affected hand [14]. Furthermore, in the former study [57], they also found that visual enlargement of the viewed hand enhanced analgesia by increasing heat-pain thresholds, while visual reduction of the viewed hand reduced analgesia. However, the opposite effect was found in clinical populations with chronic pain, in which the visual enlargement of the affected hand increased pain perception compared with visual reduction of the affected hand [14]. Furthermore, in another study, a negative body image associated with an injured-appearing hand (induced using the rubber hand illusion paradigm) reduced the pain threshold in healthy subjects, but no such increase was seen with a visually distorted (stretched) rubber hand [58]. One possible explanation for the difference is that the distorted rubber hand was not exactly co-located with the real hand of the participant, diminishing the sense of ownership of the rubber hand, as surmised by Nierula and co-authors [17].

In a previous study, Romano and Maravita [13] found that visual distortion of the hand by giving a visual minifying hand feedback increased SCR in healthy subjects, whilst a magnified visual feedback of the hand decreased SCR, which suggests that the visual size increase enhances the cognitive, anticipatory component of pain processing. In our study we also found that SCR was lower in the reddened-distorted virtual arm condition compared with normal and distorted virtual arm conditions. In line with the study from Romano and Maravita [13], we speculate that in our study the red color in the reddened-distorted virtual arm enhanced the cognitive, anticipatory component of pain processing and decreased the SCR to the subsequent threatening stimulus. In fact, it is known that by observing a reddened embodied virtual arm, we can reduce the pain threshold in healthy subjects [2]. Hence, as participants were observing the reddened virtual arm 45 s before the threatening stimulus appeared (visuo-tactile stimulation phase) at the beginning of each condition, we can speculate that the red color caused an anticipatory pain response, resulting in a reduction in SCR following the threatening stimulus being in contact or simulated contact with the virtual arm. This effect could be induced via several mechanisms: on one hand, anticipatory responses to pain could induce the activation of endogenous descending analgesic neural pathways [59], involving subcortical reticular structures that target the dorsal horns of the spinal cord grey matter, reducing afferent noxious signals. This interpretation could be explained by the principle of diffuse noxious inhibitory control, by which a noxious stimulus decreases the response (or increases the threshold) to a subsequent painful stimulus (see [60] for a review). On the other hand, the expectation of the incoming painful stimulus can induce a pre-activation of early somatosensory regions with a subsequently decreased response when the signal from the noxious stimulus arrives at the cortex [61]. Moreover, it is also known that the more certainty regarding a painful stimulus that modulates the expectancy about pain perception, the more the recruitment of attentional resources to the ascending nociceptive input [62]. Hence, one may hypothesize that changes in shape and color of an embodied virtual arm may modulate both physiological and subjective measures of pain responses.

Secondly, in our study we found a generally increased SCR and subjective measure of pain perception when the threatening stimulus touched the virtual hand, and a generally reduced SCR when the threatening stimulus approached but did not touch the virtual hand in all three virtual arm conditions. Our findings differ from those shown in the study by Romano and Maravita [13], in which they observed a reduced SCR with real contact noxious stimuli while observing a magnified hand was associated with increased anticipatory SCR when the noxious stimuli approached the skin without touching it. However, they also observed a general increase in SCR for both real and simulated contact while observing a shrunken vision of the hand. In our study we did not observe such differences in SCR between the different virtual arm conditions. One explanation for this could be the synchronous visuo-tactile stimulation that participants received in their real hand once the threatening stimulus touched the virtual hand. It is well known that through synchronous visuo-tactile stimulation we may induce a sense of ownership over a fake limb, as in the "rubber hand illusion" study [63], over a whole fake body [64] and over a virtual arm [8]. Therefore, we postulate that the fact of receiving tactile stimulation (vibration) at the same place of the real hand, at the same time that the threatening stimulus touched the embodied virtual hand, enhanced the feeling of the virtual needle hurting the virtual arm, thereby enhancing pain perception. Finally, participants experienced higher levels of ownership with the normal virtual arm condition either when the virtual needle touched or approached the virtual arm. Nevertheless, participants reported higher levels of ownership after the normal virtual arm representation in the real contact of the threatening event condition. Once again, this could be explained by the synchronous visuo-tactile stimulation that is induced when the virtual needle touches the virtual hand, which may enhance the sense of ownership over the virtual body [8]. Then, one may postulate that the observed results in the subjective pain responses and physiological responses to the threatening event may be related to the lower ownership responses towards the distorted (telescoped) virtual arm condition.

Finally, mediation effects of ownership ratings in SCR are open to several interpretations. First, this effect confirms that being embodied in a virtual body by providing a virtual body illusion can modulate physiological responses, as has been demonstrated previously [65–67]. Further, modulation of the morphological characteristics of the virtual body modulates physiological responses [68].

Our results show that changing the morphological characteristics of an embodied virtual body while being in a painful or threatening situation may modulate the physiological responses associated with pain, and these can be mediated by the feeling of ownership of the virtual body. While the use of embodiment to change body representations for pain relief has been already discussed (see [47] for a review), no mediation effects of ownership were found for the subjective pain measure (VAS ratings). One explanation of this may be because of the lower ownership ratings, compared to the normal virtual arm representation, obtained in the distorted and in the reddened-distorted virtual arm conditions. Although participants knew that the distorted virtual arm was not their real arm, it still influenced physiological responses of the participants, as has been demonstrated in previous studies [2,18,69]. Hence, even though participants felt less ownership in the distorted virtual arm conditions, physiological responses to pain were still modulated, highlighting the powerful effect of virtual embodiment in modulating body representations and their consequent impact on the modulation of physiological responses of pain responses.

5. Limitations

The present study shows a limitation regarding an unbalance in the participants' genders. It is known that females and males perceive pain differently [70], so although in this study no experimental pain was induced, the threatening event and the distortion of the virtual arm could activate both pain and anticipatory pain responses.

6. Conclusions

The present study investigated the influence of telescoping effects on the perception of pain by inducing such limb distortions in healthy people through VR. Our findings are in line with other studies in which the authors demonstrated that healthy subjects could experience the telescoped effect and the associated telescoping sensations (pain/discomfort) normally experienced by amputee patients through full virtual body illusions. Further, the results of this study demonstrate that the link between body image and pain responses is bi-directional, showing a top-down effect of body image on pain. This bi-directional link has also been reported in other studies [22,25,50,71,72]. Furthermore, our results reinforce the importance of tackling body image distortions when trying to reduce pain responses in chronic pain patients, especially in amputee patients with a telescopic limb sensation, suggesting that VR could be a powerful tool for modulating pain responses by changing the representation of the telescoped limb.

Author Contributions: Conceptualization, M.M.-G., B.N. and M.V.S.-V.; methodology, M.M.-G. and B.N.; software, M.S.; validation, M.V.S.-V.; formal analysis, M.M.-G. and M.S.; investigation, M.M.-G.; resources, M.V.S.-V. and M.S.; data curation, M.M.-G.; writing—original draft preparation, M.M.-G. and T.D.; writing—review and editing, T.D., M.V.S.-V. and M.S.; visualization, M.V.S.-V. and M.S.; supervision, M.V.S.-V.; project administration, T.D.; funding acquisition, M.V.S.-V. and M.S. All authors have read and agreed to the published version of the manuscript.

Acknowledgments: We thank Ramón Olivera from the Event-Lab for the virtual reality scenarios, and for technical support.

References

1. Martini, M.; Perez-Marcos, D.; Sanchez-Vives, M.V. Modulation of pain threshold by virtual body ownership. *Eur. J. Pain* **2014**, *18*, 1040–1048. [CrossRef]
2. Martini, M.; Perez-Marcos, D.; Sanchez-Vives, M.V. What Color is My Arm? Changes in Skin Color of an Embodied Virtual Arm Modulates Pain Threshold. *Front. Hum. Neurosci.* **2013**, *7*, 438. [CrossRef]

3. Llobera, J.; González-Franco, M.; Perez-Marcos, D.; Valls-Solé, J.; Slater, M.; Sanchez-Vives, M.V. Virtual reality for assessment of patients suffering chronic pain: A case study. *Exp. Brain Res.* **2013**, *225*, 105–117. [CrossRef] [PubMed]
4. Senkowski, D.; Heinz, A. Chronic pain and distorted body image: Implications for multisensory feedback interventions. *Neurosci. Biobehav. Rev.* **2016**, *69*, 252–259. [CrossRef]
5. Mouraux, A.; Diukova, A.; Lee, M.C.; Wise, R.G.; Iannetti, G.D. A multisensory investigation of the functional significance of the "pain matrix". *Neuroimage* **2011**, *54*, 2237–2249. [CrossRef]
6. Slater, M. Place Illusion and Plausibility Can Lead to Realistic Behaviour in Immersive Virtual Environments. *Philos. Trans. R. Soc.* **2009**, *364*, 3549–3557. [CrossRef] [PubMed]
7. Sanchez-Vives, M.V.; Slater, M. From presence to consciousness through virtual reality. *Nat. Rev. Neurosci.* **2005**, *6*, 332–339. [CrossRef]
8. Slater, M.; Perez-Marcos, D.; Ehrsson, H.H.; Sanchez-Vives, M.V. Towards a digital body: The virtual arm illusion. *Front. Hum. Neurosci.* **2008**, *2*, 6. [CrossRef] [PubMed]
9. Maister, L.; Slater, M.; Sanchez-Vives, M.V.; Tsakiris, M. Changing bodies changes minds: Owning another body affects social cognition. *Trends Cogn. Sci.* **2015**, *19*, 6–12. [CrossRef]
10. Peck, T.C.; Seinfeld, S.; Aglioti, S.M.; Slater, M. Putting yourself in the skin of a black avatar reduces implicit racial bias. *Conscious. Cogn.* **2013**, *22*, 779–787. [CrossRef]
11. Banakou, D.; Groten, R.; Slater, M. Illusory ownership of a virtual child body causes overestimation of object sizes and implicit attitude changes. *Proc. Natl. Acad. Sci. USA* **2013**, *110*, 12846–12851. [CrossRef]
12. Martini, M.; Kilteni, K.; Maselli, A.; Sanchez-Vives, M.V. The body fades away: Investigating the effects of transparency of an embodied virtual body on pain threshold and body ownership. *Sci. Rep.* **2015**, *5*, 13948. [CrossRef]
13. Romano, D.; Maravita, A. The visual size of one's own hand modulates pain anticipation and perception. *Neuropsychologia* **2014**, *57*, 93–100. [CrossRef]
14. Moseley, G.; Parsons, T.; Spence, C. Visual distortion of a limb modulates the pain and swelling evoked by movement. *Curr. Biol.* **2008**, *18*, R1047–R1048. [CrossRef]
15. Hoffman, H.G.; Patterson, D.R.; Carrougher, G.J.; Sharar, S.R. Effectiveness of virtual reality-based pain control with multiple treatments. *Clin. J. Pain* **2001**, *17*, 229–235. [CrossRef] [PubMed]
16. Hoffman, H.G.; Richards, T.L.; Coda, B.; Bills, A.R.; Blough, D.; Richards, A.L.; Sharar, S.R. Modulation of thermal pain-related brain activity with virtual reality: Evidence from fMRI. *Neuroreport* **2004**, *15*, 1245–1248. [CrossRef]
17. Nierula, B.; Martini, M.; Matamala-Gomez, M.; Slater, M.; Sanchez-Vives, M.V. Seeing an Embodied Virtual Hand is Analgesic Contingent on Colocation. *J. Pain* **2017**, *18*, 645–655. [CrossRef]
18. Romano, D.; Llobera, J.; Blanke, O. Size and viewpoint of an embodied virtual body impact the processing of painful stimuli. *J. Pain* **2015**, *17*, 350–358. [CrossRef]
19. Pozeg, P.; Palluel, E.; Ronchi, R.; Solcà, M.; Al-Khodairy, A.W.; Jordan, X.; Kassouha, A.; Blanke, O. Virtual reality improves embodiment and neuropathic pain caused by spinal cord injury. *Neurology* **2017**, *89*, 1894–1903. [CrossRef]
20. Solcà, M.; Ronchi, R.; Bello-Ruiz, J.; Schmidlin, T.; Herbelin, B.; Luthi, F.; Konzelmann, M.; Beaulieu, J.Y.; Delaquaize, F.; Schnider, A.; et al. Heartbeat-enhanced immersive virtual reality to treat complex regional pain syndrome. *Neurology* **2018**, *91*, e479–e489. [CrossRef]
21. Boesch, E.; Bellan, V.; Moseley, G.; Stanton, T. The effect of bodily illusions on clinical pain: A systematic review and meta-analysis. *Pain* **2016**, *157*, 516–529. [CrossRef]
22. Foell, J.; Bekrater-Bodmann, R.; Diers, M.; Flor, H. Mirror therapy for phantom limb pain: Brain changes and the role of body representation. *Eur. J. Pain* **2014**, *18*, 729–739. [CrossRef]
23. Giummarra, M.J.; Gibson, S.J.; Georgiou-Karistianis, N.; Bradshaw, J.L. Central mechanisms in phantom limb perception: The past, present and future. *Brain Res. Rev.* **2007**, *54*, 219–232. [CrossRef]
24. Flor, H.; Nikolajsen, L.; Staehelin Jensen, T. Phantom limb pain: A case of maladaptive CNS plasticity? *Nat. Rev. Neurosci.* **2006**, *7*, 873–881. [CrossRef]
25. Makin, T.R.; Scholz, J.; Filippini, N.; Henderson Slater, D.; Tracey, I.; Johansen-Berg, H. Phantom pain is associated with preserved structure and function in the former hand area. *Nat. Commun.* **2013**, *4*, 1570. [CrossRef]

26. Bultitude, J.H.; Rafal, R.D. Derangement of body representation in complex regional pain syndrome: Report of a case treated with mirror and prisms. *Exp. Brain Res.* **2010**, *204*, 409–418. [CrossRef]
27. Lewis, J.; Kersten, P.; McPherson, K. Wherever is my arm? Impaired upper limb position accuracy in complex regional pain syndrome. *Pain* **2010**, *149*, 463–469. [CrossRef]
28. Melzack, R. Phantom limbs and the concept of a neuromatrix. *Trends Neurosci.* **1990**, *13*, 88–92. [CrossRef]
29. Wand, B.M.; Parkitny, L.; O'Connell, N.E.; Luomajoki, H.; McAuley, J.H.; Thacker, M.; Moseley, G.L. Cortical changes in chronic low back pain: Current state of the art and implications for clinical practice. *Man. Ther.* **2011**, *16*, 15–20. [CrossRef]
30. Ramachandran, V.S.; Altschuler, E.L. The use of visual feedback, in particular mirror visual feedback, in restoring brain function. *Brain* **2009**, *132*, 1693–1710. [CrossRef]
31. Armel, K.C.; Ramachandran, V.S. Projecting sensations to external objects: Evidence from skin conductance response. *Proc. R. Soc. B Biol. Sci.* **2003**, *270*, 1499–1506. [CrossRef]
32. Moseley, G.L.; Arntz, A. The context of a noxious stimulus affects the pain it evokes. *Pain* **2007**, *133*, 64–71. [CrossRef]
33. World Medical Association World Medical Association Declaration of Helsinki: Ethical principles for medical research involving human subjects. *J. Am. Med. Assoc.* **2013**, *310*, 2191–2194. [CrossRef] [PubMed]
34. Nikolajsen, L.; Springer, J.S.; Haroutiunian, S. Phantom Limb Pain. In *Practical Management of Pain*; Elsevier Inc.: Amsterdam, The Netherlands, 2014; Chapter 26; pp. 369–377.e3. ISBN 9780323083409.
35. Price, D.D.; McGrath, P.A.; Rafii, A.; Buckingham, B. The validation of visual analogue scales as ratio scale measures for chronic and experimental pain. *Pain* **1983**, *17*, 45–56. [CrossRef]
36. Kilteni, K.; Groten, R.; Slater, M. The Sense of Embodiment in Virtual Reality. *Presence Teleoperators Virtual* **2012**, *21*, 373–387. [CrossRef]
37. Cheng, Y.; Lin, C.P.; Liu, H.L.; Hsu, Y.Y.; Lim, K.E.; Hung, D.; Decety, J. Expertise Modulates the Perception of Pain in Others. *Curr. Biol.* **2007**, *17*, 1708–1713. [CrossRef]
38. Kilteni, K.; Normand, J.-M.; Sanchez-Vives, M.V.; Slater, M. Extending body space in immersive virtual reality: A very long arm illusion. *PLoS ONE* **2012**, *7*, e40867. [CrossRef]
39. Slater, M.; Perez-Marcos, D.; Ehrsson, H.H.; Sanchez-Vives, M.V. Inducing illusory ownership of a virtual body. *Front. Neurosci.* **2009**, *3*, 214–220. [CrossRef]
40. Breimhorst, M.; Sandrock, S.; Fechir, M.; Hausenblas, N.; Geber, C.; Birklein, F. Do intensity ratings and skin conductance responses reliably discriminate between different stimulus intensities in experimentally induced pain? *J. Pain* **2011**, *12*, 61–70. [CrossRef]
41. Lykken, D.T.; Venables, P.H. Direct measurement of skin conductance: A proposal for standardization. *Psychophysiology* **1971**, *8*, 656–672. [CrossRef]
42. Rhudy, J.L.; Bartley, E.J.; Williams, A.E. Habituation, sensitization, and emotional valence modulation of pain responses. *Pain* **2010**, *148*, 320–327. [CrossRef] [PubMed]
43. Lopes-Machado, E.Z.; De Souza Crippa, J.A.; Hallak, J.E.C.; Guimarães, F.S.; Zuardi, A.W. Electrodermically nonresponsive schizophrenia patients make more errors in the stroop color word test, indicating selective attention deficit. *Schizophr. Bull.* **2002**, *28*, 459–466. [CrossRef] [PubMed]
44. Turpin, G.; Schaefer, F.; Boucsein, W. Effects of stimulus intensity, risetime, and duration on autonomic and behavioral responding: Implications for the differentiation of orienting, startle, and defense responses. *Psychophysiology* **1999**, *36*, 453–463. [CrossRef]
45. Veit, R.; Lotze, M.; Sewing, S.; Missenhardt, H.; Gaber, T.; Birbaumer, N. Aberrant social and cerebral responding in a competitive reaction time paradigm in criminal psychopaths. *Neuroimage* **2010**, *49*, 3365–3372. [CrossRef]
46. Sanchez-Vives, M.V.; Spanlang, B.; Frisoli, A.; Bergamasco, M.; Slater, M. Virtual hand illusion induced by visuomotor correlations. *PLoS ONE* **2010**, *5*, e10381. [CrossRef]
47. Matamala-Gomez, M.; Donegan, T.; Bottiroli, S.; Sandrini, G.; Sanchez-Vives, M.V.; Tassorelli, C. Immersive virtual reality and virtual embodiment for pain relief. *Front. Hum. Neurosci.* **2019**, *13*, 279. [CrossRef]
48. Moseley, G.L.; Flor, H. Targeting Cortical Representations in the Treatment of Chronic Pain. *Neurorehabil. Neural Repair* **2012**, *26*, 646–652. [CrossRef]
49. Lotze, M.; Moseley, G.L. Role of Distorted Body Image in Pain. *Curr. Rheumatol. Reports Curr. Med. Gr. LLC ISSN* **2007**, *9*, 488–496. [CrossRef]

50. Makin, T.R.; Scholz, J.; Henderson Slater, D.; Johansen-Berg, H.; Tracey, I. Reassessing cortical reorganization in the primary sensorimotor cortex following arm amputation. *Brain* **2015**, *138*, 2140–2146. [CrossRef]
51. Schott, G.D. Penfield's homunculus: A note on cerebral cartography. *J. Neurol. Neurosurg. Psychiatry* **1993**, *56*, 329–333. [CrossRef]
52. Tung, M.L.; Murphy, I.C.; Griffin, S.C.; Alphonso, A.L.; Hussey-Anderson, L.; Hughes, K.E.; Weeks, S.R.; Merritt, V.; Yetto, J.M.; Pasquina, P.F.; et al. Observation of limb movements reduces phantom limb pain in bilateral amputees. *Ann. Clin. Transl. Neurol.* **2014**, *1*, 633–638. [CrossRef] [PubMed]
53. Mercier, C.; Sirigu, A. Training With Virtual Visual Feedback to Alleviate Phantom Limb Pain. *Neurorehabil. Neural Repair* **2009**, *23*, 587–594. [CrossRef]
54. Khelemsky, Y. Acute and chronic pain management. In *Anesthesiology and Otolaryngology*; Springer: Berlin/Heidelberg, Germany, 2013; Volume 9781461441, pp. 373–391. ISBN 9781461441847.
55. Palermo, L.; Di Vita, A.; Piccardi, L.; Traballesi, M.; Guariglia, C. Bottom-up and top-down processes in body representation: A study of brain-damaged and amputee patients. *Neuropsychology* **2014**, *28*, 772–781. [CrossRef] [PubMed]
56. Moseley, G.L. I can't find it! Distorted body image and tactile dysfunction in patients with chronic back pain. *Pain* **2008**, *140*, 167–171. [CrossRef] [PubMed]
57. Mancini, F.; Longo, M.R.; Kammers, M.P.M.; Haggard, P. Visual distortion of body size modulates pain perception. *Psychol. Sci.* **2011**, *22*, 325–330. [CrossRef] [PubMed]
58. Osumi, M.; Imai, R.; Ueta, K.; Nobusako, S.; Morioka, S. Negative body image associated with changes in the visual body appearance increases pain perception. *PLoS ONE* **2014**, *9*, e107376. [CrossRef] [PubMed]
59. Fields, H.L.; Basbaum, A.I.; Heinricher, M.M. Central nervous system mechanisms of pain modulation. In *Wall and Melzack's Textbook of Pain*; Saunders: Philadelphia, PA, USA, 2006; pp. 125–142. ISBN 978-0-443-07287-1.
60. Pud, D.; Granovsky, Y.; Yarnitsky, D. The methodology of experimentally induced diffuse noxious inhibitory control (DNIC)-like effect in humans. *Pain* **2009**, *144*, 16–19. [CrossRef]
61. Porro, C.A.; Baraldi, P.; Pagnoni, G.; Serafini, M.; Facchin, P.; Maieron, M.; Nichelli, P. Does anticipation of pain affect cortical nociceptive systems? *J. Neurosci.* **2002**, *22*, 3206–3214. [CrossRef]
62. Brown, C.A.; Jones, A.K. A role for midcingulate cortex in the interruptive effects of pain anticipation on attention. *Clin. Neurophysiol.* **2008**, *119*, 2370–2379. [CrossRef]
63. Botvinick, M.; Cohen, J. Rubber hands' feel'touch that eyes see. *Nature* **1998**, *391*, 756. [CrossRef]
64. Ehrsson, H.; Petkova, V. If I were you: Perceptual illusion of body swapping. *PLoS ONE* **2008**, *3*, e3832.
65. González-Franco, M.; Peck, T.C.; Rodríguez-Fornells, A.; Slater, M. A threat to a virtual hand elicits motor cortex activation. *Exp. Brain Res.* **2014**, *232*, 875–887. [CrossRef] [PubMed]
66. Kilteni, K.; Grau-Sánchez, J.; Veciana De Las Heras, M.; Rodriguez-Fornells, A.; Slater, M. Decreased corticospinal excitability after the illusion of missing part of the arm. *Front. Hum. Neurosci.* **2016**, *10*, 3423. [CrossRef]
67. Nierula, B.; Spanlang, B.; Martini, M.; Borrell, M.; Nikulin, V.V.; Sanchez-Vives, M.V. Agency and responsibility over virtual movements controlled through different paradigms of brain−computer interface. *J. Physiol.* **2019**. [CrossRef]
68. Bergström, I.; Kilteni, K.; Slater, M. First-Person Perspective Virtual Body Posture Influences Stress: A Virtual Reality Body Ownership Study. *PLoS ONE* **2016**, *11*, e0148060. [CrossRef]
69. Romano, D.; Pfeiffer, C.; Maravita, A.; Blanke, O. Illusory self-identification with an avatar reduces arousal responses to painful stimuli. *Behav. Brain Res.* **2014**, *261*, 275–281. [CrossRef]
70. Fillingim, R.B. Sex, gender, and pain: Women and men really are different. *Curr. Rev. Pain* **2000**, *4*, 24–30. [CrossRef]
71. Schmalzl, L. "Pulling telescoped phantoms out of the stump": Manipulating the perceived position of phantom limbs using a full-body illusion. *Front. Hum. Neurosci.* **2011**, *5*, 5. [CrossRef]
72. Thøgersen, M.; Hansen, J.; Arendt-Nielsen, L.; Flor, H.; Petrini, L. Removing own-limb visual input using mixed reality (MR) produces a "telescoping" illusion in healthy individuals. *Behav. Brain Res.* **2018**, *347*, 263–271. [CrossRef]

3

The Effect of a Virtual Reality-Based Intervention Program on Cognition in Older Adults with Mild Cognitive Impairment

Ngeemasara Thapa [1,2], Hye Jin Park [1,2], Ja-Gyeong Yang [1,2], Haeun Son [1,2], Minwoo Jang [1,2], Jihyeon Lee [1], Seung Wan Kang [3], Kyung Won Park [4] and Hyuntae Park [1,2,*]

1 Department of Health Sciences, Graduate School, Dong-A University, Busan 49315, Korea; ngeemasara@gmail.com (N.T.); mihd3987@hanmail.net (H.J.P.); sky940702@naver.com (J.-G.Y.); haundl123@naver.com (H.S.); mtow0620@gmail.com (M.J.); lose0918@naver.com (J.L.)
2 Laboratory of Smart Healthcare, Dong-A University, Busan 49315, Korea
3 Data Center for Korean EEG, College of Nursing, Seoul National University, Seoul 03080, Korea; drdemian@snu.ac.kr
4 Department of Neurology, Dong-A University College of Medicine, Busan 49201, Korea; neuropark@dau.ac.kr
* Correspondence: htpark@dau.ac.kr

Abstract: This study aimed to investigate the association between a virtual reality (VR) intervention program and cognitive, brain and physical functions in high-risk older adults. In a randomized controlled trial, we enrolled 68 individuals with mild cognitive impairment (MCI). The MCI diagnosis was based on medical evaluations through a clinical interview conducted by a dementia specialist. Cognitive assessments were performed by neuropsychologists according to standardized methods, including the Mini-Mental State Examination (MMSE) and frontal cognitive function: trail making test (TMT) A & B, and symbol digit substitute test (SDST). Resting state electroencephalogram (EEG) was measured in eyes open and eyes closed conditions for 5 minutes each, with a 19-channel wireless EEG device. The VR intervention program (3 times/week, 100 min each session) comprised four types of VR game-based content to improve the attention, memory and processing speed. Analysis of the subjects for group–time interactions revealed that the intervention group exhibited a significantly improved executive function and brain function at the resting state. Additionally, gait speed and mobility were also significantly improved between and after the follow-up. The VR-based training program improved cognitive and physical function in patients with MCI relative to controls. Encouraging patients to perform VR and game-based training may be beneficial to prevent cognitive decline.

Keywords: virtual reality; dementia; mild cognitive impairment; electroencephalogram

1. Introduction

Dementia is a syndrome characterized by global cognitive impairment [1] and an estimated 50 million people worldwide have dementia [2]. It is most prevalent in individuals aged > 65 years and is considered as the greatest health challenge in the 21st century [3]. The pharmacological treatments have not yet led to an important breakthrough in the treatment of dementia, resulting in gravitation toward non-pharmacological approaches to alter the progressive course of the disease [4]. Mild cognitive impairment (MCI) is the prodromal stage of dementia [5], with around 46% progressing to dementia within 3 years [6]. Some MCI patients are stable or return to a normal state over time [7]. Thus, MCI serves as an ideal stage for preventive interventions.

The most promising non-pharmacological interventions for delaying the progression of MCI to dementia are exercise, cognitive training [8] and multicomponent intervention [9], and recently, virtual reality (VR) has also been explored for treatment and prevention of dementia [10]. A randomized control trial in normal older adults comparing physical exercise, cognitive exercise and VR exercise demonstrated that VR exercise showed significant improvements in cognitive as well as physical function, and VR exercise was more favored than physical exercise by the elderly [11]. In older adults with MCI, VR intervention has been reported to improve memory function [12]. VR is a computer-simulated environment, closely resembling real-life situations and scenarios, which provides the user with the sensation of physically "being there" [13,14]. VR can be divided into non- immersion, semi-immersion, and full immersion, based on the levels of immersion. Immersive VR provides enhanced ecological validity and the possibility to personalize the activity and environment to the needs of individuals, making VR-based training more engaging [15]. The higher level of immersion corresponds to a more realistic VR environment to the user [16]. The immersive VR has been used mostly for neurophysiological assessment, cognitive rehabilitation and the effect of VR on different cognitive domains such as executive function, attention, memory and spatial orientation is being investigated [17].

Immersive VR-based cognitive training has recently attracted attention in the research filed of MCI and dementia [18]. A recent meta-analytic study has also reported the positive effect of semi-immersive VR on cognition and physical function in individuals with MCI and dementia [19]. A fully immersive VR-based cognitive intervention study on older adults with and without dementia reported significantly higher cognitive progress in those without dementia compared to those with dementia [20]. A feasibility study using fully immersive VR cognitive training in MCI and dementia patients showed a high feeling of safety, satisfaction, reduced anxiety fatigue and low discomfort compared to pen-paper training [15]. This advantage of VR over pen-paper cognitive training can be beneficial to ensure adherence to cognitive training and when performed with caution, it has the potential to be an efficient intervention for dementia patients [15,21].

Nevertheless, immersive VR is increasingly used in health-related fields and interventions and has the potential to be a powerful tool in delaying the onset of degenerative brain and mental diseases. However, the evidence regarding the effectiveness of immersive VR in MCI and dementia is limited [22], especially the fully immersive type of VR. Several studies still rely mostly on non- and semi-immersive VR [23] and the advantages of VR with full immersion and interaction on prevention of dementia have not yet been explored to their full potential. Therefore, we aimed to investigate the effect of the fully immersive virtual reality intervention on cognitive, brain and physical function in older adults with MCI. In addition to the neurocognitive tests, we also used electroencephalography (EEG) to assess the effect of VR intervention on cognition in our study. EEG is the least invasive measure of brain electrical activity. EEG power measures are associated with memory, executive function and global cognition in patients with MCI [24].

2. Materials and Methods

2.1. Subjects

The study was announced through three regional health care centers in Busan metropolitan city, South Korea. A total of 234 participants applied and all of them underwent a screening process. The inclusion criteria were: (i) >55 and <85 years and (ii) individuals diagnosed with MCI based on medical evaluations consisting of neurological examinations and detailed neuropsychological assessments conducted by a dementia specialist. MCI was defined by the Consortium to Establish a Registry for Alzheimer's Disease Assessment Packet (CERAD) with the cut-off score developed by Chandler et al. [25]. Following some exclusion criteria, 100 out of 234 subjects were recruited to be part of this study. The exclusion criteria are explained in Figure 1. Thirty-two subjects out of 100 did not participate in the study due to personal reasons, hence our study included a total of 68 subjects who were then randomly allocated to either the control (n = 34) or VR-intervention (n = 34) group. To avoid selection bias, the random allocation was assigned via a computer-generated, fixed block randomization procedure to either the intervention or control group, generating blocks stratified by age, gender, education level, and participating center. The participants' mean age was 72.5 ± 5.32 years (mean ± standard deviation (SD)).

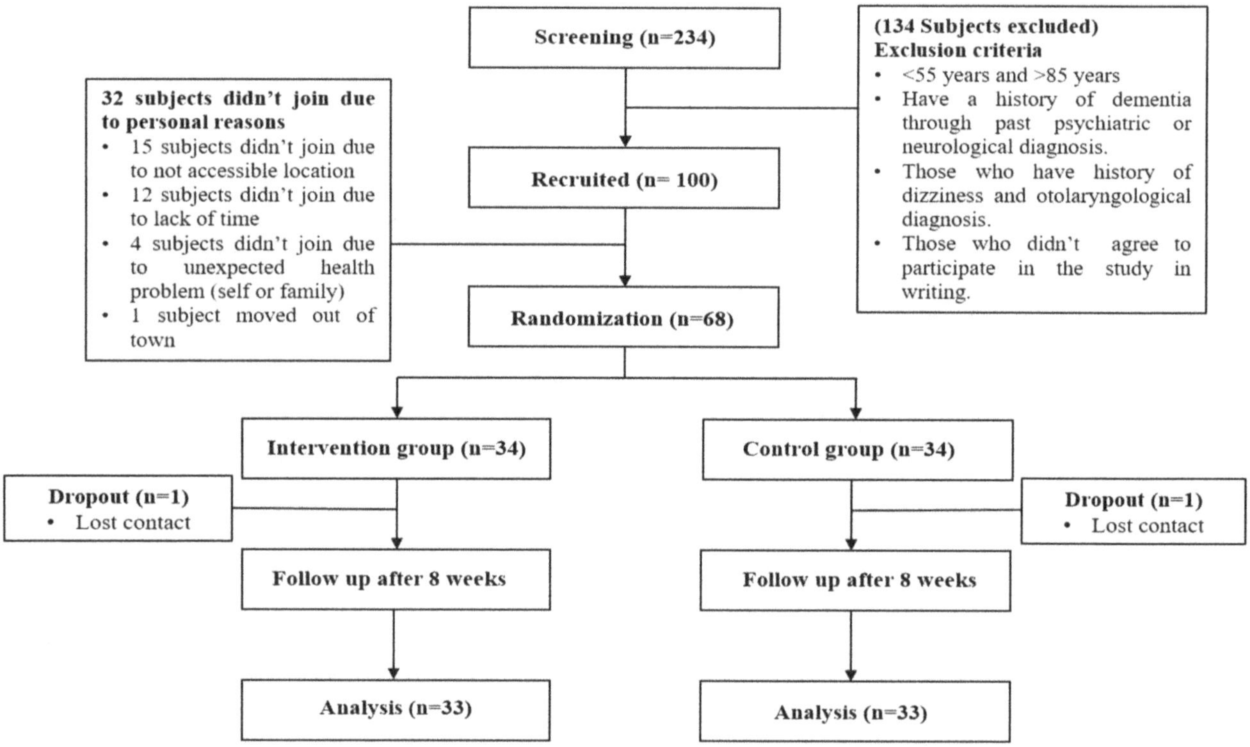

Figure 1. Flowchart of study design.

The study procedure was approved by Dong-A University Institutional Review Board on 24 October 2019 (IRB No. 2-1040709-AB-N-01-201909-HR-036-04) and all participants provided signed informed consent at the beginning of the study. This study is registered in the University Hospital Medical Information Network (UMIN) Clinical Trials Registry (Registration No. UMIN000040107).

2.2. Intervention

The intervention group performed a total of 24 sessions of VR-based cognitive training for eight weeks. Three sessions were held per week and each VR training session lasted for 100 minutes, which also included instruction regarding VR training and eye stretching exercises in between VR training, as described in Figure 2. On the other hand, the control group participated in an educational program on general health care once a week during the study intervention period (8 sessions). Each session was 30 to 50 minutes. The program was led by health professionals, an exercise specialist, a physical therapist and a nutritionist, and subjects were given information such as nutrition regarding proper diet and foods, and exercise tips to prevent geriatric diseases such as frailty, sarcopenia and dementia. In addition to VR training, the intervention group was also provided with an educational program following the same protocol as the control group.

The VR training consisted of 4 series of games. All the VR training game contents were developed by SY Innotech Inc., Busan, South Korea. The VR training was performed with an Oculus VR headset (Oculus quest headset) and two wireless hand controllers, one for each hand. The virtual reality program consists of four types (Figure 2): Juice making: This game requires the subject to pick a recipe for making a given juice in a virtual reality space, memorize the listed fruits, select the memorized material from the shelf and toss it into a container. The container is vigorously shaken until juice is made and then poured into the cup. Crow Shooting: The shooting game is set up on the beachside where the subjects are asked to shoot flying black birds. The right controller turns into a gun and the left controller into a shield. Fireworks (find the fireworks number): Three numbers are shown on the screen when the game starts and fireworks burst in a random order from the numbers. When the firework display is over, the subjects need to click the numbers in the order of which the firework exploded. Love house (d: memory object at the house): In this particular game, subjects are placed in a virtually simulated house where they were given 30 seconds to memorize the location of objects in the shelf and around the living area. The items are then misplaced, and the subjects are required to reorganize the objects in the correct location with the help of a VR hand controller.

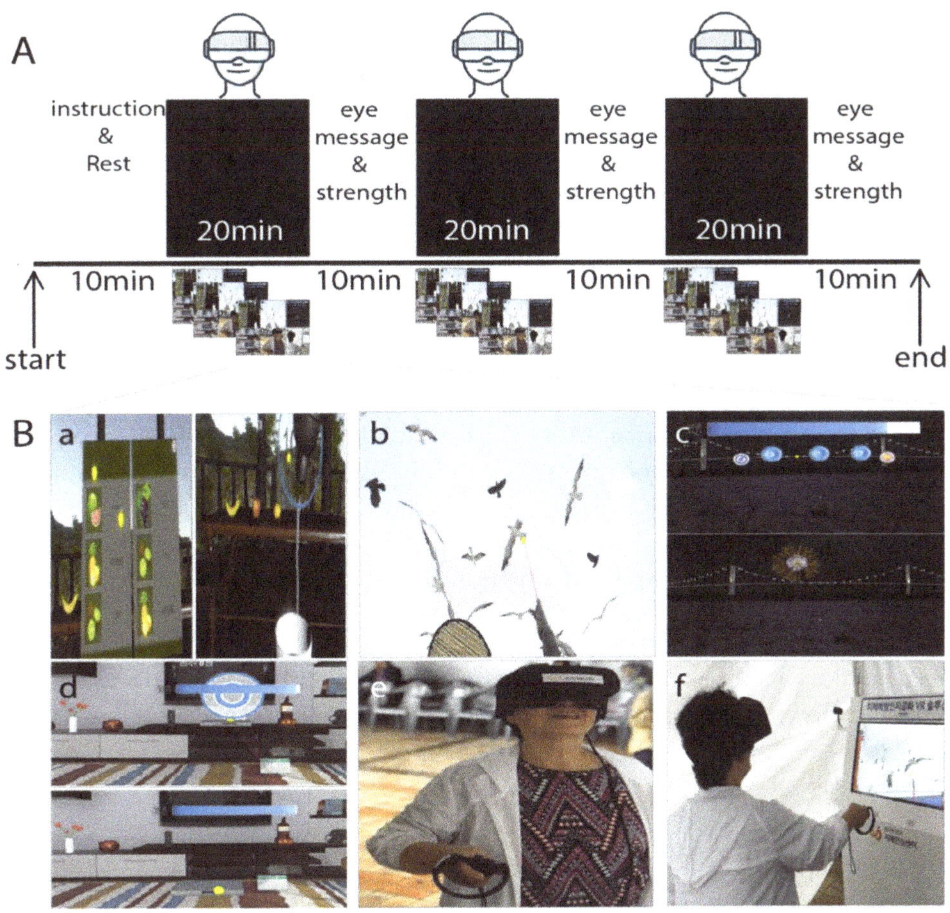

Figure 2. (**A**) This figure illustrates the design for the virtual reality (VR) training design and game contents. The total training duration was 100 minutes (three 20 min VR training sessions, and three 10 min eye massage and stretching sessions) held three times a week for 8 weeks. (**B**) The contents of the VR training games: (a) juice making, (b) crow shooting, (c) find the fireworks number, (d) memory object at the house, (e) and (f) example of subject.

2.3. Cognitive Function

Cognitive assessments were performed by neuropsychologists according to standardized methods. Global cognitive function was assessed with the Korean version of the Mini-Mental State Examination-Dementia screening test (MMSE-DS) [26]. From the National Center for Geriatrics and Gerontology Functional Assessment Tool (NCGG-FAT), the trail making test (TMT) A & B, and symbol digit substitution test (SDST) in the form of an electronic tablet were used to assess cognitive function [27]. In TMT A, the subjects were instructed to touch the target number in consecutive order of 1–15 shown in the tablet as quickly as possible. In TMT B, the subjects were instructed to touch numbers and letters alternatively in consecutive order. In SDST, 9 pairs of numbers and symbols were shown in the top half of the tablet display, and the subjects were asked to match the symbols to their corresponding numbers displayed in the bottom half of the display. TMT and SDST were both timed, and shorter time taken to complete the test indicated better cognitive function.

2.4. EEG Recording and Data Acquisition

The EEG was recorded in a dimly lit and quiet room with a Cognionics Quick-20 (Cognionics Inc., San Diego, CA, USA) dry EEG headset. The EEG headset had a built-in design based on the international 10–20 system (Fp1, Fp2, F7, F3, Fz, F4, F8, T3, C3, Cz, C4, T4, T5, P3, Pz, P4, T6, O1 and O2) positioned according to the international 10–20 system [28]. The resting state EEG data of 5 minutes was recorded with the eyes closed condition. The subjects were instructed to keep their eyes closed but stay awake during EEG recordings. The EEG was recorded at a sampling rate of 500 Hz and filtered through a band-pass of 0.53–120 Hz. The electrodes impedance was kept under 500 kΩ. The artifact removal was conducted with independent component analysis (ICA) individually for each channel. The EEG brain power ratio-theta/beta ratio (TBR), theta/alpha ratio (TAR) and delta/alpha ratio (DAR) between baseline and follow-up data (within the VR intervention and control groups) were analyzed in iSyncBrain software, v.2.1, 2018 (iMediSync, Inc., Seoul, South Korea) and the difference was observed with paired t-test. The EEG band power was shown in a topographic map (Topo map) plotted with the built-in sLoreta function in iSyncBrain software v.2.1. The differences were observed with paired t-test.

2.5. Physical Function

Physical function was assessed by gait speed test, mobility test and handgrip strength. The gait speed test was 7 m long, which included a 1.5 m acceleration distance, a 4 m "preferred walking speed" followed by a 1.5 m deceleration distance. Only the 4 m walk was timed. The 8-feet Up and Go test of 2.44 m was used to assess mobility. Handgrip strength (HGS) of the non-dominant hand was measured with a digital hand dynamometer (TKK 5101 Grip-D Takei, Tokyo, Japan). The HGS was measured twice and the mean value was used for statistical analysis. During the test, participants were instructed to maintain their shoulders slightly apart from their body, and hold the dynamometer pointing to the ground.

Socio-demographic variables such as education, age, medication intake and smoking were acquired through interviews by trained researchers.

2.6. Statistical Analysis

All comparisons were two-sided, with an alpha level of 0.05. All statistical analyses were analyzed using the IBM SPSS Statistics, version 25.0, 2017 software package for Windows (SPSS Inc., Chicago, IL, USA). The Shapiro–Wilk test was used to determine the normality of the data distribution. The independent t-test or the chi-square test was used to assess differences in the baseline (beginning of the intervention) variables. We used the intention-to-treat approach, and between-group comparisons of continuous variables were conducted using a repeated measures analysis of variance (ANOVA) model after adjusting for the potential covariates (age, sex and years of education) for primary and secondary endpoint outcome. Time was treated as a categorical variable, and the models included group, time and group-by-time interaction as fixed effects. The conclusions about the effectiveness of the VR intervention were based on between-group comparisons of change in global and prefrontal cognitive function (working memory, processing and executive function) from baseline to 8 weeks after, as assessed with the MMSE, TMT A & B, SDST and other physical function determined by the time-by-group interaction of the model.

3. Result

In Table 1, the demographics of the study population along with baseline physical functions and global cognitive functions are described. There are no significant differences in parameters between the intervention and control groups at the baseline.

Table 1. Selected anthropometric, cognitive and physical function characteristics of the subjects at the baseline.

Variables	VR Intervention	Control
n (male)	34 (6)	34 (10)
Age (years)	72.6 ± 5.4	72.7 ± 5.6
Education (years)	9.3 ± 4.0	8.4 ± 3.5
Height (m)	1.58 ± 0.08	1.58 ± 0.08
No. of medication intake (n)	2.3 ± 1.4	2.12 ± 1.4
Weight (kg)	60.7 ± 9.8	61.3 ± 9.1
BMI (kg/m^2)	24.3 ± 3.0	24.5 ± 2.7
SBP (mg/hg)	129.6 ± 15.8	129.6 ± 17.9
DBP (mg/hg)	74.8 ± 11.3	69.5 ± 11.8
Grip strength (kg)	22.2 ± 6.3	23.4 ± 5.7
Gait speed (s)	1.15 ± 0.33	1.18 ± 0.21
8-feet Up and Go (s)	6.27 ± 1.48	7.04 ± 2.02
MMSE (score)	26.0 ± 1.8	26.3 ± 3.3
TMT A (s)	26.3 ± 7.3	27.9 ± 9.2
TMT B (s)	56.6 ± 25.0	58.5 ± 28.1
SDST (score)	33.4 ± 9.0	32.4 ± 8.2

BMI: Body mass index, SPB: Systolic blood pressure, DBP: Diastolic blood pressure, MMSE: Mini mental state examination, TMT A: Trail making test A, TMT B: Trail making test B, SDST: Symbol digit substitution test. The values are expressed in mean and standard deviation (mean ± SD). All variables have no significant differences measured by independent t- test or chi-square test.

In Table 2, TMT B time decreased significantly in the intervention group compared to the control group ($p = 0.03$). Similarly, small, but not significant, positive changes were observed in MMSE and SDST. The physical function such as gait speed ($p = 0.02$) and 8-feet Up and Go were significantly improved ($p = 0.03$) in the intervention group.

Table 2. The comparison of physical function and global cognitive function between baseline and post intervention in the VR intervention and the control groups.

Variables	VR Intervention			Control			Group x Time Interaction	
	Baseline	Follow Up	*p*-Value [a]	Baseline	Follow Up	*p*-Value [a]	*p*-Value [b]	Effect Size
Grip strength (kg)	22.2 ± 6.3	24.4 ± 5.3	0.03	23.4 ± 5.7	23.9 ± 5.7	n.s.	n.s.	-
Gait speed (m/s)	1.15 ± 0.33	1.19 ± 0.37	0.04	1.18 ± 0.21	1.12 ± 0.26 *	0.01	0.02	0.143
8-feet Up and go (s)	6.77 ± 1.48	6.32 ± 1.92	0.02	7.04 ± 2.02	7.06 ± 1.87 *	n.s.	0.03	0.107
MMSE (score)	26.0 ± 1.8	26.9 ± 2.0	n.s.	26.3 ± 3.3	26.4 ± 2.7	n.s.	n.s.	-
TMT A (s)	26.3 ±7.3	24.2 ± 5.3	0.04	27.9 ± 9.2	27.8 ± 8.1	n.s.	n.s.	-
TMT B (s)	56.6 ± 25.0	51.3 ± 24.8	0.03	58.5 ± 28.1	63.2 ± 25.1 *	0.01	0.03	0.208
SDST (score)	33.4 ± 9.0	39.6 ± 9.5	0.02	32.4 ± 8.2	21.8 ± 8.2	< 0.01	0.03	0.264

The values are expressed in mean and standard deviation (mean ± SD). [a] Paired t-test between baseline and follow-up assessment. [b] Repeated-measures analysis of variance (ANOVA) testing interaction of intervention (VR intervention versus control) by time (baseline versus follow-up) for each outcome, adjusted for age, gender and years of education. Effect size is partial eta squared for group by time. * Represents a significant difference between the intervention and control group. n.s. = not significant, MMSE: Mini mental state examination, TMT A: Trail making test A, TMT B: Trail making test B, SDST: Symbol digit substitution test.

3.1. EEG

3.1.1. Band Power

In the elderly, increased Theta wave (>3.5 to <8 Hz) is associated with the risk of developing cognitive impairment [29,30]. The theta has been observed to be significantly decreased around the parietal ($p = 0.013$) and temporal ($p = 0.036$) regions at follow up (G2) compared to baseline (G1) in the VR intervention group (Figure 3).

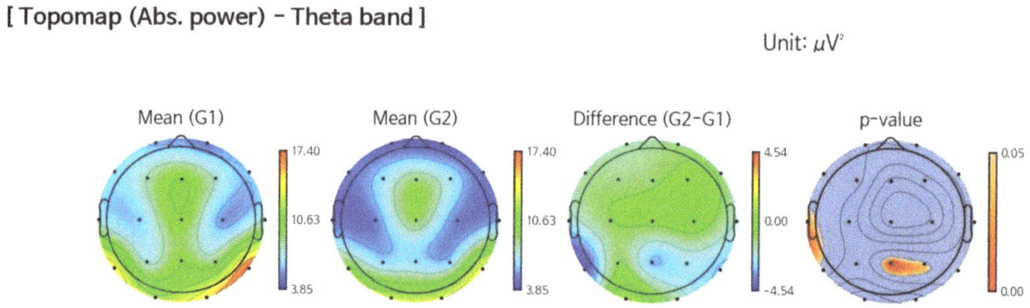

Figure 3. This figure shows a significant decrease in Theta power in the parietal ($p = 0.013$) and temporal areas ($p = 0.036$) at follow up (G2) compared to baseline (G1) in the VR intervention group.

3.1.2. Power Ratio

The higher TBR is related to mind wandering, which is considered to be associated with reduced attention [31]. In the VR intervention group, the Theta/Beta ratio (TBR) is decreased in the temporal ($p = 0.035$) and parietal ($p = 0.027$) regions at follow up (Figure 4). In the control group, all power ratios did not show any changes.

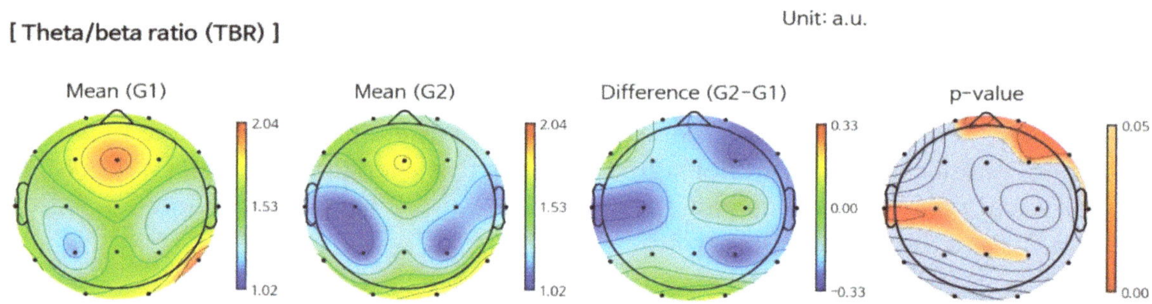

Figure 4. This figure shows a significant decrease in the Theta/Beta power ratio ($p = 0.027$) at follow up (G2) compared to baseline (G1) in the VR intervention group.

4. Discussion

Our study examined the effect of a VR game intervention on cognitive and brain activity in older adults with MCI. Our findings show that the VR game intervention is an effective way to improve cognitive and frontal brain function in MCI patients. The improvements in the 8-feet Up and Go test and gait speed were also observed in the intervention group.

Over the past decade, technology-based cognitive interventions have gained immense interest worldwide. Our study results show positive effects for the VR intervention on key outcome variables, such as cognitive and physical function. The VR intervention effect in the cognition category is consistent with the result of a systematic review by Coyle et al. [32]. Coyle and colleagues showed that the VR intervention moderately improved the cognitive function of participants with cognitive impairment. A recent VR study has reported improvements in executive functions [33] after the VR intervention, similar to our study results. TMT is often used as a measure of executive function [34]. TMT A measures psychomotor speed and visual scanning, while TMT B reflects working memory [35–37]. However, our results showed significant positive improvements in TMT B but not in TMT A. The contents of our VR training consisted of games such as love home, juice making and fireworks, which required subjects to memorize objects, recipes and numbers respectively, highly involving use of working memory along with other cognitive functions, such as attention and processing speed. This could explain the significant change in TMT B score. In addition, we also measured brain electrical activity during the resting state of mind. The theta power was observed to be decreased in the VR intervention at follow up. Increased theta, in the elderly, is associated with the risk of developing cognitive impairment [29,30]. Our study also a showed significant decrease in TBR in the temporal and parietal regions of the brain. The higher TBR was observed to be related to mind wandering, which is considered to be associated with reduced attention [31]. However, detailed studies over a longer period on each EEG rhythm are required to draw its strong relationship with VR training.

Studies have also shown that VR intervention is effective to improve physical function and walking speed of community-dwelling patients who had a stroke [38–40]. Our study results further expand this data as significant improvements in physical function, especially gait speed and the 8-feet Up and Go test, in MCI patients were observed after 8 weeks of VR training. Several studies have found physical functions such as handgrip strength [41–43] and gait speed [44] to be associated with cognitive decline in older adults. Gait speed has been reported to rely on motor function and cognitive processes, which includes executive function and attention [45], which may explain the relationship between gait speed and cognition. Furthermore, improved brain function may be due to health promoting behaviors, such as physical activity and nutrition, and health literacy [46]. However, further studies are needed in order to evaluate the bidirectional relationship between the improvement of cognition and physical function.

VR provides an artificial interactive environment closely representing reality. Older adults with dementia can experience various sensory stimulation in a comfortable and safe virtually simulated environment, which could lead to a boost in functional learning and transfer of learned functions [47]. Unlike computerized computer training, VR is immersive and closely mimics reality, intensifying ecological legitimacy, offering greater potential for transfer to activities of daily life (ADL) [48]. We performed fully immersive VR training in order to examine the effectiveness of using VR intervention on cognitive, brain and physical function in MCI patients. The VR contents in our study used real life locations. Fully immersive VR corresponds more to feeling like the individual is experiencing real-life scenarios [23]. A functional magnetic resonance imaging study showed that the virtual reality-generated environment activates the associated brain areas, similar to the real environment [49].

Our study yielded a positive effect of fully immersive VR training on cognitive as well as physical function in older adults with MCI. The subjects in the VR intervention group strongly adhered to the training and the dropout number was low (n = 1). One of the limitations of our study was that there was no follow up in the middle of the intervention period or some period after the study was over, due to which the short- and long-term effect of the VR intervention on cognition and physical function were not observed. Secondly, the VR intervention program group had more sessions (n = 24) compared to the control group (n = 8) and hence, the intervention group had more interaction with each other and their supervising health professionals. The increased social interaction has been associated with preventing cognitive decline [50,51]. This could have somewhat contributed to positive results in the intervention group. The participants of our study were predominantly women (n = 52), compared to men (n = 16), and future studies regarding gender differences on the effect of the VR intervention are necessary.

5. Conclusions

In summary, our results show that VR-based cognitive training has a positive effect on cognition in MCI patients. Although the global cognitive function did not change significantly, we observed significant improvement in executive function, and some physical functions such as gait speed and the 8-feet Up and Go test. Moreover, the EEG test showed a positive change in brain activity related to attention after the intervention period. Nevertheless, further work is needed in this area to confirm the long-term effectiveness and feasibility.

Author Contributions: Conceptualization, H.P.; methodology, J.-G.Y., H.J.P. and M.J.; software, N.T., J.-G.Y., S.W.K. and J.L.; formal analysis, H.S., K.W.P. and N.T.; investigation, N.T., M.J., J.L., H.J.P. and J.-G.Y.; writing—original draft preparation, N.T. and H.P.; writing—review and editing, N.T., H.P.; visualization, N.T. and H.P.; supervision, H.P.; project administration, H.P.; funding acquisition, H.P. All authors have read and agreed to the published version of the manuscript.

Acknowledgments: The authors would like to thank the CEO Yeanhwa Lee and Sujin Seo of SY Inotech Inc., who provided VR contents for this study and helped us in operating the program. We thank the patients for participating in the Busan Metropolitan HealthCare Center. We also thank Dave (DaeKeun) Kim and other technical staff of iMediSync Inc. for the support in EEG data analysis and data filtering. We would also like to thank Hansol Kim for providing the administrative support.

References

1. National Collaborating Centre for Mental Health (UK). Dementia. In *Dementia: A NICE-SCIE Guideline on Supporting People With Dementia and Their Carers in Health and Social Care*; British Psychological Society: Lester, UK, 2007.
2. World Health Organization. Dementia. Available online: https://www.who.int/news-room/fact-sheets/detail/dementia (accessed on 26 February 2020).
3. Livingston, G.; Sommerlad, A.; Orgeta, V.; Costafreda, S.G.; Huntley, J.; Ames, D.; Ballard, C.; Banerjee, S.; Burns, A.; Cohen-Mansfield, J. Dementia prevention, intervention, and care. *Lancet* **2017**, *390*, 2673–2734. [CrossRef]
4. D'Cunha, N.M.; Georgousopoulou, E.N.; Dadigamuwage, L.; Kellett, J.; Panagiotakos, D.B.; Thomas, J.; McKune, A.J.; Mellor, D.D.; Naumovski, N. Effect of long-term nutraceutical and dietary supplement use on cognition in the elderly: A 10-year systematic review of randomised controlled trials. *Br. J. Nutr.* **2018**, *119*, 280–298. [CrossRef]
5. Albert, M.S.; DeKosky, S.T.; Dickson, D.; Dubois, B.; Feldman, H.H.; Fox, N.C.; Gamst, A.; Holtzman, D.M.; Jagust, W.J.; Petersen, R.C. The diagnosis of mild cognitive impairment due to Alzheimer's disease: Recommendations from the National Institute on Aging-Alzheimer's Association workgroups on diagnostic guidelines for Alzheimer's disease. *Alzheimer's Dement.* **2011**, *7*, 270–279. [CrossRef] [PubMed]
6. Pal, K.; Mukadam, N.; Petersen, I.; Cooper, C. Mild cognitive impairment and progression to dementia in people with diabetes, prediabetes and metabolic syndrome: A systematic review and meta-analysis. *Soc. Psychiatry Psychiatr. Epidemiol.* **2018**, *53*, 1149–1160. [CrossRef]
7. Gauthier, S.; Reisberg, B.; Zaudig, M.; Petersen, R.C.; Ritchie, K.; Broich, K.; Belleville, S.; Brodaty, H.; Bennett, D.; Chertkow, H. Mild cognitive impairment. *Lancet* **2006**, *367*, 1262–1270. [CrossRef]
8. Daviglus, M.L.; Bell, C.C.; Berrettini, W.; Bowen, P.E.; Connolly, E.S.; Cox, N.J.; Dunbar-Jacob, J.M.; Granieri, E.C.; Hunt, G.; McGarry, K. National Institutes of Health State-of-the-Science Conference statement: Preventing Alzheimer disease and cognitive decline. *Ann. Intern. Med.* **2010**, *153*, 176–181. [CrossRef] [PubMed]
9. Park, H.; Park, J.H.; Na, H.R.; Hiroyuki, S.; Kim, G.M.; Jung, M.K.; Kim, W.K.; Park, K.W. Combined Intervention of Physical Activity, Aerobic Exercise, and Cognitive Exercise Intervention to Prevent Cognitive Decline for Patients with Mild Cognitive Impairment: A Randomized Controlled Clinical Study. *J. Clin. Med.* **2019**, *8*, 940. [CrossRef]
10. Zucchella, C.; Sinforiani, E.; Tamburin, S.; Federico, A.; Mantovani, E.; Bernini, S.; Casale, R.; Bartolo, M. The multidisciplinary approach to Alzheimer's disease and dementia. A narrative review of non-pharmacological treatment. *Front. Neurol.* **2018**, *9*, 1058. [CrossRef] [PubMed]
11. Htut, T.Z.C.; Hiengkaew, V.; Jalayondeja, C.; Vongsirinavarat, M. Effects of physical, virtual reality-based, and brain exercise on physical, cognition, and preference in older persons: A randomized controlled trial. *Eur. Rev. Aging Phys. Act.* **2018**, *15*, 1–12. [CrossRef]
12. Optale, G.; Urgesi, C.; Busato, V.; Marin, S.; Piron, L.; Priftis, K.; Gamberini, L.; Capodieci, S.; Bordin, A. Controlling memory impairment in elderly adults using virtual reality memory training: A randomized controlled pilot study. *Neurorehabilit. Neural Repair* **2010**, *24*, 348–357. [CrossRef]
13. Baus, O.; Bouchard, S. Moving from Virtual Reality Exposure-Based Therapy to Augmented Reality Exposure-Based Therapy: A Review. *Front. Hum. Neurosci.* **2014**, 8. [CrossRef]
14. Moreno, A.; Wall, K.J.; Thangavelu, K.; Craven, L.; Ward, E.; Dissanayaka, N.N. A systematic review of the use of virtual reality and its effects on cognition in individuals with neurocognitive disorders. *Alzheimer's Dement. Transl. Res. Clin. Interv.* **2019**, *5*, 834–850. [CrossRef] [PubMed]

15. Manera, V.; Chapoulie, E.; Bourgeois, J.; Guerchouche, R.; David, R.; Ondrej, J.; Drettakis, G.; Robert, P. A feasibility study with image-based rendered virtual reality in patients with mild cognitive impairment and dementia. *PLoS ONE* **2016**, *11*, e0151487.
16. Gatica-Rojas, V.; Méndez-Rebolledo, G. Virtual reality interface devices in the reorganization of neural networks in the brain of patients with neurological diseases. *Neural Regen. Res.* **2014**, *9*, 888. [CrossRef] [PubMed]
17. Garcia-Betances, R.I.; Jiménez-Mixco, V.; Arredondo, M.T.; Cabrera-Umpiérrez, M.F. Using virtual reality for cognitive training of the elderly. *Am. J. Alzheimer's Dis. Other Demen.* **2015**, *30*, 49–54. [CrossRef]
18. Rizzo, A.S.; Kim, G.J. A SWOT analysis of the field of virtual reality rehabilitation and therapy. *Presence Teleoperators Virtual Environ.* **2005**, *14*, 119–146. [CrossRef]
19. Kim, O.; Pang, Y.; Kim, J.-H. The effectiveness of virtual reality for people with mild cognitive impairment or dementia: A meta-analysis. *BMC Psychiatry* **2019**, *19*, 219. [CrossRef]
20. Zając-Lamparska, L.; Wiłkość-Dębczyńska, M.; Wojciechowski, A.; Podhorecka, M.; Polak-Szabela, A.; Warchoł, Ł.; Kędziora-Kornatowska, K.; Araszkiewicz, A.; Izdebski, P. Effects of virtual reality-based cognitive training in older adults living without and with mild dementia: A pretest–posttest design pilot study. *BMC Res. Notes* **2019**, *12*, 776. [CrossRef]
21. Weniger, G.; Ruhleder, M.; Lange, C.; Wolf, S.; Irle, E. Egocentric and allocentric memory as assessed by virtual reality in individuals with amnestic mild cognitive impairment. *Neuropsychologia* **2011**, *49*, 518–527. [CrossRef]
22. Sayma, M.; Tuijt, R.; Cooper, C.; Walters, K. Are We There Yet? Immersive Virtual Reality to Improve Cognitive Function in Dementia and Mild Cognitive Impairment. *Gerontologist* **2019**. [CrossRef]
23. García-Betances, R.I.; Arredondo Waldmeyer, M.T.; Fico, G.; Cabrera-Umpiérrez, M.F. A succinct overview of virtual reality technology use in Alzheimer's disease. *Front. Aging Neurosci.* **2015**, *7*, 80. [PubMed]
24. Van der Hiele, K.; Vein, A.; Reijntjes, R.; Westendorp, R.; Bollen, E.; Van Buchem, M.; Van Dijk, J.; Middelkoop, H. EEG correlates in the spectrum of cognitive decline. *Clin. Neurophysiol.* **2007**, *118*, 1931–1939. [CrossRef]
25. Chandler, M.J.; Lacritz, L.; Hynan, L.; Barnard, H.; Allen, G.; Deschner, M.; Weiner, M.; Cullum, C. A total score for the CERAD neuropsychological battery. *Neurology* **2005**, *65*, 102–106. [CrossRef] [PubMed]
26. Kim, T.H.; Jhoo, J.H.; Park, J.H.; Kim, J.L.; Ryu, S.H.; Moon, S.W.; Choo, I.H.; Lee, D.W.; Yoon, J.C.; Do, Y.J. Korean version of mini mental status examination for dementia screening and its' short form. *Psychiatry Investig.* **2010**, *7*, 102. [CrossRef] [PubMed]
27. Makizako, H.; Shimada, H.; Park, H.; Doi, T.; Yoshida, D.; Uemura, K.; Tsutsumimoto, K.; Suzuki, T. Evaluation of multidimensional neurocognitive function using a tablet personal computer: Test–retest reliability and validity in community-dwelling older adults. *Geriatr. Gerontol. Int.* **2013**, *13*, 860–866. [CrossRef] [PubMed]
28. Klem, G.H.; Lüders, H.O.; Jasper, H.; Elger, C. The ten-twenty electrode system of the International Federation. *Electroencephalogr. Clin. Neurophysiol.* **1999**, *52*, 3–6.
29. Prichep, L.; John, E.; Ferris, S.; Rausch, L.; Fang, Z.; Cancro, R.; Torossian, C.; Reisberg, B. Prediction of longitudinal cognitive decline in normal elderly with subjective complaints using electrophysiological imaging. *Neurobiol. Aging* **2006**, *27*, 471–481. [CrossRef]
30. Sánchez-Moguel, S.M.; Alatorre-Cruz, G.C.; Silva-Pereyra, J.; González-Salinas, S.; Sanchez-Lopez, J.; Otero-Ojeda, G.A.; Fernández, T. Two Different Populations within the Healthy Elderly: Lack of Conflict Detection in Those at Risk of Cognitive Decline. *Front. Hum. Neurosci.* **2018**, *11*, 658. [CrossRef]
31. Van Son, D.; De Blasio, F.M.; Fogarty, J.S.; Angelidis, A.; Barry, R.J.; Putman, P. Frontal EEG theta/beta ratio during mind wandering episodes. *Biol. Psychol.* **2019**, *140*, 19–27. [CrossRef]
32. Coyle, H.; Traynor, V.; Solowij, N. Computerized and virtual reality cognitive training for individuals at high risk of cognitive decline: Systematic review of the literature. *Am. J. Geriatr. Psychiatry* **2015**, *23*, 335–359. [CrossRef]
33. Liao, Y.-Y.; Chen, I.-H.; Lin, Y.-J.; Chen, Y.; Hsu, W.-C. Effects of Virtual Reality-Based Physical and Cognitive Training on Executive Function and Dual-Task Gait Performance in Older Adults with Mild Cognitive Impairment: A Randomized Control Trial. *Front. Aging Neurosci.* **2019**, *11*, 162. [CrossRef] [PubMed]

34. Mahurin, R.K.; Velligan, D.I.; Hazleton, B.; Mark Davis, J.; Eckert, S.; Miller, A.L. Trail making test errors and executive function in schizophrenia and depression. *Clin. Neuropsychol.* **2006**, *20*, 271–288. [CrossRef] [PubMed]
35. Sánchez-Cubillo, I.; Perianez, J.; Adrover-Roig, D.; Rodriguez-Sanchez, J.; Rios-Lago, M.; Tirapu, J.; Barcelo, F. Construct validity of the Trail Making Test: Role of task-switching, working memory, inhibition/interference control, and visuomotor abilities. *J. Int. Neuropsychol. Soc.* **2009**, *15*, 438–450. [CrossRef] [PubMed]
36. Budson, A.E.; Solomon, P.R. Memory Loss, Alzheimer's disease, and dementia e-book: A practical guide for clinicians. *Elsevier Health Sci.* **2015**, 5–38.
37. Llinàs-Reglà, J.; Vilalta-Franch, J.; López-Pousa, S.; Calvó-Perxas, L.; Torrents Rodas, D.; Garre-Olmo, J. The trail making test: Association with other neuropsychological measures and normative values for adults aged 55 years and older from a Spanish-Speaking Population-based sample. *Assessment* **2017**, *24*, 183–196. [CrossRef]
38. Neri, S.G.; Cardoso, J.R.; Cruz, L.; Lima, R.M.; De Oliveira, R.J.; Iversen, M.D.; Carregaro, R.L. Do virtual reality games improve mobility skills and balance measurements in community-dwelling older adults? Systematic review and meta-analysis. *Clin. Rehabil.* **2017**, *31*, 1292–1304. [CrossRef]
39. Rodrigues-Baroni, J.M.; Nascimento, L.R.; Ada, L.; Teixeira-Salmela, L.F. Walking training associated with virtual reality-based training increases walking speed of individuals with chronic stroke: Systematic review with meta-analysis. *Braz. J. Phys. Ther.* **2014**, *18*, 502–512. [CrossRef]
40. Van Schaik, P.; Martyr, A.; Blackman, T.; Robinson, J. Involving persons with dementia in the evaluation of outdoor environments. *Cyberpsychol. Behav.* **2008**, *11*, 415–424. [CrossRef]
41. Fritz, N.E.; McCarthy, C.J.; Adamo, D.E. Handgrip strength as a means of monitoring progression of cognitive decline—A scoping review. *Ageing Res. Rev.* **2017**, *35*, 112–123. [CrossRef]
42. Sternäng, O.; Reynolds, C.A.; Finkel, D.; Ernsth-Bravell, M.; Pedersen, N.L.; Dahl Aslan, A.K. Grip strength and cognitive abilities: Associations in old age. *J. Gerontol. Ser. B Psychol. Sci. Soc. Sci.* **2016**, *71*, 841–848.
43. Vancampfort, D.; Stubbs, B.; Firth, J.; Smith, L.; Swinnen, N.; Koyanagi, A. Associations between handgrip strength and mild cognitive impairment in middle-aged and older adults in six low-and middle-income countries. *Int. J. Geriatr. Psychiatry* **2019**, *34*, 609–616. [CrossRef] [PubMed]
44. Best, J.R.; Liu-Ambrose, T.; Boudreau, R.M.; Ayonayon, H.N.; Satterfield, S.; Simonsick, E.M.; Studenski, S.; Yaffe, K.; Newman, A.B.; Rosano, C. An evaluation of the longitudinal, bidirectional associations between gait speed and cognition in older women and men. *J. Gerontol. A Biol. Sci. Med. Sci.* **2016**, *71*, 1616–1623. [CrossRef] [PubMed]
45. Buracchio, T.; Dodge, H.H.; Howieson, D.; Wasserman, D.; Kaye, J. The trajectory of gait speed preceding mild cognitive impairment. *Arch. Neurol.* **2010**, *67*, 980–986. [CrossRef] [PubMed]
46. Rasmussen, L.J.H.; Caspi, A.; Ambler, A.; Broadbent, J.M.; Cohen, H.J.; D'Arbeloff, T.; Elliott, M.; Hancox, R.J.; Harrington, H.; Hogan, S. Association of neurocognitive and physical function with gait speed in midlife. *JAMA Netw. Open* **2019**, *2*, e1913123. [CrossRef] [PubMed]
47. Sánchez, A.; Millán-Calenti, J.C.; Lorenzo-López, L.; Maseda, A. Multisensory stimulation for people with dementia: A review of the literature. *Am. J. Alzheimer's Dis. Other Demen.* **2013**, *28*, 7–14.
48. Rose, F.D.; Attree, E.A.; Brooks, B.M.; Andrews, T.K. Learning and memory in virtual environments: A role in neurorehabilitation? Questions (and occasional answers) from the University of East London. *Presence Teleoperators Virtual Environ.* **2001**, *10*, 345–358. [CrossRef]
49. Clemente, M.; Rey, B.; Rodriguez-Pujadas, A.; Breton-Lopez, J.; Barros-Loscertales, A.; Baños, R.M.; Botella, C.; Alcañiz, M.; Avila, C. A functional magnetic resonance imaging assessment of small animals' phobia using virtual reality as a stimulus. *JMIR Serious Games* **2014**, *2*, e6. [CrossRef]
50. Hikichi, H.; Kondo, K.; Takeda, T.; Kawachi, I. Social interaction and cognitive decline: Results of a 7-year community intervention. *Alzheimer's Dement. Transl. Res. Clin. Interv.* **2017**, *3*, 23–32. [CrossRef]
51. Zunzunegui, M.-V.; Alvarado, B.E.; Del Ser, T.; Otero, A. Social networks, social integration, and social engagement determine cognitive decline in community-dwelling Spanish older adults. *J. Gerontol. B Psychol. Sci. Soc. Sci.* **2003**, *58*, S93–S100. [CrossRef]

4

The Equivalence between Virtual and Real Feared Stimuli in a Phobic Adult Sample: A Neuroimaging Study

Wenceslao Peñate [1], Francisco Rivero [1], Conrado Viña [1], Manuel Herrero [1], Moisés Betancort [1], Juan De la Fuente [2], Yolanda Álvarez-Pérez [2] and Ascensión Fumero [1,*]

1. Universidad de La Laguna, 38200 La Laguna, Spain; wpenate@ull.edu.es (W.P.); friverop@ull.edu.es (F.R.); cmvinalo@ull.edu.es (C.V.); mherrero@ull.edu.es (M.H.); moibemo@ull.edu.es (M.B.)
2. Servicio Canario de la Salud, 38004 S.C. Tenerife, Spain; jafuente@ull.es (J.D.l.F.); yolanda.alvarezperez@sescs.es (Y.Á.-P.)

* Correspondence: afumero@ull.es

Abstract: The clinical use of virtual reality (VR) has proven its efficacy, especially when used as an exposure technique. A prominent property of VR's utility is its equivalence with the reality it represents. In this study, we explored this equivalence in a clinical context using neuroimaging. A sample of 32 adults with specific phobias (i.e., to cockroaches, spiders, or lizards) was divided into two groups: One was exposed to phobic stimuli using VR and the other was exposed to real phobic images (RI). We used brain activations as a dependent measure, focusing specifically on brain areas usually associated with fear processing. Whole-brain analysis detected higher activations for RI in the hippocampus, occipital, and calcarine areas. A specific analysis of the amygdala and insula also detected higher activations and extensions in response to RI, but VR stimuli also activated those areas in a significant manner. These results suggest that even in those cases where RI stimuli activate all of the brain's fear-processing circuits, VR stimuli do so as well. This implies that VR can be useful as an exposure technique similar to RI and applied as more than a mere training mechanism.

Keywords: virtual reality; real phobic images; anxiety disorders; specific phobia; fMRI; neuroimaging

---

1. Introduction

The use of virtual reality (VR) as a tool for psychological treatment has grown since it was first employed [1] as an exposure procedure for the treatment of phobic disorders. Since then, many studies have been conducted with VR as the main therapeutic resource, which has maintained interest in this topic over the years [2]. Although VR has been employed in several therapeutic approaches, it most often takes the form of "virtual reality exposure therapy" (VRET) [3].

The efficacy and efficiency of VRET have been proven in a considerable number of clinical trials and experimental designs, as shown by several systematic reviews and meta-analyses [3–6]. There are several reasons for this efficacy: VR is an intermediate step in graduated exposure, a safe condition in which to train patients to cope with real stimuli. VR also enhances exposure when VRET is combined with in vivo exposure [5–10]. Interestingly, two processes in the functioning of VR can be inferred from these explanations: VR accurately represents real stimuli (exposure process [8]), and VR is an opportunity to cope with a distressing stimulus (training process [11,12]).

The efficacy of VRET has a prerequisite related to the physical properties of the virtual scenarios used. The key concept here is immersive technology. This concept is related to VR's property of "enveloping" participants and making them feel as if they are "actually there". There are several definitions of immersive technology [13]. These definitions share the idea that the more similar a virtual context is to a real one, the greater its immersive power. Technical characteristics (e.g., environments, distinctness, movements) and the type of presentation (i.e., 3D) are physical attributes that can shape a more immersive and consequently more effective VR [14]. Implicitly, the fact that VR scenarios are "immersive" also means that they are processed similarly to real ones. However, this property of sensation of presence, being a prerequisite, is not sufficient to explain the efficacy of VRET [15]. This efficacy seems to be supported in the property of VR to stimulate a brain representation to create an embodied simulation of the body in the world, including main informational processes: Visceral/autonomic, sensory, and motor information [15]. As a consequence, observed brain activations as a function of VRET need to reflect this embodied simulation.

Functional magnetic resonance imaging (fMRI) studies have shed light on how patients with phobias process phobic stimuli. According to systematic reviews and meta-analyses [16–20], the presence of phobic stimuli is associated with greater activation of the left amygdala and insular cortex than of other brain areas. Other structures involved in phobic responses are the fusiform gyrus, the left dorsolateral prefrontal cortex, and the left cingulate cortex. Compared to the limbic areas, frontal areas have been found to be less consistent and less stable in processing phobic stimuli. These findings are congruent with the existence of a dual-route functional network in processing feared stimuli [21–24]: Wave1, a short/unconscious route that involves a direct link between the thalamus and the amygdala; and Wave2, a long/conscious route that involves the thalamus-sensory and cortex-entorhinal cortex–hippocampus–subiculum–amygdala.

Given that therapeutic exposure is related to how patients process phobic stimuli, the activation of these routes can have direct implications for exposure efficacy: Conscious routes imply more complex processing and a better opportunity for patients to change the significance of a phobic stimulus and develop a more adaptive response. In this regard, the present study was aimed at testing whether exposure to virtual phobic stimuli in a group of patients with specific phobias (i.e., to small animals) could activate the same brain regions as exposure to real image stimuli. We also intended to test whether virtual stimuli could also facilitate the activation of the conscious Wave2 route in processing phobic stimuli (as real image stimuli do) and to consider the implications of these data for the efficacy of exposure techniques. Specifically, we planned to compare activity in empirically supported brain regions associated with phobic stimulus processing.

2. Materials and Methods

2.1. Participants

The sample was composed of 32 adults. There were 26 (real phobic images (RI): 40.6%; VR: 40.6%) female and 6 (RI: 9.4%; VR: 9.4%) male participants. Sixteen participants (mean age 35.25 years, SD 12.17) were exposed to real images of small animals (i.e., cockroaches, spiders, or lizards), and 16 participants (mean age 33.43 years, SD 10.26) watched films of virtual images of such animals. The phobic stimulus matched the individual's phobia.

All participants were right-handed and had normal vision. The main inclusion criterion was being an adult with a diagnosis of specific phobia. The phobia had to be a primary psychological disorder and not be explained by another health condition. Other inclusion criteria for participants included not receiving any treatment for a specific phobia at the time of the study and not having any impediment to undergoing a magnetic resonance imaging session.

2.2. Instruments

The Composite International Diagnostic Interview (CIDI), Version 2.1 (WHO, Geneve, Switzerland) [25] was used to verify the diagnosis of phobia. The CIDI is a structured interview for major mental disorders according to the CIE-10 criteria [26]. For the purposes of this study, questions related to a specific phobia, social phobia, agoraphobia, and panic attacks were selected. Participants diagnosed with a specific small-animal phobia were included (F40.218; [26]).

The S–R Inventory of Anxiousness [27] is a 14-item inventory with a 5-point Likert-type scale that assesses physiological, cognitive, and behavioral anxiety symptoms associated with an anxiety-inducing situation. The phobic stimulus target is pointed out prior to the participant's response. The inventory has shown high internal consistency (0.95) and adequate convergent validity [27,28]. For the current study, Cronbach's alpha was 0.79.

The Beck Anxiety Inventory (BAI) [29] is a 21-item self-report instrument for assessing the severity of anxiety states. Participants are asked to rate the severity of each symptom using a 4-point Likert-type scale ranging from 0 ("Not at all") to 3 ("Severely—I could barely stand it"). Total scores range from 0 to 63. Scores of 26–63 represent severe anxiety [29]. Cronbach's alpha for the current study was high (0.93).

Hand preference was assessed with the Edinburgh Handedness Inventory (EHI) [30]. This inventory consists of ten items: Writing, drawing, throwing, using scissors, toothbrush, knife (without fork), spoon, broom, striking a match, and opening a box. Participants indicated the strength of their hand preference for each of the 10 items by putting one or two ticks in the appropriate column, or one tick in each column if they were indifferent about that item. The EHI provides a Laterality Quotient ranging from +100 (totally right-handed) to −100 (totally left-handed).

2.3. Design

A 2 × 2 factor design was used: The first independent variable was "stimulus format" with two levels (real images and virtual reality), and the second independent variable was "type of stimulus" (phobic and neutral stimulus).

The stimuli consisted of small animals in motion. These were filmed in 3D video for the real images. To control the presentation modality effects, 3D recorded movies were used as the models to create the virtual reality stimuli. The arousal properties of these virtual reality stimuli were tested by measuring activations of the brain regions of interest (ROIs) at the initial fMRI session. Because the virtual stimuli were directly related to each specific phobia (i.e., participants with a spider phobia received only spider stimuli), stimulus valence was not assessed. All participants were informed about the stimulus format (virtual or real images).

Both the real image and virtual reality formats included both phobic stimuli (i.e., cockroaches, spiders, or lizards) and neutral stimuli (i.e., wooden balls). All images were presented before an identical white background. Stimuli were presented in 3D virtual reality video format (VR group) and 3D real image video format (RI group). Figure 1 shows examples of the RI and VR stimuli.

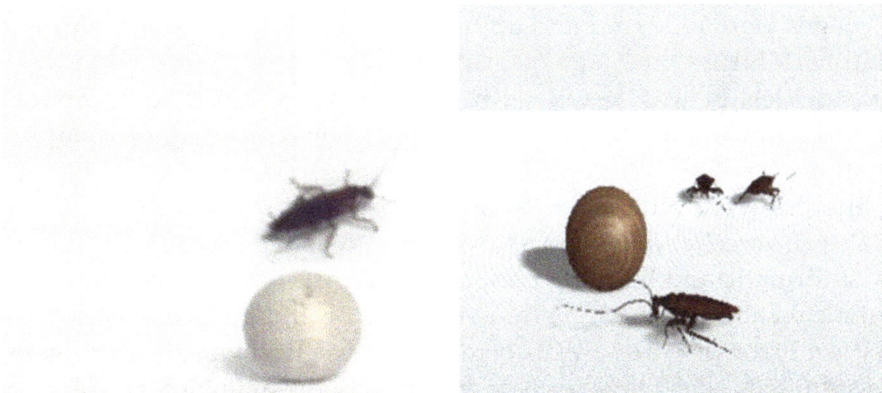

Figure 1. Example of the real image (RI) and virtual reality (VR) stimuli.

Participants were randomly assigned (direct method) to one of two groups: One received the stimuli in virtual reality format (VR group) and the other received them as real images (RI group). Participants were exposed to two different conditions: Phobic stimuli and neutral stimuli (i.e., wooden balls).

We used neuroimaging activations as dependent variables. The images were filtered for ROI, taking into account previous results with patients with phobias [16–20]. Nine regions were selected for both hemispheres: Amygdala, hippocampus, insula, fusiform gyrus, occipital cortex (inferior, medial, and superior), calcarine area, and thalamus.

Stimuli were recorded in 3D and projected in the MRI scanner in stereoscopic 3D video using Visual Stim digital MRI-compatible 3D glasses (graphics card: GeForce 8600GT), (Resonance Technology Inc., Northridge, CA, US). We presented the stimuli using a block design. Each participant was randomly presented with 16 blocks of phobic images and 16 blocks of images of wooden balls. The duration of each block was 20 seconds.

2.4. Procedure

The study was conducted from April to July 2016. Phobic participants were recruited through various media (i.e., website, press, flyers, radio, TV, and newspapers). Next, an e-mail with the inventories was sent to possible participants. The initial diagnosis of specific phobia according to participants' inventory scores was corroborated by a semistructured interview. Those who did not meet the inclusion criteria (or met the exclusion criteria) were excluded. In addition, due to the interference with the fMRI analysis, participants with nonremovable metal devices were excluded. Participants signed an informed consent form included in the study that had been approved by the Ethics Committee for Research and Animal Welfare of the University of La Laguna (CEIBA2012-0033). After their participation, subjects were entitled to receive as payment an eight-session free psychological treatment for specific animal phobia.

2.5. fMRI Data Acquisition

Functional MRI data were collected with a 3T General Electric Signa Excite scan (General Electric, Madrid, Spain). The BOLD signal was measured with an echo planar imaging sequence with 30 ms of echo time, 2000 ms of repetition time, 25.6 of field of view, and 75° of flip angle. The image dimensions were $64 \times 64 \times 32$ mm with $4 \times 4 \times 4$ mm voxel dimensions.

2.6. fMRI and Data Analysis

Brain images were analyzed with Statistical Parametric Mapping (SPM 12) software (London University College, London, UK). Preprocessing procedures included realigning, coregistering, segmenting (with forward deformation fields), normalizing (structural images with a $1 \times 1 \times 1$ mm voxel size and functional images with a $4 \times 4 \times 4$ mm voxel size), and smoothing (Gaussian Kernel of 8 mm, FWHM). Images were rendered and adjusted to the standard brain template of the Montreal Neurological Institute (MNI).

The 2×2 factor design was tested with a two-way ANOVA to compare the main effects of image format and stimuli and the interaction effect between image format and stimuli on the whole-brain activation.

In addition, images were filtered for ROIs (amygdala, hippocampus, insula, fusiform gyrus, occipital cortex, calcarine area, and thalamus). All these ROIs were extracted from the WFU Pickatlas 3.0.5b (Radiology Informatic and Imaging Laboratory, Winston-Salem, NC, US) for SPM 12 with the Automated Anatomical Labeling (AAL2) brain atlas and Brodmann areas atlas.

The Family-Wise Error ($p < 0.05$ FWE corrected) correction was used. However, noncorrected probabilities were admitted when they were congruent with the biological model of phobias (but never higher than 0.001 uncorrected). The error was corrected considering that there was activation when the activated area was equal to or greater than a 3-voxel cluster with a voxel size of $4 \times 4 \times 4$ mm.

3. Results

An initial statistical analysis was performed to test the comparability between the VR group and RI group in anxiety measures (S–R and BAI scores). No significant differences (see Figure 2) were found between the two groups in these variables ((S–R: VR group M = 7.75, SD = 2.7; RI group M = 6.4, SD = 4.22) (BAI: VR group M = 18.0, SD = 14.14; RI group M = 16.3, SD = 11.95)).

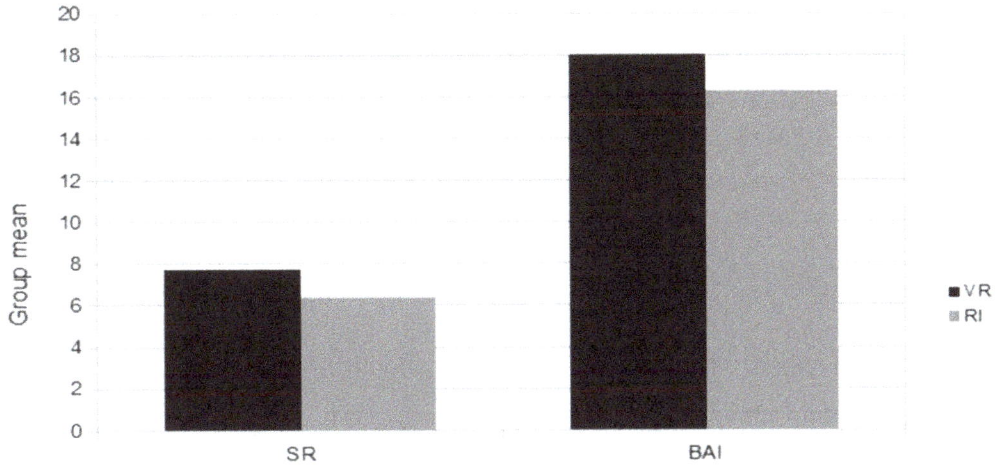

Figure 2. Anxiety measures.

After that, a two-way ANOVA (whole-brain analysis) was conducted with image format (virtual, real) and type of stimulus (phobic, neutral) as independent variables. The whole-brain activations are shown in Figure 3. The interaction effect was significant (F (1.60) = 25.22, $p < 0.05$). This value was considered as the F score threshold. Moreover, an overall main effect was found for type of stimulus (F (1.60) = 26.78, $p < 0.05$). This main effect revealed a significant difference between phobic stimuli and neutral stimuli in brain activity: Fear-related stimuli generated higher brain activation than neutral stimuli. There were no differences in brain activity according to the image format factor (virtual vs. real phobic stimuli).

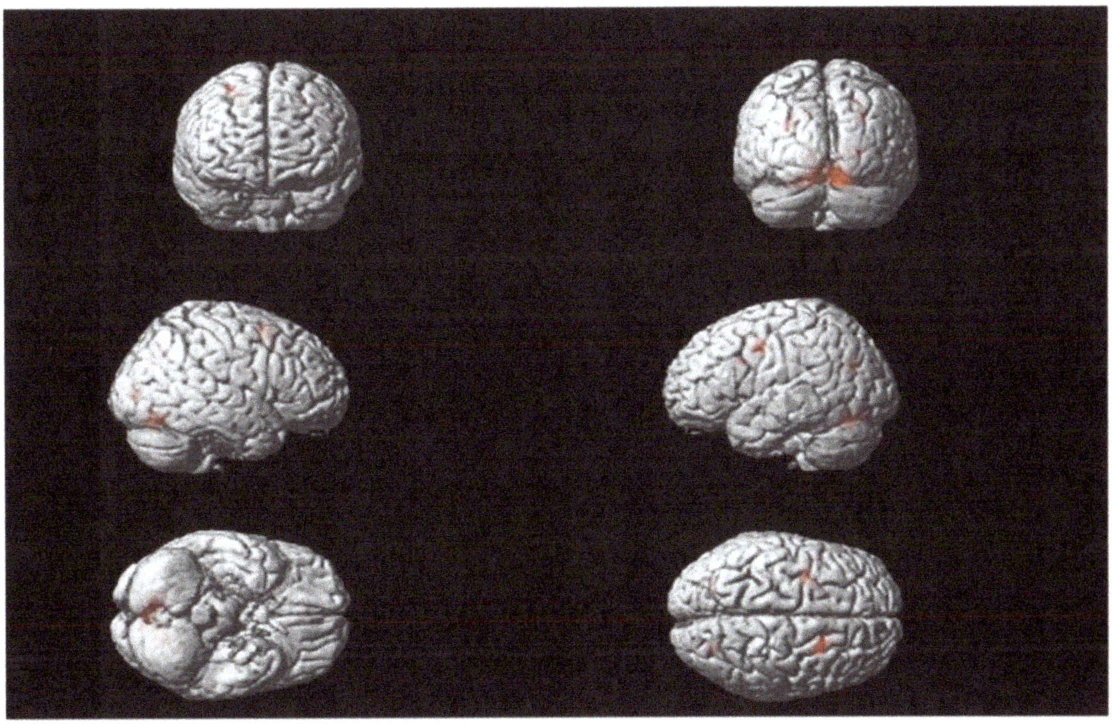

Figure 3. Whole-brain interaction effect. F (1.60) = 25.22, $p < 0.05$ (Family Wise Estimation (FWE)).

The following analyses were performed on the brain areas selected as ROIs. For exploratory reasons, a significance threshold of $p \leq 0.001$, uncorrected $k \geq 3$, was used to detect subtle changes in brain activation. In addition, to reduce the probability of false positive results, we set a contiguity threshold for cluster volumes of at least 20 voxels with a size of 2 × 2 × 2 mm [31] and did not consider clusters with a Z lower than 3.00. The fMRI comparisons between the RI group and the VR group in ROI brain areas are summarized in Table 1. These results showed significantly higher activations with real images in the hippocampus (R: $F(1.60) = 25.77$, $p < 0.001$; L: $F(1.60) = 23.74$, $p < 0.001$), fusiform gyrus ($F(1.60) = 48.44$, $p < 0.000$), bilateral middle occipital cortex (R: $F(1.60) = 41.25$, $p < 0.000$; L: $F(1.60) = 46.09$, p < 0.000), bilateral superior occipital cortex (R: $F(1.60) = 44.78$, $p < 0.000$; L: $F(1.60) = 37.34$, $p < 0.00$), and bilateral calcarine area (R: $F(1.60) = 32.07$, $p < 0.01$; L: $F(1.60) = 29.53$, $p < 0.01$). No differences were observed in the amygdala, insula, bilateral inferior occipital cortex, or thalamus in RI compared to VR.

Table 1. fMRI comparisons between the RI group and the VR group in brain regions of interest (ROIs).

AREA	Coordinates	Hemisphere	*K*	*Z*	*P*
Real Image > VR Phobics					
Amygdala		Right/Left			n.s.
Hippocampus	22, −28, −6	Right	4	3.4	0.0001
Insula		Right/Left			n.s.
Fusiform gyrus	38, −72, −18	Right	11	4.54	0.0001
	22, −64, 14	Right	3	4.51	0.0001
	−34, -52, −22	Left	18	3.92	0.0001
	−26, −68, −6	Left	-	3.51	0.0001
	34, −48, −14	Right	4	3.37	0.0001
Occipital cortex					
Inferior		Right			n.s.
Middle	26, −88, 6	Right	49	4.29	0.0001
Superior	26, −72,34	Right	28	4.42	0.0001
Inferior		Left			n.s.
Middle	−30, −72, 26	Left	38	4.47	0.0001
Superior		Left			n.s.
Calcarine area	−14, −76, 1	Left	10	3.7	0.0001
Thalamus		Right/Left			n.s.

n.s.: Not significant. RI: Real Image; VR: Virtual Reality; AREA: Brain region, K: Voxel's number, Z: Tipical score.

A new and specific ROI analysis was performed separately for the amygdala and insula as two brain areas usually associated with the processing of anxiety-related stimuli, taking virtual vs. real image phobic stimuli as an independent variable. Figure 4 shows the activation observed in the amygdala. The response to real image stimuli was significant in a cluster in both the right amygdala (18, 0, −14) and left amygdala (−26, −4, −22), which both exhibited intense activity (t mean = 6.21; t SD = 0.20 right side, and t mean = 4.98; t SD = 0.54 left side). For VR stimuli, significant activity occurred in both the right (18, 0, −14) and left clusters (−26, 0, −22), which showed similar intensity (t mean = 4.59; t SD = 0.27 right side, and t mean = 4.40; t SD = 0.19 left side). These data revealed that stimulus processing was greater and more extensive in the real image format than in virtual reality.

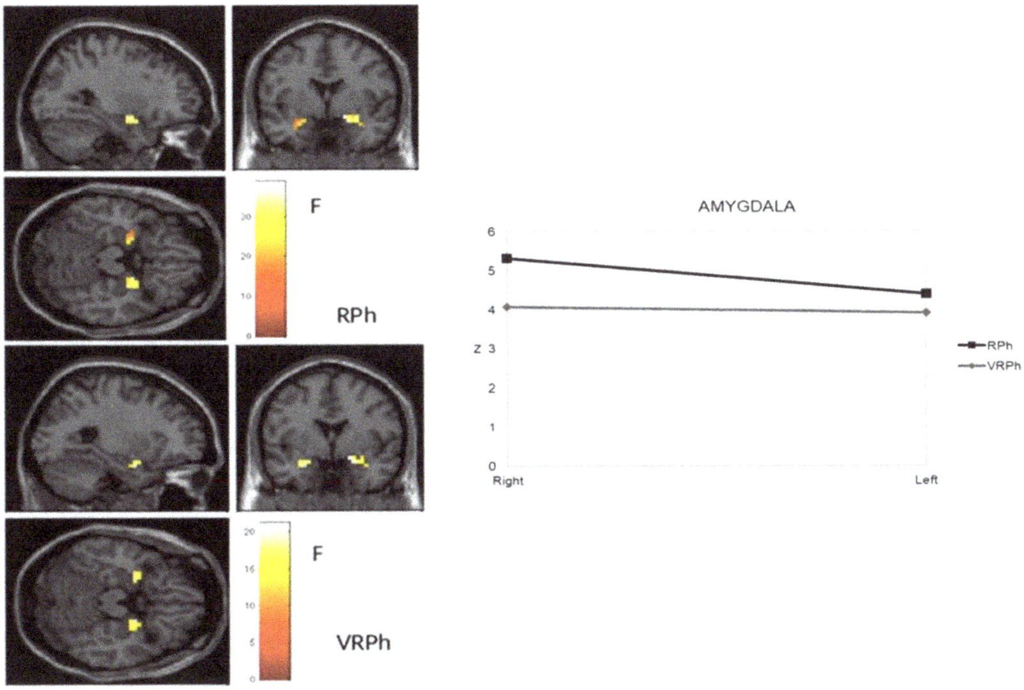

Figure 4. Amygdala activation of phobic stimuli processing (virtual and real format) in an adult sample with a specific phobia. RPh: Phobic real image; VRPh: Phobic virtual reality image.

Figure 5 shows activation of the insula. A similar activation was found in the right insula (42, 24, 2) with both real and virtual images. Yet, in the left insula, real images were associated with greater intensity ($Z = 7.10$; $p < 0.000$; $Z = 6.22$; $p < 0.000$; $Z = 5.47$; $p < 0.000$; $Z = 5.45$; $p < 0.000$) and extension (42, 24, 2; −46, 12, −6; −30, −28, 22; 38, −28, 22). These data suggest that fear-related (compared to neutral) images preferentially activated many of the regions involved in a hierarchical system responsible for organizing defensive behavior in both virtual and real image formats.

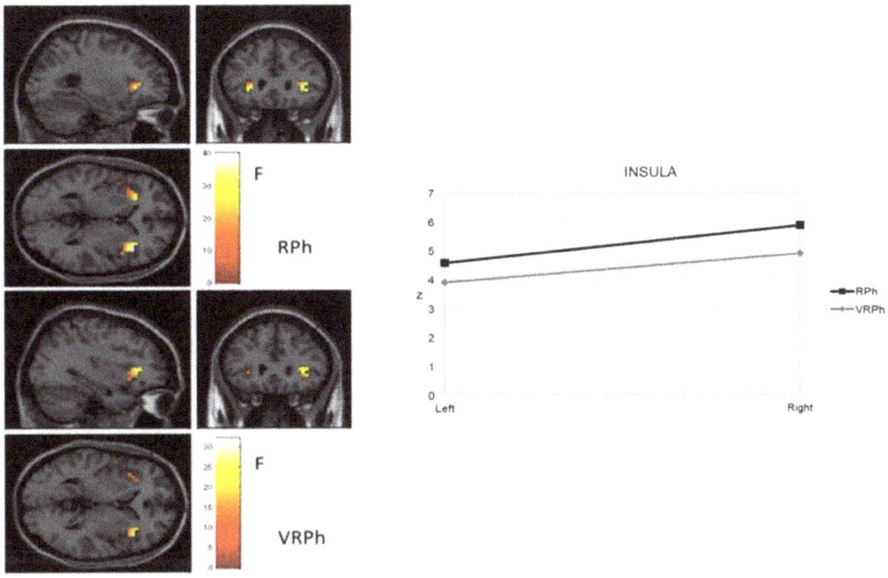

Figure 5. Insula activation of phobic stimuli processing (virtual and real format) in an adult sample with specific phobia.

Finally, to test the research objective related to the functional processing of Wave2 with virtual or real image phobic stimuli, new ROI analyses were performed: We explored the involvement of visual and limbic brain areas and their connectivity, selecting the Brodmann visual area and the amygdala for study. The insula was also selected because of its functional relationship in processing interceptive inputs. Figure 6 shows the results obtained. Initial data showed that visual processing of the stimuli started similarly for both groups. The primary visual activity associated with phobic stimulus processing (BA17) was similar in the RI and VR groups. However, there were differences in the associative visual cortex (BA18 and BA19). Specifically, the real image was significant in a cluster (46, −72, −6) of the right occipital cortex with very extensive (52 BA18 voxels and 59 BA19 voxels) and intense activity (BA18 t mean = 4.75; t SD = 2.85 and BA19 t mean = 5.72; t SD = 3.82). In the VR group, significant activity occurred in both right and left clusters. In the right cluster (46, −72, −6), it was observed in the same coordinate with similar intensity (BA18 t mean = 5.71; t SD = 2.02 and BA19 t mean = 4.90; t SD = 3.33), but was less extensive (4 BA18 voxels and 11 BA19 voxels). In the left cluster (−30, −88, −18), significant activity was observed in the associative visual areas with the same extension in BA18 and BA19 (15 voxels) and stronger intensity (BA18 t mean = 5.51; t SD = 2.96 and BA19 t mean = 4.44; t SD = 1.80). These results suggested differential Wave2 phobic stimulus processing according to the image format.

Phobic Real image Phobic VR image

Figure 6. Visual activation of phobic stimuli processing (virtual and real format) in an adult sample with a specific phobia.

4. Discussion

In the present study, we attempted to test whether exposure to virtual phobic stimuli activated the same brain areas as exposure to real image stimuli in a group of patients with phobias to small animals. This was explored specifically in regions usually associated with phobic stimulus processing: Amygdala, hippocampus, insula, fusiform gyrus, occipital cortex, calcarine area, and thalamus.

As pointed out by previous systematic reviews and meta-analyses, greater activations were found in the areas traditionally involved in fear processing [16–20]. These activations were found regardless of whether participants were exposed to virtual stimuli or real image stimuli. The absence of a main effect of image format supports the idea that virtual reality activates similar brain areas to those that real images do, including the regions involved in both Wave1 and Wave2 phobic stimulus processing. Main differences between VR and RI phobic stimuli were observed in activation intensity: Real images generated greater intensity in the hemodynamic response than virtual images. These data support an idea that is simple, but has clear implications for exposure technique: Real phobic images produce higher anxiety responses, but virtual stimuli also produce significant levels of anxiety [32]. These results can be understood as an initial endorsement of the use of VR as an exposure procedure [8] and not as a mere training opportunity [11,12].

As mentioned above, both VR and RI activated the two fear processing routes, but greater activation of the visual areas (inferior, medial, and superior occipital cortex and calcarine area) was observed with RI stimuli. The differences between real and virtual images were not found in the primary visual area (BA17), but in the associative visual areas (BA18 and BA19). The calcarine area has been found to play a main role in the visual network associated with the conditioning of fear [33,34]. These data indicate a greater activation of the Wave2/conscious route when participants are exposed to real image phobic stimuli. This greater involvement of associative visual processing has also been observed when the stimulus resembles the experience of the individual, as happens with in vivo exposure to the phobic stimulus [35,36]. These results support the idea that real images activate more areas from the Wave2 processing of phobic stimuli than VR and could be a therapeutic resource. Brain activation with feared stimuli produces higher levels of distress, and maintaining exposure to real images eventually starts to reduce anxiety. Consequently, the more patients become accustomed to facing the feared stimulus, the less anxious they will be when they face it again and, therefore, the less they will associate it with the expected negative response.

The study of the interaction between the independent variables in the various brain areas selected for their involvement in phobia processing, as shown by the ANOVA, revealed differences in the brain activation of cortical perceptual regions, but not in the limbic system regions. However, the differences in the ROI analysis observed in the amygdala and insula indicate that fear-related stimuli produced higher and more extensive brain activation when real images were processed compared to images presented in virtual reality. As shown by the data, there was also a greater activation (and extension) in the left insula when participants were exposed to RI compared to VR stimuli. It has been proposed that the insula integrates bottom-up interoceptive signals with top-down information [37]. Specifically, a signal is activated when affective visual stimuli are processed and this signal is guided by certain top-down requirements. The presence of feared stimuli represents an excellent opportunity for these requirements. Subsequently, this signal can be conveyed to control regions such as the prefrontal cortex for appropriate behavioral output. This "appropriate" behavior may take the form of an escape behavior for patients with phobias. In fact, the higher intensity of insula activation during real phobic stimulus presentation can be associated with more escape behaviors [38]. In addition, VR stimuli may be more suitable for the exposure procedure because they are less likely to activate escape behaviors.

As virtual stimuli affect ROIs that are usually related to brain responses to phobias, VR produces a significant subjective experience and generates a sense of presence. Thus, virtual phobic stimuli can produce a significant level of anxiety. Yet, as shown by the differences in brain activation, the immersive properties of virtual stimuli are lower than those of real images, but VR also activates a complex neural connectivity, including several associative areas, far from a mere activation of fear circuitry. Does this imply that VR can initiate an embodied simulation, aside from a rigorous representation of fear stimuli? As cited [15], embodied simulation is being proposed as the key mechanism for why VRET is effective, because VR provides a mental internal model, as a predictive coding regulating the body in its context effectively. As a result, more thorough experimental designs (with precise brain measures regarding embodiment) are needed.

Meanwhile, in practice, exposure to real phobic images produces higher activations and it also may require a greater effort to voluntarily inhibit emotional activation than exposure to virtual stimuli and consequently may lead to more escape behaviors. Although there are no conclusive data on this [39], given that VR phobic stimulus exposure activates fewer escape behaviors, lower attrition rates and more therapeutic adherence can be expected, as reported by other studies [7,9,39,40]. For this, according to our data, virtual phobic stimuli require two paradoxical properties: They must be as similar as possible to real stimuli to activate the mechanisms associated with fear responses, but at the same time, participants need to be able to identify them as virtual.

This study has several limitations. First, the small sample size may have affected the reliability of the results [41]. In addition, also due to sample size, sex differences could not be taken into account. Furthermore, this study only used one type of specific phobia (i.e., small animal phobia) with few experimental stimulation conditions: Data about comorbid phobias and evolution time were not taken into account, and these data can affect results. Moreover, we did not assess participants' level of disgust as an emotional state different to fear/phobia [42], nor did we measure their escape behavior. However, the role of neural activity with escape/avoidance behavior is well established [43]. To add, we used 3D filmed real phobic stimuli as a representative condition to in vivo exposure, but this equivalence was not tested. Finally, we did not establish if the results were due to a phobic condition or could also be observed in anxious nonphobic individuals.

5. Conclusions

In short, the small animal images filmed in both real image and virtual reality formats generated the functional activation of the brain regions involved in the emotional processing of fear—thalamus, amygdala, hippocampus, fusiform gyrus, insula and occipital cingulate, and prefrontal cortices—in phobic individuals. However, real images produced more intense brain activations and a different pattern of hemodynamic responses than those elicited by virtual reality stimuli. This notwithstanding, these differences do not preclude the use of VR as an exposure resource, as the virtual images provided a sufficiently intense distress response in phobic individuals, activated a conscious process pathway, and, furthermore, led to fewer escape behaviors. These data support the use of virtual reality as an exposure procedure in the treatment of phobia disorders with similar properties to activate underlying mechanisms of exposure techniques.

Author Contributions: Conceptualization, methodology, formal analysis, and original draft preparation: W.P., F.R., C.V., M.H., M.B., J.D.L.F., and A.F.; writing—review and editing, W.P., F.R., Y.A.-P. and A.F.; Editing the final version, W.P, F.R., Y.A.-P. and A.F.

Acknowledgments: Thank you to the Servicio General de Apoyo a la Investigación de la Universidad de La Laguna (SEGAI).

References

1. North, M.; North, S. Virtual environments and psychological disorders. *Electron. J. Virtual Cult.* **1994**, *2*, 37–42.
2. Powers, M.B.; Rothbaum, B.O. Recent advances in virtual reality therapy for anxiety and related disorders: Introduction to the special issue. *J. Anxiety Disord.* **2019**, *61*, 1–2. [CrossRef] [PubMed]
3. Krijn, M.; Emmelkamp, P.M.G.; Olafsson, R.P.; Biemond, R. Virtual reality exposure therapy of anxiety disorders: A review. *Clin. Psychol. Rev.* **2004**, *24*, 259–281. [CrossRef] [PubMed]
4. De Carvalho, M.R.; Freire, R.C.; Nardi, A.E. Virtual reality as a mechanism for exposure therapy. *World J. Biol. Psychiat.* **2010**, *11*, 220–230. [CrossRef]
5. Opriş, D.; Pintea, S.; García-Palacios, A.; Botella, C.; Szamosközi, Ş.; David, D. Virtual reality exposure therapy in anxiety disorders: A quantitative meta-analysis. *Depress. Anxiety* **2012**, *29*, 85–93. [CrossRef]
6. Powers, M.B.; Emmelkamp, P.M.G. Virtual reality exposure therapy for anxiety disorders: A meta-analysis. *J. Anxiety Disord.* **2008**, *22*, 561–569. [CrossRef]
7. Carl, E.; Stein, A.T.; Levihn-Coon, A.; Pogue, J.R.; Rothbaum, B.; Emmelkamp, P.; Asmundson, G.J.G.; Carlbring, P.; Powers, M.B. Virtual reality exposure therapy for anxiety and related disorders: A meta-analysis of randomized controlled trials. *J. Anxiety Disord.* **2019**, *61*, 27–36. [CrossRef]
8. Botella, C.; Fernández-Álvarez, J.; Guillén, V.; García-Palacios, A.; Baños, R. Recent progress in virtual reality exposure therapy for phobias: A systematic review. *Curr. Psychiat. Rep.* **2017**, *19*, 42. [CrossRef]
9. Fernández-Álvarez, J.; Rozental, A.; Carlbring, P.; Colombo, D.; Riva, G.; Anderson, P.L.; Baños, R.M.; Benbow, A.A.; Bouchard, S.; Bretón-López, J.M.; et al. Deterioration rates in Virtual Reality Therapy: An individual patient data level meta-analysis. *J. Anxiety Disord.* **2019**, *61*, 3–17. [CrossRef]
10. Morina, N.; Ijntema, H.; Meyerbröker, K.; Emmelkamp, P.M.G. Can virtual reality exposure therapy gains be generalized to real-life? A meta-analysis ofstudies applying behavioral assessments. *Behav. Res. Ther.* **2015**, *74*, 18–24. [CrossRef]
11. Pasco, D. The potential of using virtual reality technology in physical activity settings. *Quest* **2013**, *65*, 429–441. [CrossRef]
12. Zeng, N.; Pope, Z.; Lee, J.E.; Gao, Z. Virtual Reality Exercise for anxiety and depression: A preliminary review of current research in an emerging field. *J. Clin. Med.* **2018**, *7*, 42. [CrossRef]
13. Suh, A.; Prophet, J. The state of immersive technology research: A literature analysis. *Comput. Hum. Behav.* **2018**, *86*, 77–90. [CrossRef]

14. Rubio-Tamayo, J.L.; Gertrudix-Barrio, M.; García-García, F. Immersive environments and virtual reality: Systematic review and advances in communication, interaction and simulation. *Multimodal Technol. Interact.* **2017**, *1*, 21. [CrossRef]
15. Riva, G.; Wiederhold, B.K.; Mantovani, F. Neuroscience of virtual reality: From virtual exposure to embodied medicine. *Cyberpsychol. Behav. Soc. Netw.* **2019**, *22*, 82–96. [CrossRef] [PubMed]
16. Del Casale, A.; Ferracuti, S.; Rapinesi, C.; Serata, D.; Piccirilli, M.; Savoja, V.; Kotzalidis, G.D.; Manfredi, G.; Angeletti, G.; Tatarelli, R.; et al. Functional neuroimaging in specific phobia. *Psychiatr. Res. Neuroimaging* **2012**, *202*, 181–197. [CrossRef]
17. Fullana, M.A.; Harrison, B.J.; Soriano-Mas, C.; Vervliet, B.; Cardoner, N.; Ávila-Parcet, A.; Radua, J. Neural signatures of human fear conditioning: An updated and extended meta-analysis of fMRI studies. *Mol. Psychiatr.* **2016**, *21*, 500–508. [CrossRef]
18. Peñate, W.; Fumero, A.; Viña, C.; Herrero, M.; Marrero, R.J.; Rivero, F. A meta-analytic review of neuroimaging studies of specific phobia to small animals. *Eur. J. Psychiat.* **2017**, *31*, 23–36. [CrossRef]
19. Linares, I.M.P.; Trzesniak, C.; Chagas, M.H.N.; Hallak, J.E.C.; Nardi, A.E.; Crippa, J.A.S. Neuroimaging in specific phobia disorder: A systematic review of the literature. *Rev. Bras. Psiquiatr.* **2012**, *34*, 101–111. [CrossRef]
20. Ipser, J.C.; Singh, L.; Stein, D.J. Meta-analysis of functional brain imaging in specific phobia. *Psychiat. Clin. Neurosci.* **2013**, *67*, 311–322. [CrossRef]
21. Das, T.; Padakannaya, P.; Pugh, K.R.; Singh, N.C. Neuroimaging reveals dual routes to reading in simultaneous proficient readers of two orthographies. *Neuroimage* **2011**, *54*, 1476–1487. [CrossRef] [PubMed]
22. Granziera, C.; Hadjikhani, N.; Arzy, S.; Seeck, M.; Meuli, R.; Krueger, G. In-vivo magnetic resonance imaging of the structural core of the Papez circuit in humans. *Neuroreport* **2011**, *22*, 227–231. [CrossRef] [PubMed]
23. Papez, J.W. A proposed mechanism of emotion. 1937. *J. Neuropsychi. Clin. N.* **1995**, *7*, 103–112. [CrossRef]
24. Rivero, R.; Herrero, M.; Viña, C.; Álvarez-Pérez, Y.; Peñate, W. Neuroimaging in cockroach phobia: An experimental study. *Int. J. Clin. Health Psych.* **2017**, *17*, 207–215. [CrossRef]
25. Kessler, R.C.; Üstün, T.B. The world mental health (WMH) survey initiative version of the world health organization (WHO) composite international diagnostic interview (CIDI). *Int. J. Meth. Psych. Res.* **2004**, *13*, 93–121. [CrossRef] [PubMed]
26. World Health Organization. *The ICD-10 Classification of Mental and Behavioural Disorders: Clinical Descriptions and Diagnostic Guidelines*; WHO: Geneva, Switzerland, 1992.
27. Endler, N.S.; Hunt, J.M.C.V.; Rosenstein, A.J. An S-R Inventory of Anxiousness. *Psychol. Monogr.* **1962**, *76*, 143–146. [CrossRef]
28. Kameoka, V.A.; Tanaka-Matsumi, J. The appropriateness of using the S-R Inventory of Anxiousness to measure sources of behavioral variability. *Appl. Psych. Meas.* **1981**, *5*, 229–235. [CrossRef]
29. Beck, A.T.; Epstein, N.; Brown, G.; Steer, R.A. An inventory for measuring clinical anxiety: Psychometric properties. *J. Consult. Clin. Psych.* **1988**, *56*, 893. [CrossRef]
30. Oldfield, R.C. The assessment and analysis of handedness: The Edinburgh inventory. *Neuropsychologia* **1971**, *9*, 97–113. [CrossRef]
31. Forman, S.D.; Cohen, J.D.; Fitzgerald, M.; Eddy, W.F.; Mintun, M.A.; Noll, D.C. Improved assessment of significant activation in functional magnetic resonance imaging (fMRI): Use of a cluster-size threshold. *Magn. Reson. Med.* **1995**, *33*, 636–647. [CrossRef]
32. Juan, M.C.; Baños, R.; Botella, C.; Pérez, D.; Alcaníiz, M.; Monserrat, C. An augmented reality system for the treatment of acrophobia: The sense of presence using immersive photography. *Presence Teleop. Virt.* **2006**, *15*, 393–402. [CrossRef]
33. Lithari, C.; Moratti, S.; Weisz, N. Limbic areas are functionally decoupled and visual cortex takes a more central role during fear conditioning in humans. *Sci. Rep.* **2016**, *6*, 29220. [CrossRef] [PubMed]
34. Silverstein, D.N.; Ingvar, M. A multi-pathway hypothesis for human visual fear signaling. *Front. Syst. Neurosci.* **2015**, *9*, 101. [CrossRef] [PubMed]
35. Paquette, V.; Lévesque, J.; Mensour, B.; Leroux, J.M.; Beaudoin, G.; Bourgouin, P.; Beauregard, M. Change the mind and you change the brain: Effects of cognitive-behavioral therapy on the neural correlates of spider phobia. *NeuroImage* **2003**, *18*, 401–409. [CrossRef]
36. Weiner, K.S.; Zilles, K. The anatomical and functional specialization of the fusiform gyrus. *Neuropsychologia* **2016**, *83*, 48–62. [CrossRef]

37. Gu, X.; Hof, P.R.; Friston, K.J.; Fan, J. Anterior insular cortex and emotional awareness. *J. Comp. Neurol.* **2013**, *521*, 3371–3388. [CrossRef]
38. Palminteri, S.; Justo, D.; Jauffret, C.; Pavlicek, B.; Dauta, A.; Delmaire, C.; Czernecki, V.; Karachi, C.; Capelle, L.; Durr, A.; et al. Critical roles for anterior insula and dorsal striatum in punishment-based avoidance learning. *Neuron* **2012**, *76*, 998–1009. [CrossRef]
39. Benbow, A.A.; Anderson, P.L. A meta-analytic examination of attrition in virtual reality exposure therapy for anxiety disorders. *J. Anxiety Disord.* **2019**, *61*, 18–26. [CrossRef]
40. Peñate, W.; Roca, M.J.R.; Pitti, C.T.; Bethencourt, J.M.; de la Fuente, J.A.; Gracia, R.G. Cognitive-behavioral treatment and antidepressants combined with virtual reality exposure for patients with chronic agoraphobia. *Int. J. Clin. Hlth. Psych.* **2014**, *14*, 9–17. [CrossRef]
41. Button, K.S.; Ioannidis, J.P.; Mokrysz, C.; Nosek, B.A.; Flint, J.; Robinson, E.S.; Munafò, M.R. Power failure: Why small sample size undermines the reliability of neuroscience. *Nat. Rev. Neurosci.* **2013**, *14*, 365. [CrossRef]
42. Bareither, I.; Hasler, F.; Strasser, A. Nueve ideas para mejorar la neurociencia. *Mente Cereb.* **2015**, *73*, 48–51.
43. Gogolla, N. The insular cortex. *Curr. Biol.* **2017**, *27*, R580–R586. [CrossRef] [PubMed]

5

Virtual Enactment Effect on Memory in Young and Aged Populations

Cosimo Tuena [1,*], Silvia Serino [2], Léo Dutriaux [3], Giuseppe Riva [1,4] and Pascale Piolino [5,6,7]

1 Applied Technology for Neuro-Psychology Lab, IRCCS Istituto Auxologico Italiano, 20149 Milan, Italy
2 MySpace Lab, Department of Clinical Neurosciences, University Hospital Lausanne (CHUV), CH-1011 Lausanne, Switzerland; silvia.serino@chuv.ch
3 Institute of Neuroscience and Psychology, University of Glasgow, Glasgow G12 8QB, UK; leo.dutriaux@glasgow.ac.uk
4 Department of Psychology, Catholic University of the Sacred Heart, 20123 Milan, Italy; giuseppe.riva@unicatt.it
5 Memory and Cognition Laboratory, Institute of Psychology, Paris Descartes University, Sorbonne Paris Cité, 92774 Boulogne-Billancourt, France; pascale.piolino@parisdescartes.fr
6 INSERM UMR S894, Center for Psychiatry and Neurosciences, 75014 Paris, France
7 Institut Universitaire de France (IUF), 75231 Paris, France
* Correspondence: cosimotuena@gmail.com

Abstract: Background: Spatial cognition is a critical aspect of episodic memory, as it provides the scaffold for events and enables successful retrieval. Virtual enactment (sensorimotor and cognitive interaction) by means of input devices within virtual environments provides an excellent opportunity to enhance encoding and to support memory retrieval with useful traces in the brain compared to passive observation. Methods: We conducted a systematic review with Preferred Reporting Items for Systematic Reviews and Meta-Analysis (PRISMA) guidelines concerning the virtual enactment effect on spatial and episodic memory in young and aged populations. We aim at giving guidelines for virtual enactment studies, especially in the context of aging, where spatial and episodic memory decline. Results: Our findings reveal a positive effect on spatial and episodic memory in the young population and promising outcomes in aging. Several cognitive factors (e.g., executive function, decision-making, and visual components) mediate memory performances. Findings should be taken into account for future interventions in aging. Conclusions: The present review sheds light on the key role of the sensorimotor and cognitive systems for memory rehabilitation by means of a more ecological tool such as virtual reality and stresses the importance of the body for cognition, endorsing the view of an embodied mind.

Keywords: spatial memory; episodic memory; virtual reality; enactment; memory rehabilitation; embodied cognition; aging

---

1. Introduction

When we think of an event, we commonly see with our mind's eye where this event occurred and what temporal, perceptual, and affective details were associated with it; indeed, this spatial scaffold influences the specificity, richness, and vividness of events we retrieve from the memory [1]. When not defined in its schematic representation of the topography, this ability is considered as the ability to visualize the detailed spatial context (e.g., street, room, park) of specific episodes [2]. In its topographical definition, spatial memory [3] is a complex ability devoted to the encoding and storage of different types of information from our surroundings for successful orientation and navigation. Spatial information is represented and used in our brain with two frames of reference [4]:

egocentric (self-to-object) and allocentric (object-to-object), respectively located in the parietal and medial temporal regions with the retrosplenial cortex, playing a critical role in switching between these representations [5]. Spatial information can be divided into survey (e.g., maps, wayfinding, and pointing task), route (e.g., dynamic sequencing of landmarks), and landmark knowledge (e.g., landmark recognition) [6]. Survey knowledge refers to an allocentric map of the spatial layout, whereas route and landmark knowledge are based on an egocentric representation of the space.

On the other hand, episodic memory is a neurocognitive system that allows people to remember the *what*, *where*, and *when* of a personally experienced event [7]. Binding [8–10] is a key feature of this system; it is the process that binds the *what* with the other contextual features (i.e., *when*, *where*, and *details* such as perceptual and affective details). These elements are crucial for the so-called "autonoetic consciousness", or the feeling of mentally travelling back to the spatiotemporal and phenomenal features of the experienced event [7,11,12].

The hippocampus is known to play a crucial role in spatial cognition [4,13,14], episodic memory [15,16], and recognition [17]; this structure binds cognitive, bodily and emotional information [18–20] and connects to cortical representations facilitating the retrieval of episodes [21]. In particular, according to Nadel and colleagues [13,22] the hippocampus provides the allocentric spatial scaffold for episodes binding neocortial representations of the event (i.e., Multiple Trace Theory). The link between spatial cognition and episodic memory is also highlighted by the fact that egocentric spatial updating with self-motion cues (i.e., path integration of dynamic bodily signals) plays a critical role during retrieval (recall and recognition) of dynamically encoded scenes [23], confirming the role of egocentric information in manipulating and translating allocentric long-term representations of events [24,25]. Despite the crucial role of medial temporal lobes during encoding, storage, and retrieval [26], the parietal and frontal lobes have been also identified as a crucial substrate of episodic memory, absolving different declarative memory functions such as encoding, retrieval, storage, and monitoring [27–30] (for a meta-analysis of navigation and episodic memory brain network, see [31]).

Recent insights from philosophy, psychology, and neuroscience have drawn attention to the essential role of the body in cognition [32,33]. The framework known as the "embodied cognition" theory provided a fresh and innovative way to conceptualize the relationship between these two long-debated components of human psychology. Indeed, psychological processes are influenced by body morphology and sensorimotor systems [34]. There is growing interest and evidence on how the body affects several cognitive domains, including memory [35,36]. However, the concept of memory can be expanded to take into account the whole body as crucial in encoding, storage, and retrieval [37]. These assumptions have great relevance in the context of normal and pathological aging, where physiological changes modify regions of the brain involved in memory formation, leaving primary cortices spared [38–40].

Indeed, sensorimotor involvement may leave traces that are useful for memory retrieval [41–43], and encoding strategies are among the most effective methods to enhance memory [8]. The encoding specificity principle states that recollection is facilitated when an overlap occurs between the elements of the retrieval context and those of the encoding context [44]. Retrieval is possible thanks to a cue, and a memory trace is mediated by the same cognitive operations that occurred during encoding [45]. From a neuroanatomical point of view, there is growing theoretical and empirical evidence indicating how retrieval may be considered an overlapping process [46,47] that reactivates the same brain regions at encoding [21,48,49], including primary cortices [50–52].

Interestingly, active navigation in virtual environments (VEs) by means of input tools can be considered a form of enactment able to enhance spatial [41] and episodic [8] performance. According to Wilson and colleagues [53], active navigation in VEs can be divided into physical activity (motor control) and psychological activity (decision-making). More precisely, the manipulation of spatial information is not the only process involved in navigation; rather, motor commands, proprioceptive information, vestibular information, decision-making, and allocation of attentional resources are all also essential parts of what is called "active spatial learning" in everyday life, whereas passive navigation involves visual information only [6]. We define the virtual enactment effect as the effect provided by one or more of these components on memory retrieval compared to the virtual passive observation of the environment. Virtual reality (VR) allows individuals to interact with the environment thanks to multimodal stimulation, providing a rich embodied experience [54] that can be used to enhance memory in elders [55]. Indeed, technological devices (e.g., joysticks or 3D visors) require the subject to process psychological information, as well as idiothetic (i.e., motor commands, proprioception, and vestibular information) and allothetic information (e.g., landmarks and boundaries). The aim of this work is to review the potential of the virtual enactment effect (i.e., the role of active components of virtual navigation compared to passive observation) in order to contribute to a better understanding of its beneficial effect on spatial and episodic memory. This contribution will provide research and clinical guidelines for future studies within the context of VR memory rehabilitation and enhancement. In order to provide a complete overview of the results, we will cluster findings according to spatial memory (survey and route and landmark knowledge; respectively allocentric and egocentric frames) and episodic memory tasks (episodic features, such as *what*, *where*, *when*, *details*, and binding; episodic functioning, like learning, forgetting, and strategic processing; and item recognition).

2. Method

Preferred Reporting Items for Systematic Reviews and Meta-Analysis (PRISMA) guidelines were followed [56].

2.1. Search Strategy

Two high-profile databases (PubMed and Web of Science) were used to perform the computer-based research on the 25 January 2019. The string used to carry out the search (Title/Abstract for PubMed and Topic for Web of Science) was as follows: ("active" OR "enactment") AND ("spatial memory" OR "spatial knowledge" OR "episodic memory") AND ("virtual reality" OR "environment*). The search resulted in 647 articles for Web of Science and 94 for PubMed (total of 741). We made a first selection by reading titles and abstracts after removing duplicates. Four papers were identified through other sources. A total of 35 manuscripts were chosen for full-text screening. This procedure resulted in 31 experimental studies. See the flow diagram (Figure 1) for the paper selection procedure.

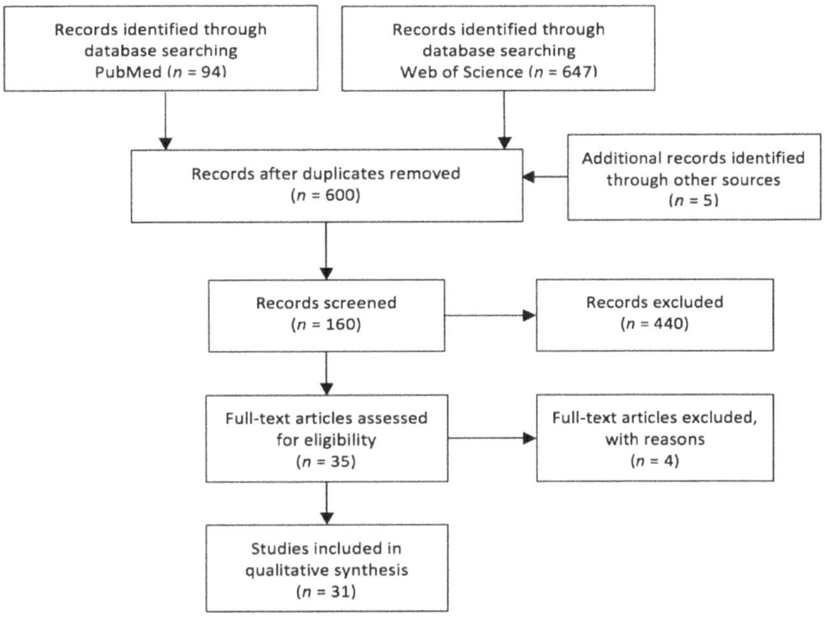

Figure 1. PRISMA flow chart.

2.2. *Selection Criteria*

Studies on the role of active navigation and enactment on spatial and episodic memory in young and aged populations (healthy and pathological) were included. We also included studies in languages other than English and excluded studies which did not follow our aims (non-age-related diseases, developmental studies, active- or passive-only conditions, active vs. passive conditions not related to the context of active navigation and action). We excluded articles for which the full text was not available or for which the abstract lacked basic information for review. Reviews, meeting abstracts, notes, case reports, letters to the editor, research protocols, patents, editorials and other editorial materials were also excluded. Five studies [57–61] did not appear during our search but were in line with our inclusion criteria; therefore, they were added to the included studies.

2.3. *Quality Assessment and Data Abstraction*

PRISMA guidelines were strictly followed; search results found by the first author (C.T.) were shared with the review authors for individual selection of papers in order to reduce the risk of bias, and disagreements were resolved through consensus. The data extracted from each included study were as follows: reference, year, sample(s), conditions, design (for the navigation condition), virtual apparatus, memory assessment, and primary outcomes.

3. Results

Several studies have been conducted to assess the role of active navigation in human memory. However, the growing interest in virtual reality (VR) has led researchers to question how the different aspects of navigation interact with the virtual environment. In particular, sensorimotor involvement, which is known for its positive effect on memory enhancement, seems to be one of the most investigated virtual enactment form. In our review, we aim at discovering whether this beneficial effect could also be observed when the subjects interact with technology devices.

To satisfy our aim, six clusters will be discussed: (1) the target population; (2) virtual apparatus; (3) conditions manipulated during navigation; (4) memory tasks; (5) the role of action and its effects on memory; and (6) cognitive domains underlying active navigation and memory performances. A synthesis of the results is reported in Table 1. Nine studies in Table 1 are reported with each sub-experiment; among these, only the experiments (e.g., Exp. 1, Exp. 2) that aim specifically at studying spatial or episodic memory appear in the table.

Table 1. Summary of the included studies. VE: virtual environment; HMD: head-mounted display; VR: virtual reality; OA: older adults; YA: young adults; aMCI: amnestic mild cognitive impairment; AD: Alzheimer's disease; HNC: high navigation control; LNC: low navigation control; IC: itinerary control; Exp.: experiment; //: same as above; 1A: first trial apartment; 2A: second trial apartment; B: third trial apartment.

Ref.	Sample (s)	Conditions	Design (Navigation)	Virtual Apparatus	Memory Assessment	Primary Outcomes
[62]	48 YA (age range: 21–38; 24 males)	Effect of active (no decisional level) vs. passive (prerecorded travel) vs. snapshot exploration (static condition) on scene recognition and memory of displacements. Intentional encoding.	Within	Non-immersive (CaTS driving simulator); input device: joystick.	Scene recognition (route snapshots); Pointing toward the origin test using the joystick; drawing test (shape of the path).	Path shape task benefitted from active condition, whereas recognition and pointing task were not affected by the exploring conditions.
[41] Exp. 1	30 YA (mean age = 27.1; 14 males)	Effect of active vs. passive (recorded navigation) navigation on spatial memory. No intentional encoding. Participants could freely navigate the apartment.	Between (yoked)	Non-immersive; input device: joystick; house apartment navigation.	Spatial layout test (spatial layout drawing of the VE); recall test (location and objects name on VE map).	Active group showed better spatial layout scores. No effect on recall test.
[41] Exp. 2	40 YA (mean age = 26; 18 males)	Effect of active vs. passive (recorded navigation) navigation on spatial memory. No intentional encoding. Participants could freely navigate the apartment.	//	Non-immersive; input device: joystick; house apartment navigation.	Spatial layout test (spatial layout drawing of the VE); recognition task (objects); object location test.	Spatial layout recall replicated for active condition. No effect on other tasks.
[63]	30 YA (age range = 18–30) and 30 OA (age range = 58–72)	Role of active vs. passive (pre-recorded video) motor exploration in spatial memory and wayfinding. Intentional encoding. No decision-making.	Between	Non-immersive; input device: joystick; virtual replica of Bordeaux.	Wayfinding task (replication of the path; use of spatial representation, errors and stops were calculated); spatial memory task (map drawing + picture classification; route and survey representations).	Active condition worsened survey knowledge (spatial map) in both groups, led to better wayfinding scores in YA and worsened in OA. Executive functions have a crucial role during active navigation.
[64] Exp. 1	22 undergraduates (14 males)	Exploring the role of motion control vs. passive condition (VE tour) on spatial learning. Intentional encoding (learning phase before test phase). Navigation instructions were given.	Between	Non-immersive; input device: keyboard; VE of a research lab.	Spatial learning test (indicate position and direction of egocentric pictures on a lab map; object location test).	View positioning test was better for active participants, no significant difference between the conditions was observed for object location task. Active navigation contributes partially to survey representation.
[64] Exp. 2	80 undergraduates (49 males)	Exploring the role of optical flow (action with object in active condition) vs. passive navigation vs. static condition on spatial learning between active. Intentional encoding (learning phase before test phase). Navigation instructions were given.	//	Non-immersive; input device: keyboard; VE of a research lab.	Spatial learning test (indicate position and direction of egocentric pictures on a lab map; object location test).	Active participants performed better in object locations task and passive condition performed better than static condition. No difference among the conditions was observed for the first task.
[65] Exp. 1	82 university students (age range: 19–33; 43 males)	Effect of intentional vs. incidental encoding vs. active vs. passive navigation (observing the participant navigating) on spatial memory. Auditory route instructions were given (no decision-making).	Between (yoked)	Non-immersive; input devices: keyboard and mouse; virtual city.	Spatial memory test (landmark recognition task, pointing task and path-sketching, route navigation task; respectively, landmark, survey and route knowledge).	Active navigation led to better landmark and route knowledge performances. No effect on survey knowledge. No effect of encoding.

Table 1. *Cont.*

Ref.	Sample (s)	Conditions	Design (Navigation)	Virtual Apparatus	Memory Assessment	Primary Outcomes
[65] Exp. 2	88 university students (age range: 18–33; 10 males)	Effect of movement (active navigation vs. passive) vs. instruction control (instructing vs. listening) vs. instruction specificity (landmark information vs. layout information) on spatial memory. Navigation instructions were written (no decision-making).	//	Non-immersive; input devices: keyboard and mouse; apartment with rooms.	Spatial memory test (landmark recognition task, tour integration task, route navigation task).	Landmark knowledge, tour integration and route knowledge benefited from self-contained condition. Effect on performance was mediate by instruction specificity and control in the latest task.
[65] Exp. 3	102 students (age range: 19–41; 21 males)	Effect of active vs. passive navigation vs. decision-making (map) vs. less decision-making (map with suggested path) vs. no-map condition on spatial memory. Participants were asked to find the shortest possible route.	//	Non-immersive; input devices: keyboard and mouse; apartment with rooms.	Spatial memory test (landmark recognition task and tour integration task; route navigation task).	Active navigation led to better landmark recognition performance. Decision-making helped participants in observed movement condition and less decision-making worsened route knowledge.
[66]	24 undergraduates (age range: 18–21; 7 males)	Effect of active free navigation (with decision-making) vs. passive on object-memory. Intentional encoding.	Between (yoked)	Non-immersive; input device: keyboard; virtual city.	Object task (locate objects) and recognition task.	No difference between the two conditions in the tasks.
[53] Exp. 1	72 undergraduates (age range: 18–27; 22 males)	Effect of psychological activity (decision-making vs. no decision-making on directions) and physical activity (motor control vs. no motor control on keyboard) vs. control group on spatial performance. No intentional encoding (explore VE).	Between	Non-immersive; input device: keyboard; virtual city.	Orientation task (direction test + map drawing).	No difference was observed between the conditions manipulated.
[53] Exp. 2	36 undergraduates (age range: 18–42)	Effect of active exploration vs. passive observation of navigation vs. control (no exploration of VE) on wayfinding. No intentional encoding (explore VE).	Between	Non-immersive; input device: keyboard; virtual arena.	Wayfinding task.	No difference was observed between the conditions manipulated.
[67]	18 YA (age range: 20–39; 9 males)	Effect of active (with decision-making) vs. passive dynamic (recorded video) vs. passive static (slide-like scenes) free exploration on spatial layout performances. Intentional encoding.	Within	Non-immersive; input device: joystick; virtual arena with cubes.	Target location test (8 trials; score, time, orientation and verbal or drawing description of the strategies used to reach a given target were calculated).	Active participants performed better than the two passive conditions in the task (scores, time, verbal and layout descriptions but no orientation task). Active motor behaviour with active perception is crucial to extract invariants in the VE.
[68]	30 YA (age range = 18–25) and 30 OA (age range = 60–81)	Active (with decision-making) vs. passive (computer-guided tour) free navigation effects on memory for everyday objects. Intentional encoding.	Between	Non-immersive; input devices: keyboard and mouse; VR-based Human Objects Memories from Everyday Scenes (HOMES).	Free recall and recognition (learning, proactive interference, semantic clustering, recognition hits, and false recognitions). VE 1A followed by free recall task + VE 2A followed by free recall task + VE B followed by recognition task.	Active navigation had a beneficial effect on recognition hits only, in both YA and OA compared with passive mode. Active mode reduced false recognitions in YA but increased these in OA. Active navigation enhanced memory in older adults when to not demanding.

Table 1. *Cont.*

Ref.	Sample (s)	Conditions	Design (Navigation)	Virtual Apparatus	Memory Assessment	Primary Outcomes
[69]	44 students (mean age = 21.94, SD = 2.13; 21 males)	Active (with decision-making) vs. passive (computer-guided tour) free navigation effects on memory for everyday objects. Intentional encoding.	Between	Non-immersive; input devices: keyboard and mouse; VR-based HOMES.	Free recall and recognition (learning, proactive interference, semantic clustering, recognition hits, and false recognitions). VE 1A followed by free recall task + VE 2A followed by free recall task + VE B followed by recognition task.	Active navigation led to better recognition hits performances compared to passive condition. Active participants had less source-based false recognition compared with passive participants. Active navigation was useful to enrich visuomotor details of episodic memory traces but had no effect on semantic relational processing.
[9] Exp. 3	41 participants (age range: 18–34; 12 males)	Active vs. passive (recorded actions; no motor response) selection affects memory for object. Intentional encoding. Instructions.	Between	Non-immersive; input device: keyboard; WWW (*what–where–when*) variation built with Second Life arena.	Object name cued recall (full episodic recall: *what* + *where* + *when*; non-episodic: *where* + *what* or *when* + *what* or *what* only).	Active condition reduced distractor encoding compared to the passive viewing of the action of the avatar.
[43]	72 Psychology students (mean age = 22.23, SD = 3.94; 36 males)	Interaction condition (motor trace in memory, no decision on itinerary) vs. planning condition (no control of the vehicle; decisional level) vs. passive (recorded video). Intentional encoding.	Between	Non-immersive; input devices: steering wheel and pedals; virtual city.	Free recall of elements; visuospatial memory test (draw map + locate elements); visuospatial cued recall (locate elements on a prepared map); recognition test (elements, locations and navigation directions after seeing the elements).	Interaction enhanced memory recall, in particular spatial memory test (no effect on influence on visuospatial cued recall or recognition); however, interaction worsened elements recognition compared with passive condition; planning condition boosted visuospatial recalls. Both interaction and planning had an effect on episodic memory.
[70]	21 healthy OA (4 males), 15 aMCI (7 males) and 15 AD (2 males)	Active vs. passive (recorded video) encoding influences episodic memory. Intentional encoding. Predetermined route.	Between	Non-immersive; input devices: steering wheel and pedals; two virtual cities.	Immediate free recall (*what, details, when,* egocentric *where*, allocentric *where*, binding); recognition (elements, spatial and temporal relations between elements; remember/know paradigm); delayed free recall (same as immediate free recall).	Active exploration led in OA, aMCI, and AD groups to better recall of elements, allocentric spatial information and binding. Procedural skills and self-involvement may be crucial for episodic performances in aMCI and AD patients.
[71]	113 psychology students (mean age = 21.57, SD = 2.99) and 45 OA	Effect of active vs. passive navigation and intentional vs. incidental encoding on episodic memory. Predetermined route.	Between	Non-immersive; input devices: steering wheel and pedals; virtual city.	Free recall (*what*, verbal *where*, visuospatial *where*, *when*, *details*); recognition test (elements).	Encoding conditions affect differently episodic features in YA and OA. However, any effect due to sensorimotor implication emerged in the study.
[8]	64 YA and 64 OA (32 males)	HNC (real-life driving conditions) vs. LNC (only pedals; no enactment associated with direction) vs. IC (verbal instructions without driving; decisional level only) vs. passive (no driving no decision) effect on episodic memory performance. Intentional encoding.	Between	Non-immersive; input devices: steering wheel and pedals; virtual city.	Immediate free recall (*what* and *details*; binding: *what* + *where* + *when*; remember/know paradigm); visuospatial recall test (*what, where, when* on real map); delayed free recall test (*what, details, where,* and *when*); recognition test (elements).	Binding, regardless of age-groups, was enhanced by LNC and IC; HNC and passive conditions did not help episodic memory performance in both groups. Interestingly, Remember responses were boosted in older adults by IC condition. Active condition may be helpful when do not overload cognitive resources.
[72]	90 students (average age of 20; 45 males)	Passive VE (recorded route) vs. active VE vs. real environment (navigate the environment with instructions) and immediate vs. 48-h recall. Predetermined route.	Between	Non-immersive; input device: joystick; virtual replica of the Bordeaux area.	Immediate or 48-h recall task: real world wayfinding (replication of the real route), freehand sketch (directional changes) and photograph classification (picture in chronological order).	Transfer and sketch task are efficient after 48 h of retention and it is efficient for the two paper-pencil tasks. Active navigation led to benefits in wayfinding task, irrespective of the delay retention.

Table 1. *Cont.*

Ref.	Sample (s)	Conditions	Design (Navigation)	Virtual Apparatus	Memory Assessment	Primary Outcomes
[73]	59 YA (age range: 19–29; 19 males)	Effect of active vs. passive free exploration on object recognition in VEs.	Between	Immersive; input device: keyboard; virtual rooms with objects.	Recognition task (objects).	Active navigation led to higher hit and lower miss responses than the passive condition. Active navigation has an important role in landmark recognition.
[74] Exp. 1	32 YA (age range: 18–34; 16 males)	Active vs. passive free navigation with four trials with different virtual maze.	Between	Non-immersive with static navigation; input devices: keyboard and mouse; virtual maze.	"Active" test: number of moves and time.	Navigational knowledge is represented regardless the kind of exploration condition.
[58]	20 male students (age range: 20–26)	Active (self-governed) vs. passive (avatar-guided) free exploration. Four exploring sessions. Intentional encoding.	Between	Immersive (HMD); input device: joystick; virtual school.	Wayfinding task (short route to starting point); pointing task (orienting to the starting point); sketch-map (local accuracy or survey-type organization).	Self-governed explorers were better in completing the wayfinding task. Sketch-map accuracy was similar in both groups, whereas self-governed group had better survey-type organization. No differences were shown in pointing task. Self-governed participants organize their knowledge in survey mode.
[75]	34 YA (age range: 18–38; 7 males)	Active vs. passive (passenger condition) condition. Participants were before divided in driver and non-drivers. Intentional encoding and decision-making.	Between	Non-immersive: input devices: steering wheel and pedals; virtual city.	Survey knowledge: pointing error scores (street-level view) and map placement error scores (bird's eye view); route knowledge: route scores (shortest route).	Driver had better route scores during active navigation compared with drivers in passive and non-driver in active conditions. Drivers showed better map scores (no condition effect). Active navigators do not learn more spatial layout knowledge and dual task effect may affect scores in non-drivers.
[59]	54 students (9 males)	Active vs. passive (passenger condition). Three exposures (3, 10, or 15 times). No intentional encoding. Predetermined path.	Between (yoked)	Non-immersive: input devices: steering wheel and pedals; virtual city.	Survey knowledge (map sketch drawing and map rates' score), route knowledge (travel directions) and landmark knowledge (landmarks recall).	Passengers recalled more landmarks across exposure conditions. Survey errors reduced between 5 and 15 times in both conditions. Exposure led to better map reliability especially for the passive condition. Attentional resources could have led to worst performance in active drivers.
[76] Exp. 3	41 undergraduates (age range: 18–24; 20 males)	VE active vs. VE passive (watch experimenter navigation) vs. VE + line (active with path to follow; no free exploration) vs. control (no VE training; real -world wayfinding).	Between	Non-immersive. Input device: keyboard; virtual replica of an office.	Real world transfer task (balloons wayfinding times and errors from virtual to real places); training task (wayfinding time and errors in VE conditions).	Times for active condition were lower compared with control condition and active and VE + line led to fewer errors than control condition. Virtual real transfer occurs thanks to virtual interaction.

Table 1. *Cont.*

Ref.	Sample (s)	Conditions	Design (Navigation)	Virtual Apparatus	Memory Assessment	Primary Outcomes
[60]	64 students (average age of 20; 32 males)	Ground vs. areal point of view and active vs. passive navigation. Predetermined route	Between	Non-immersive; input device: joystick; virtual replica of the Bordeaux area.	Real world wayfinding task (replication of the real route; error scores), sketch-drawing task (directional changes; errors and omissions scores) and scene-sorting task (errors).	Active navigation boosted sketch-mapping task and worsened wayfinding and picture-sorting scores. Grounded-level condition improved performance in wayfinding and picture-sorting tasks, whereas aerial-level in sketch-mapping task. Active navigation and grounded-level interaction had a positive effect in the wayfinding and picture-sorting tasks, whereas passive and aerial-level condition improved sketch-mapping scores. Egocentric information and motor information create a correct perception-action coupling.
[77]	64 students (average age of 20; 32 males)	Detailed vs. undetailed visual fidelity and active vs. passive navigation. Predetermined route.	Between	Non-immersive; input device: joystick; virtual replica of the Bordeaux area.	Real-world wayfinding task (replication of the real route; errors and hesitations scores), sketch-mapping task (directional changes; errors and omissions scores), and scene-sorting task (errors).	Results highlighted better performance for each spatial task in both active and detailed condition. Interaction effect (active and detailed) led to better scores for sketch task and active condition combined with undetailed VE worsened scene-sorting task. Perceptual-motor information is crucial in spatial knowledge. Visual fidelity has positive effect for allocentric representation but not for route knowledge.
[78] Exp. 1 & 2	28 students (age range: 18–23; 9 males)	Active exploration (experiment 1) vs. passive exploration (experiment 2; video of active exploration). Predetermined route of familiar environment.	Between	Non-immersive; input device: keyboard; university building.	Orientation test trials of external cues from four virtual rooms (internal visited and unvisited, external visited and unvisited).	There is no difference in the two conditions.
[78] Exp. 3	54 visitors (mean age = 17.55, SD = 1.14; 19 males)	Active exploration vs. passive exploration. Predetermined route of unfamiliar environment.	Between	Non-immersive; input device: keyboard; university building.	Orientation test trials of external cues from four virtual rooms (internal visited and unvisited, external visited and unvisited).	No effect of unfamiliarity for active participants. Passive participants had greater error for the internal unvisited room. Active exploration enhances survey knowledge for unfamiliar environments.
[79]	60 adults (mean age = 25.2, SD = 4.5; males 49)	Active exploration vs. passive exploration (video of passive exploration) and immersive vs. computer screen. Predetermined rout of Gowanus canal. Intentional encoding. An allocentric map of the canal was provided in all conditions.	Within	Immersive (Emotiv EPOC headset) and non-immersive; input device: mouse and headset gyroscope; Gowanus Canal.	Elements recognition task	No difference between the two navigation conditions. However, active navigation with the mouse has higher level of engagement.

Table 1. *Cont.*

Ref.	Sample (s)	Conditions	Design (Navigation)	Virtual Apparatus	Memory Assessment	Primary Outcomes
[80] Exp. 1 and 2		3D active exploration (Exp. 1) vs. 2D passive snapshots presentation (Exp. 2). Free exploration and intentional encoding.	Between	Immersive (nVisor SX111) and non-immersive; input device: Wiimote; virtual apartment.	Search trials of geometric and contextual objects.	Search task improved in both conditions but in the immersive condition initial fixations and time spent in the incorrect rooms and better selection of the correct room indicate higher use of memory.
[81]	28 YA (mean age = 25.6, SD = 5.4; 17 males)	Active navigation vs. passive navigation (video). Immediate (intentional encoding) and 24 h delayed (naïve) recall. Participants could freely navigate the environment.	Between	Non-immersive; input device: keyboard and mouse; virtual city.	Immediate and delayed free recall of semantically linked images of 3D objects placed in the town.	No effect of navigation types on spatial memory.
[57]	14 YA (mean age = 22, SD = 2.08; 7 males)	Full condition (full control over the navigation) vs. medium condition (participants move but do not control pre-recorded navigation) vs. low condition (watch pre-recorded navigation).	Within	Immersive (Oculus Rift DK2); input device: Kinect for legs and arms movement detection; virtual city.	Immediate free recall (*what*, egocentric *where*, *details*, *when*, *binding*) and item recognition (source memory, remember/know/guess paradigm), egocentric, allocentric and temporal recognition.	Any significance was found among the conditions. However, the full and medium (virtual embodiment) conditions were more immersive than the passive one.
[82]	16 students (females = 16)	Active navigation vs. passive (watching the navigation of the active participant). Free exploration.	Between (yoked)	Non-immersive (46-inch touchscreen monitor); input device: joystick; virtual rooms	Immediate memory recognition for objects manipulated in each room).	Both passive and active navigation had a significant negative effect on memory of object, with active navigation having a greater effect compared to passive.
[61]	22 YA (mean age = 19.71, SD = 2.19; females = 11) and 22 OA (mean age = 74.55, SD = 7.82; females = 10)	Active navigation vs. passive. Free exploration.	Within (yoked)	Immersive (cardboard) mobile application (input device: button headset and head movements); VE (city, park, mall)	Encoding-Retrieval route overlap accuracy	Active encoding leads to better spatial memory in OA; accuracy is predicted by age, active exploration and visuospatial abilities.

3.1. What Populations Have Been Included?

From our systematic search, it emerged that the majority of the experiments included healthy participants, mainly young adults (YA), but also older adults (OA). Studies focused on spatial domain; however, a cluster of seven studies investigated episodic memory and its subcomponents in healthy populations (YA and OA). Nevertheless, age ranges varied across the studies for YA and OA, and for the "student" samples the age information was vague. Importantly, in six studies no gender information [53,63,68,71] or matching [58,82] were reported. Only one study recruited clinical populations of Alzheimer's disease (AD) pathology: 15 AD patients and 15 amnestic mild cognitive impairment (aMCI) patients compared to 21 healthy OA were included in the study of Plancher and colleagues [70] to assess the effect of active and passive virtual navigation on episodic performance. A synthesis of populations (YA, OA, AD, and aMCI), with mean age and standard deviation and number of males/females, is reported in Table 1.

3.2. What Virtual Apparatus Have Been Used?

For the purposes of our review, it is essential to summarize the apparatus been used in each experiment. Ecological virtual environments (VEs) have been used to assess the virtual enactment effect regardless of the domain (spatial or episodic memory); specifically, cities or apartments were used to evaluate the effect of active interaction (e.g., input device interaction)—namely, the "virtual enactment effect"—on memory recall, while four experiments [9,53,67,74] used basic virtual scenarios with poor ecological validity (e.g., virtual arenas). Concerning the input devices, researchers mainly used joysticks and keyboards to navigate the VEs, whereas five studies used a steering wheel and pedals to control a virtual car. The use of these controllers is linked to the type of immersion; indeed, the vast majority of the experiments' apparatus were non-immersive (PC screen or projectors). Only six experiments [57,58,61,73,79,80] used head-mounted display (HMD) to assess the role of active navigation on spatial performances and only one study used immersive virtual reality to assess the effect of full body involvement during encoding on episodic retrieval.

3.3. What are the Navigation Conditions in the Included Studies?

In the following paragraph, studies will be discussed in terms of navigation condition, degree of decision-making, and type of encoding. Active navigation studies used classic dynamic navigation, whereas non-dynamic navigation (e.g., snapshots or teleporting) were added as the comparison condition [62,67,80]. The former might be more suitable compared to static navigation if we consider the role of constant mapping provided by the hippocampus (i.e., place cells) in building the map of the environment [83]. Passive navigation in the studies included in the review consisted of a yoked condition or pre-recorded navigations. Navigational decision-making, or free exploration, is another crucial aspect of active navigation and spatial knowledge [84]; however, in 17 experiments [9,59–65,70–72,77–79], researchers gave a predetermined route or instructions to follow. Moreover, decision-making is a crucial aspect of the virtual enactment effect when older participants are involved in active navigation [8] due to overload on the frontal lobes and the executive functions capacity on memory encoding [68], which are known to decline with aging [85]. Indeed, Jebara and colleagues [8] found that navigational decision-making, intended as a form of virtual enactment effect, is more effective in OA compared to the active motor condition due to executive function overload at encoding [8,63,68]. Another aspect to consider is the point of view (areal vs. egocentric). The egocentric point of view along combined with the active motor condition improves allocentric and egocentric memory, whereas the areal point of view with passive navigation improves allocentric memory only [60]. Graphic realism when building VEs should take into account the fact that a detailed environment positively affects memory performances [77]. Other elements that neuroscientists in the field of VR and memory should consider are the type of encoding (incidental vs. intentional); although the authors of [62] showed no effect of encoding, in our review intentional encoding leads to better performance across the populations and the type of memory assessed [8,9,43,58,59,67–70,75,80]. Crucially, only one study [72] compared active VR vs. passive VR vs. real-world navigation, with real-world navigation and active VR leading to better spatial recall, in this order, compared to passive VR. Lastly, from a methodological point of view, researchers are encouraged to evaluate the consequences of using between or within condition. In our review, the majority of the studies included between navigation conditions, while only five studies [57,61,62,67,79] used within conditions. Researchers should consider strengths and weaknesses of within and between designs with potential biases in the light of the objectives of their study [86], as explained in the discussion paragraph.

3.4. How Has Memory Performance Been Measured?

Several VEs (cities, rooms, mazes, and arenas) were used in the reviewed experiments in order to test two main memory clusters: spatial memory and episodic memory (event and object memory). The evaluation included for spatial memory tasks involved survey knowledge (maps, pointing and wayfinding tasks), route knowledge (chronological order tasks), and item recognition/recall for landmark knowledge (see Table 1 for a summary of these tasks).

To investigate the role of active navigation in episodic memory, six studies used a similar navigation paradigm in a virtual city in which events occurred [10,43,57,70,71]. Participants were tested on events encountered, landmarks and spatial layout of the cities. These paradigms aim at assessing *what′ where* (egocentric and allocentric), *when*, *details*, and binding among elements in ecological VEs with free recall, delayed recall, and recognition. Laurent et al. [9] studied the different components of episodic memory; a variation of the WWW (*what–when–where*) task was used in order to study the binding of contextual aspects to objects. Finally, Sauzéon and colleagues [68,69] used free recall (learning, proactive interference, semantic clustering based on the California Verbal Learning Test (CVLT) [87]) and a recognition task (recognition hits and false recognitions); object recognition memory was also used to assess event memory in Pettijohn and Radvansky [82]. Interestingly, Pacheco and Verschure [81] assessed their samples on an immediate and delayed free recall task of images semantically associated with an object they found in the virtual town. For a summary of these tasks, see Table 1.

3.5. Do "Virtual" Actions Have a "Real" Effect on Spatial and Episodic Memory?

In the following subsection, memory performance will be clustered by the different components taken into consideration in the included study of the review: spatial memory, episodic memory, and recognition memory of both spatial and episodic studies (Figure 2). The Primary Outcomes column in Table 1 provides in detail the virtual enactment effect on each task/measure. Using the correct task to target specific sub-components is crucial for the researchers; we suggest future research to put effort into designing and conceptualizing the task and test method to tap memory processes.

In the present review, we found a general positive effect of virtual enactment in young adults for spatial memory; however, further studies need to assess this in older adults as spatial enhancement in OA is controversial [61,63]. In particular for spatial scores in aging, active navigation involving an overloading task during encoding affected retrieval [63]; decision-making in active navigation appeared to be more suitable in this sample [8].

Similarly, experiments investigating episodic memory showed initial support for a virtual enactment effect in young adults (Figure 2); although findings are few, encouraging results come from studies of neurodegenerative conditions that may benefit from virtual enactment, whereas non-spatial features of episodic memory are influenced by demanding tasks during encoding (Figure 2). These findings could also confirm the embodied nature of episodic memory as a cognitive and bodily experience [18,20,35,88–90].

Initial recognition scores in spatial and memory performance results are controversial and need further investigation. Although past research on enactment showed a positive effect on recognition memory [91], recognition scores in spatial and memory performance results are controversial. A possible explanation for this could be that recognition occurs in the brain at different degrees [92,93] such as visual recognition, guessing (Guess responses), familiarity (Know responses), and source recognition and recollection (Remember responses); the latter, with source memory, is thought to be related to recollective aspects of episodic memory linked with autonoesis and full detailed recall. As a consequence, it is important to adopt a recognition paradigm that is able to grasp perceptual and sensory elements of the memory traces at retrieval.

(No effect was found in these spatial studies [53,66,74,78,79], and on episodic memory scores *what*, verbal *where*, visuospatial *where*, *when*, and *details* in the works of Plancher et al. [71] and Tuena and colleagues [57]), or on object recognition memory in the work of Pacheco and Verschure [81]. Finally, although results are encouraging, some studies showed passive enhancement (see Figure 2); therefore, results of the review are preliminary, and future studies need to deepen the virtual enactment effect in order to confirm the enhancing effect from which different populations might benefit.

It is well known that active navigation promotes better learning performance [6]. We found confirmations of how the body shapes memories and how it can be used as a medium to enhance learning by means of input tools as an extension of previous research on the enactment effect with ecological scenarios and items [42,88,94,95].

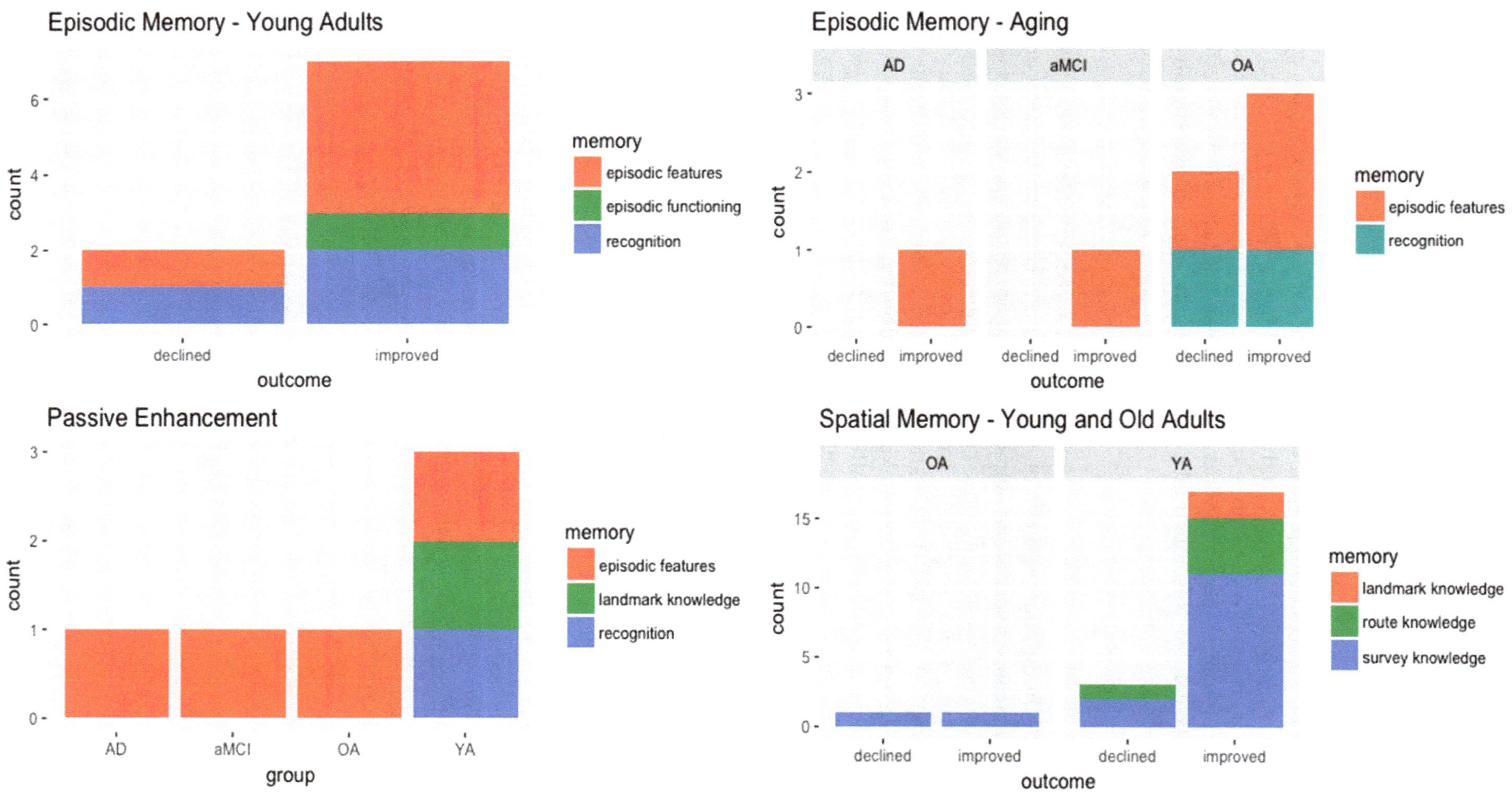

Figure 2. Summary of virtual enactment effect and passive enhancement in the samples. YA: young adults; OA: older adults; aMCI: amnestic mild cognitive impairment; AD: Alzheimer's disease.

3.6. What Are the Cognitive Factors Mediating Active Navigation and Memory Performance?

Among the included studies, cognitive factors underlying navigation have been studied in the same healthy population [74], whereas neuropsychological factors were used to evaluate the effect of active navigation on memory in YA vs. OA [8,63]. In particular, visuospatial abilities and especially executive function seem to be crucial for spatial memory [63,74] and for episodic memory functioning [68] and features [70,71]; in particular, executive function and attention appear to influence performance [8,69].

Cutmore et al. [74] conducted four experiments in order to evaluate the effect of gender, visuospatial abilities, cognitive style, and cerebral asymmetry during static active navigation (teleporting). Males showed faster results in finding the exit of the virtual maze compared with females, while both groups benefited from a landmark cue condition (landmark associated with a room). Moreover, males were more accurate; in this case, a compass cue condition (compass heading cue) led to better performance compared to a landmark condition. Visuospatial abilities were evaluated with the Wechsler Adult Intelligence Scale—Revised (WAIS-R) [96]. The high visuospatial group was better at Euclidean (survey knowledge) distance estimation compared with the low group. Participants' cognitive styles (verbal-sequential vs. visuospatial) were evaluated with the same test. The visuospatial group showed better navigation performance; moreover, this effect was shown for static navigation when compared with verbal-sequential participants. The visuospatial group was also better in navigating the maze backward. Finally, Cutemore and colleagues [74] used electroencephalography to observe cerebral asymmetry: the verbal-sequential group showed a greater right hemisphere activation (effort computing spatial problem solving) compared with the visuospatial group. However, only females were recruited for the last three experiments, since a gender effect was found in the second experiment. The authors wanted to evaluate whether navigation is related to superior spatial skills in a sample of females, but von Stülpnagel [88] found that sense of orientation abilities affected false alarms and route navigation performance regardless of gender.

Taillade et al. [63] found that YA were better than OA in terms of executive function, visuospatial abilities, and memory. In particular, wayfinding tasks (survey knowledge) seemed to be affected by executive function. Jebara et al. [8] correlated the binding scores with age and neuropsychological tests. An effect of age was found in all the navigation conditions. Binding score was significantly correlated with visual memory and working memory in high navigation control (HNC; motor trace and decision-making), low navigation control (LNC; motor trace only), and itinerary condition (IC; decision-making only) conditions. Shifting (executive function) negatively affected the VR binding scores for LNC and HNC but not for the passive condition and IC. When controlling for age, the scores in HNC were still significantly affected by executive function. Verbal memory correlated positively only with the IC condition. Similarly, Sauzéon and colleagues found a positive correlation between recognition hits and episodic memory (CVLT [87]) and executive function (mental rotation and Stroop color-word task; [97,98]) in the active but not the passive navigation condition. Total false recognitions (source-based and gist-based) were correlated with episodic memory and executive function tests. An age effect on false recognition was also found. In particular, executive function, after partial correlation between age and false recognitions, contributed to recognition performance under the active navigation condition [68].

It is also worth reporting that cognitive differences among the populations emerged in terms of gender, age and pathology. Plancher and colleagues [70] found differences among individuals with AD, aMCI, and OA in their episodic memory task. The same performance pattern (AD < aMCI < OA) emerged for *what*, *details*, egocentric and allocentric *where*, and recognition. AD and aMCI individuals had less recollection compared to controls. AD patients' binding was lower than that of aMCI patients and OA, whereas aMCI patients had a delayed recall deficit compared to OA. *When* scores were lower for the AD group compared with the aMCI group and OA, while AD and aMCI individuals presented a difference between immediate and delayed recall. Moreover, the authors found better *what* recognition in OA, aMCI, and AD compared to other episodic recognitions. Plancher and colleagues found that

AD and aMCI patients had worse recognition than OA; similarly, OA performed better in terms of recollection rates than aMCI and AD.

Tasks revealed an age effect in different studies [8,61,63,71,80] as well as a gender effect [43,65,80]. The findings of Jebara and co-authors [8] revealed an age effect for *what* (immediate and delayed), binding (immediate and delayed), visuospatial recall, and recognition total score. An age effect on spatial memory and recognition was found by other studies. Sauzéon and co-authors [68] showed that OA have worse learning, proactive interference, and false recognition compared with YA. Taillade and colleagues [63] found that YA fared better in a wayfinding task than OA, but this pattern did not emerge for spatial memory tasks. An age effect emerged in the first study of Plancher and colleagues [71]. Young participants were better compared to OA in terms of verbal and visuospatial *where*, *when*, and *details*. Moreover, findings showed a main effect of intentional encoding for *what*, verbal *where*, visuospatial *where*, *when*, and *details*. In an active navigation condition, OA had better *what* recall in incidental encoding, while YA had better recognition, *when*, verbal *where*, and visuospatial *where* on intentional encoding compared with OA. Finally, Plancher and co-authors [56] found that women performed better (statistical tendency) on the recognition task, whereas men had better scores for the cued visuospatial task. No effect of condition emerged. Von Stülpnagel and Steffens [65] showed that women had more false alarms than men, who were faster in a route navigation task; moreover, women revealed a lower sense of orientation and computer experience than men. Findings of Dalgarno et al. [64] were not affected by gender. Lastly, recall decreased with age [68] for both immediate and delayed recall [6]. Taillade et al. [63] highlighted an age effect for a wayfinding task but not for a spatial memory task. Recognitions decreased with age [8], but the same was not found by Sauzéon and co-authors [68], who showed more false recognition for OA.

The following neuropsychological tests were correlated with memory tasks [71]. Trail Making Test (TMT) A and B [99] was used to evaluate executive functions and attention in OA and was negatively correlated with *what* and *where* and sustained attention scores were associated with *where* responses; lastly, the Cognitive Difficulties Scale [70,71] was significantly associated with episodic scores in normal and pathological aging.

Von Stülpnagel and Steffens [65] found different interactions with the movement (self-contained vs. observed) condition. In the second experiment, providing layout and landmark information along with self-contained movement led to better route knowledge (tour integration task), whereas for the route navigation task better scores were obtained when self-contained movements were associated with reading instructions. In the last of their experiments, recognition performance was enhanced when any allocentric map was given, whereas the tour integration task benefited by a map with path to follow and not by self-contained condition. Finally, in the route navigation, the map with a path to follow worsened the scores, whereas the active map helped participants in the observed movement condition. Farrell and colleagues [76], in their first experiment, found that active navigation with or without an allocentric map led to better virtual to real world transfer of spatial knowledge compared to control (real-world wayfinding) and this is true also for active virtual exploration with a path to follow (no decision-making). In their second experiment, virtual exploration with the map did not lead to better transfer compared to the allocentric map studying condition without real or virtual exploration.

Other relevant effects that interact with cognition are reported. In particular, dynamic active navigation generally led to better results, as noted by three studies [62,67,80]; however contradictory (path shape but not orientation and recognition; [62]) were also reported. Some authors [62,64,80] have highlighted the importance of optic flow for spatial learning in VE. Visual fidelity is also crucial for both survey and route knowledge [77], and the first-person perspective of the virtual environment boosted wayfinding and route knowledge, whereas an aerial-view improved allocentric representation [60]. Three-dimensional virtual reality seems to stimulate memory due to higher body involvement but also reduced energy consumption [74]; however, Palermo and co-authors [79] found that immersive interaction with a gyroscope, although reported as interesting, could be frustrating and showed a minor degree of engagement compared to classic active interaction with a mouse. Finally, a trial effect emerged confirming the positive effect of repetition on performance (e.g., [59]). Interestingly, exposure times led to better survey representation for passive participants, as noted by Sandamas and Foreman [59]. Wallet et al. [72] found better delayed recall, but not Pacheco and Verschure [81], in their 24-h delayed recall, for active participants after 48 h for spatial memory. Similarly, Jebara et al. [6] found YA, but not OA, had better delayed (20-min) as compared to immediate recall for episodic recall (item information and binding). No effect of condition emerged in the latter study. With regard to expertise, Sandamas and Foreman [75] found that drivers, regardless of the navigation condition, were better in the map task (survey knowledge). Moreover, different studies aimed at balancing driving [6,43,75] and technology experience (e.g., [60,65]), since these could influence the performance.

In addition to age, gender, skills, and cognitive functioning, it is crucial for neuropsychology research to consider the roles of consolidation, repetition, and dynamic changes in order to build effective and ergonomic training for memory rehabilitation and enhancement.

4. Discussion

In the present review, we provided initial positive results concerning the virtual enactment effect on spatial and episodic memory performance, highlighting the embodied potential of virtual reality (VR). For each of the questions presented (see Section 3 subsection headings), we provided theoretical and practical solutions to guide future studies within the context of the virtual enactment effect and its use in aging. To summarize, the virtual enactment effect on memory is: (1) present in the young population; (2) possible in aging but needs further investigation; (3) mediated by neurocognitive factors, especially in aging; and (4) dependent on the use of technological devices and their interaction characteristics.

In general, we suggest that future research should aim at designing experiments for older people and pathological aging, in both spatial and episodic memory in order to test the virtual enactment effect. Moreover, we encourage further research on episodic memory involving young participants to consolidate or extend the findings we reported in this systematic review. Innovative cognitive rehabilitative systems are needed to slow down or prevent memory decline in neurodegenerative conditions, and VR provides a powerful tool to stimulate brain plasticity in Alzheimer's disease and aging [100,101].

We highly recommend that researchers take into account these elements and consider the use of immersive apparatus by means of head-mounted display (HMD). The main limits of non-immersive studies reported in the review are that they do not grasp the full experience of active navigation, since they do not involve bodily-based (e.g., idiothetic) components [6], and the motor traces used while using controllers might be too weak to have an impact on memory traces [71]. Therefore, researchers should consider the use of a HMD. For instance, with an HMD it is possible to walk around a small area with trackers detecting movements and interact with the scenario with controllers. Moreover, VR enables the user to experience an "egocentric space" [102], which is a critical aspect of spatial processing as it occurs in everyday life [4]. Researchers should not forget the role of interaction (e.g., intentions and actions) on the sense of presence, which is considered to impact more on presence rather than graphic realism [103]. Another critical aspect of memory performance is the type of encoding of virtual scenarios. In real-life situations, episodic memory encoding occurs non-intentionally [10], whereas with spatial learning a certain amount of information is encoded incidentally and with procedural memory [104,105]. However, when planning interventions that exploit the virtual enactment effect, clinicians and neuroscientists are encouraged to design instructions according to the sample; for instance, aging is known to affect incidental rather than intentional encoding, with attentional and executive components playing a critical role in encoding and storage in the former [106]. Lastly, from a methodological point of view, we encourage the use of within-interaction conditions: first, within-subject studies have greater statistical power compared to between-subjects designs; second, they allow the researcher to control variables (e.g., gender) that may affect memory performance (e.g., gender effect on spatial memory [80]), thus providing balanced groups; finally, within-subject designs permit the researcher to assess source memory by asking the participants to recall the context in which an event occurred (see [57]). However, within-subjects studies might overload or confound memory traces if the tasks are too complex or numerous. Researchers should consider the strengths and weaknesses of within and between subjects designs with potential biases in light of the objectives of their studies [86].

Assessment of performance is a critical aspect of research and clinical practice in order to evaluate and analyse what the researcher really wants to achieve. We highly recommend defining tasks based on strong theoretical and empirical considerations when assessing the complexity of memory within the context of virtual enactment. In the context of spatial memory, we suggest using egocentric and allocentric measures to tap spatial cognition features [4]; this can be achieved using landmarks, boundaries and maps with paper-and-pencil, computerized or VR tasks. However, in the present review, this is especially true when the spatial layout is considered within the context of episodic memory (e.g., [8,57]). When research focused on schematic/topographical representation [2], papers mainly used spatial levels of knowledge of the space (survey, route and landmark); therefore, we applied these levels to the cluster spatial task (Figure 2). Nevertheless, recent discoveries in cognitive neuroscience and clinical neuropsychology support the crucial role of spatial frames of reference in representing the space [5,14,83]; moreover, survey knowledge and landmark knowledge resemble, respectively, allocentric and egocentric representation, whereas route knowledge appears to be related to procedural memory due to landmark-based navigation [105,107]. For episodic memory, we strongly encourage the paradigms that tap the elements described by Tulving [7] as central aspects of this type of memory (i.e., event, spatiotemporal details, and emotional and perceptual details). The advent of VR enables neuroscientists to study in an ecological, standardized, and realistic way a complex function such as episodic memory [8,108].

Concerning the virtual enactment effect on spatial memory, the young population reported more positive outcomes on survey knowledge compared to route and landmark knowledge; nevertheless, findings in general are promising. Young adults and both the healthy and pathological aged population showed improvements on episodic item memory, spatial context and binding. However, further studies need to evaluate this effect on aging and neurodegenerative disorders in the domains of both spatial and episodic memory. It might be of interest to deepen our understanding of in which situations passive enhancement is present and why (Figure 2). Moreover, we suggest that future studies include real-world navigation conditions; while all of the studies had a passive control condition, only one [72] used a real-world control condition. Finally concerning mediating factors, although visuospatial abilities are crucial for spatial memory [74], executive functions have a great impact on spatial and episodic performances, and this is especially true for older people [8,63,68]. Other variables such as age, gender, expertise (e.g., videogames, driving), dynamic navigation, virtual realism, and delayed testing influence memory performance.

Findings are promising in the light of memory decline in aging. An age-dependent decrease is normally observed in these crucial cognitive domains [109], and the decline in spatial and episodic memory is accompanied by neural changes in the medial temporal lobe, hippocampus and prefrontal cortex in the aged population [110–112]. Aging is accompanied by spatial memory decline [113]. Indeed, Colombo and colleagues [114] recently shown that older people have specific allocentric impairments and difficulty in switching between the egocentric and the allocentric frame of reference; the translation from the allocentric to the egocentric frame of reference is possible thanks to the activity of the retrosplenial cortex, which converts neural representations of the medial temporal lobe to parietal and vice versa [5,115].

In particular, spatiotemporal details, along with associative (i.e., medial temporal binding processes) and strategic (i.e., frontal monitoring during encoding and retrieval) information, decline with aging [8]. Aging is also accompanied by differences in the encoding and retrieval of episodic memories [10,11]. Piolino and colleagues [11] showed that this was particularly true for autobiographical events in recent periods, with more responses (less spatiotemporal information, details, familiarity and third-person perspective) associated with reduced autonoesis for older adults (OA) compared to young adults (YA).

Memory impairments due to medial temporal lobe degeneration are classic features of Alzheimer's disease (AD) [116], mild cognitive impairment (MCI) [117], and amnestic mild cognitive impairment (aMCI) [118], which are considered part of the prodromal stage of dementia and in particular AD [119]. Deactivation and decreased functional connectivity of the default mode network is shown in healthy aging, MCI, and AD [120–122]. Retrosplenial cortex hypoactivity occurs in both AD and MCI and may explain episodic and navigation deficits in these patients [5]. Spatial disorientation in AD and aMCI is thought to be the result of degenerative processes taking place in the hippocampus and in deficient spatial frame synchronization [123]. Indeed, early markers of AD can be the switching abilities in aMCI and AD individuals [124]: allocentric impairments are present in aMCI and AD patients and moreover a deficit in the switch from egocentric to allocentric was found in these groups. Concerning episodic memory, these neurological conditions lead to deficits in the spatiotemporal and binding components of episodic recall [70], as well as autonoetic consciousness [125,126].

Finally, the present findings stress the essential role of the body in cognition, and memory in particular, as claimed by embodied cognition researchers. The virtual enactment effect could be used to study how the different levels of active and passive virtual navigation contribute to spatial and episodic performance and could potentially be used as a way to enhance memory in aging.

Author Contributions: Conceptualization: C.T., S.S. and P.P.; methodology: C.T., L.D. and S.S.; writing—review and editing: C.T., S.S., L.D., G.R.; supervision: P.P.; funding acquisition: G.R.

References

1. Robin, J. Spatial scaffold effects in event memory and imagination. *Wiley Interdiscip. Rev. Cogn. Sci.* **2018**, *9*, e1462. [CrossRef] [PubMed]
2. Moscovitch, M.; Rosenbaum, R.S.; Gilboa, A.; Addis, D.R.; Westmacott, R.; Grady, C.; McAndrews, M.P.; Levine, L.; Black, S.; Winocur, G.; et al. Functional neuroanatomy of remote episodic, semantic and spatial memory: A unified account based on multiple trace theory. *J. Anat.* **2005**, *207*, 35–66. [CrossRef] [PubMed]
3. American Psychological Association. *APA Dictionary of Psychology*; American Psychological Association: Washington, DC, USA, 2007.
4. Burgess, N. Spatial cognition and the brain. *Ann. N. Y. Acad. Sci.* **2008**, *1124*, 77–97. [CrossRef]
5. Vann, S.D.; Aggleton, J.P.; Maguire, E.A. What does the retrosplenial cortex do? *Nat. Rev. Neurosci.* **2009**, *10*, 792–802. [CrossRef] [PubMed]
6. Chrastil, E.R.; Warren, W.H. Active and passive contributions to spatial learning. *Psychon. Bull. Rev.* **2012**, *19*, 1–23. [CrossRef] [PubMed]
7. Tulving, E. Episodic Memory: From Mind to Brain. *Annu. Rev. Psychol.* **2002**, *53*, 1–25. [PubMed]
8. Jebara, N.; Orriols, E.; Zaoui, M.; Berthoz, A.; Piolino, P. Effects of enactment in episodic memory: A pilot virtual reality study with young and elderly adults. *Front. Aging Neurosci.* **2014**, *6*, 338. [CrossRef] [PubMed]
9. Laurent, X.; Ensslin, A.; Marí-Beffa, P. An Action to an Object Does Not Improve Its Episodic Encoding but Removes Distraction. *J. Exp. Psychol. Hum. Percept. Perform.* **2016**, *42*, 494–507.
10. Plancher, G.; Gyselinck, V.; Nicolas, S.; Piolino, P. Age effect on components of episodic memory and feature binding: A virtual reality study. *Neuropsychology* **2010**, *24*, 379–390. [CrossRef] [PubMed]
11. Piolino, P.; Desgranges, B.; Clarys, D.; Guillery-Girard, B.; Taconnat, L.; Isingrini, M.; Eustache, F. Autobiographical memory, autonoetic consciousness, and self-perspective in aging. *Psychol. Aging* **2006**, *21*, 510–525. [CrossRef] [PubMed]
12. Prebble, S.C.; Addis, D.R.; Tippett, L.J. Autobiographical memory and sense of self. *Psychol. Bull.* **2013**, *139*, 815–840. [CrossRef]
13. O'Keefe, L.; Nadel, J. *The Hippocampus as a Cognitive Map*; Clarendon Press: Oxford, UK, 1978.

14. Hartley, T.; Lever, C.; Burgess, N.; O'Keefe, J. Space in the brain: How the hippocampal formation supports spatial cognition. *Philos. Trans. R. Soc. Lond. B Biol. Sci.* **2014**, *369*, 20120510. [CrossRef] [PubMed]
15. Burgess, N.; Maguire, E.A.; O'Keefe, J. The human hippocampus and spatial and episodic memory. *Neuron* **2002**, *35*, 625–641. [CrossRef]
16. Kühn, S.; Gallinat, J. Segregating cognitive functions within hippocampal formation: A quantitative meta-analysis on spatial navigation and episodic memory. *Hum. Brain Mapp.* **2014**, *35*, 1129–1142. [CrossRef] [PubMed]
17. Manus, J.R.; Hopkins, R.O.; Reed, J.M.; Kitchener, E.G.; Squire, L.R. Recognition memory and the human hippocampus. *Neuron* **2003**, *37*, 171–180. [CrossRef]
18. Bergouignan, L.; Nyberg, L.; Ehrsson, H.H. Out-of-body–induced hippocampal amnesia. *Proc. Natl. Acad. Sci. USA* **2014**, *111*, 4421–4426. [CrossRef]
19. Eichenbaum, H. Time cells in the hippocampus: A new dimension for mapping memories. *Nat. Rev. Neruosci.* **2014**, *15*, 732–744. [CrossRef]
20. Glenberg, A.M.; Hayes, J. Contribution of embodiment to solving the riddle of infantile amnesia. *Front. Psychol.* **2016**, *7*, 10. [CrossRef] [PubMed]
21. Ritchey, M.; Wing, E.A.; Labar, K.S.; Cabeza, R. Neural Similarity Between Encoding and Retrieval is Related to Memory Via Hippocampal Interactions. *Cereb. Cortex* **2012**, *23*, 2818–2828. [CrossRef] [PubMed]
22. Nadel, L.; Winocur, G.; Ryan, L.; Moscovitch, M. Systems consolidation and hippocampus: Two views. *Debates Neurosci.* **2007**, *1*, 55–66. [CrossRef]
23. Gomez, A.; Rousset, S.; Baciu, M. Egocentric-updating during navigation facilitates episodic memory retrieval. *Acta Psychol.* **2009**, *132*, 221–227. [CrossRef]
24. Burgess, N. The hippocampus, space, and view points in episodic memory. *Q. J. Exp. Psychol.* **2002**, *55A*, 1057–1080. [CrossRef]
25. Gomez, A.; Rousset, S.; Charnallet, A. Spatial deficits in an amnesic patient with hippocampal damage: Questioning the multiple trace theory. *Hippocampus* **2012**, *22*, 1313–1324. [CrossRef]
26. Tromp, D.; Dufour, A.; Lithfous, S.; Pebayle, T.; Després, O. Episodic memory in normal aging and Alzheimer disease: Insights from imaging and behavioral studies. *Ageing Res. Rev.* **2015**, *24*, 232–262. [CrossRef] [PubMed]
27. Wheeler, M.A.; Stuss, D.T.; Tulving, E. Toward a theory of episodic memory: The frontal lobes and autonoetic consciousness. *Psychol. Bull.* **1997**, *121*, 331–354. [CrossRef] [PubMed]
28. Habib, R.; Nyberg, L.; Tulving, E. Hemispheric asymmetries of memory: The HERA model revisited. *Trends Cogn. Sci.* **2003**, *7*, 241–245. [CrossRef]
29. Lepage, M.; Ghaffar, O.; Nyberg, L.; Tulving, E. Prefrontal cortex and episodic memory retrieval mode. *Proc. Natl. Acad. Sci. USA* **2000**, *97*, 506–511. [CrossRef]
30. Burgess, N.; Maguire, E.A.; Spiers, H.J.; O'Keefe, J. A temporoparietal and prefrontal network for retrieving the spatial context of lifelike events. *Neuroimage* **2001**, *14*, 439–453. [CrossRef] [PubMed]
31. Spreng, R.N.; Mar, R.A.; Kim, A.S.N. The Common Neural Basis of Autobiographical Memory, Prospection, Navigation, Theory of Mind, and the Default Mode: A Quantitative Meta-analysis. *J. Cogn. Neurosci.* **2008**, *21*, 489–510. [CrossRef]
32. Clark, A. An embodied cognitive science? *Trends Cogn. Sci.* **1999**, *3*, 345–351. [CrossRef]
33. Wilson, M. Six views of embodied cognition. *Psychon. Bull. Rev.* **2002**, *9*, 625–636. [CrossRef] [PubMed]
34. Glenberg, A.M. Embodiment as a unifying perspective for psychology. *Wiley Interdiscip. Rev. Cogn. Sci.* **2010**, *1*, 586–596. [CrossRef] [PubMed]
35. Dijkstra, K.; Post, L. Mechanisms of embodiment. *Front. Psychol.* **2015**, *6*, 1525. [CrossRef] [PubMed]
36. Vallet, G.T. Embodied cognition of aging. *Front. Psychol.* **2015**, *6*, 463. [CrossRef]
37. Spackman, J.S.; Yanchar, S.C. Embodied Cognition, Representationalism, and Mechanism: A Review and Analysis. *J. Theory Soc. Behav.* **2014**, *44*, 46–79. [CrossRef]
38. Braak, H.; Braak, E. Neuropathological stageing of Alzheimer-related changes. *Acta Neuropathol.* **1991**, *82*, 239–259. [CrossRef]
39. Fjell, A.M.; Westlye, L.T.; Amlien, I.; Espeseth, T.; Reinvang, I.; Raz, N.; Agartz, I.; Salat, D.H.; Greve, D.N.; Fischl, B.; et al. High consistency of regional cortical thinning in aging across multiple samples. *Cereb. Cortex* **2009**, *19*, 2001–2012. [CrossRef]

40. Braak, H.; Braak, E. Staging of alzheimer's disease-related neurofibrillary changes. *Neurobiol. Aging* **1995**, *16*, 271–278. [CrossRef]
41. Brooks, B.M.; Attree, E.A.; Rose, F.D.; Clifford, B.R.; Leadbetter, A.G. The Specificity of Memory Enhancement During Interaction with a Virtual Environment. *Memory* **1999**, *7*, 65–78. [CrossRef]
42. Engelkamp, J. *Memory for Actions*; Psychology Press/Taylor & Francis: London, UK, 1998.
43. Plancher, G.; Barra, J.; Orriols, E.; Piolino, P. The influence of action on episodic memory: A virtual reality study. *Q. J. Exp. Psychol.* **2013**, *66*, 895–909. [CrossRef]
44. Tulving, E. Ecphoric process in episodic memory. *Philos. Trans. R. Soc. Lond. B* **1983**, *1110*, 361–370. [CrossRef]
45. Rugg, M.D.; Wilding, E.L. Retrieval processing and episodic memory. *Trends Cogn. Sci.* **2000**, *4*, 108–115. [CrossRef]
46. Kent, C.; Lamberts, K. The encoding-retrieval relationship: Retrieval as mental simulation. *Trends Cogn. Sci.* **2008**, *12*, 92–98. [CrossRef]
47. Meyer, K.; Damasio, A. Convergence and divergence in a neural architecture for recognition and memory. *Trends Neurosci.* **2009**, *32*, 376–382. [CrossRef]
48. Johnson, J.D.; Price, M.H.; Leiker, E.K. Episodic retrieval involves early and sustained effects of reactivating information from encoding. *Neuroimage* **2015**, *106*, 300–310. [CrossRef] [PubMed]
49. Rugg, M.D.; Johnson, J.D.; Park, H.; Uncapher, M.R. Encoding-retrieval overlap in human episodic memory: A functional neuroimaging perspective. *Prog. Brain Res.* **2008**, *169*, 339–352. [PubMed]
50. Danker, J.F.; Anderson, J.R. The ghosts of brain states past: Remembering reactivates the brain regions engaged during encoding. *Psychol. Bull.* **2010**, *136*, 87–102. [CrossRef] [PubMed]
51. Nyberg, L.; Habib, R.; McIntosh, A.R.; Tulving, E. Reactivation of encoding-related brain activity during memory retrieval. *Proc. Natl. Acad. Sci. USA* **2000**, *97*, 11120–11124. [CrossRef]
52. Wheeler, M.; Petersen, S.; Buckner, R. Memory's Echo: Vivid Remembering Reactivates Sensory-Specific Cortex. *Proc. Natl. Acad. Sci. USA* **2000**, *97*, 11125–11129. [CrossRef]
53. Wilson, P.N.; Foreman, N.; Gillett, R.; Stanton, D. Active Versus Passive Processing of Spatial Information in a Computer- Simulated Environment. *Ecol. Psychol.* **1997**, *9*, 37–41. [CrossRef]
54. Riva, G. From virtual to real body: Virtual reality as embodied technology. *J. Cyber Ther. Rehabil.* **2008**, *1*, 7–22.
55. Repetto, C.; Serino, S.; Macedonia, M.; Riva, G. Virtual Reality as an Embodied Tool to Enhance Episodic Memory in Elderly. *Front. Psychol.* **2016**, *7*, 1839. [CrossRef]
56. Moher, D.; Liberati, A.; Tetzlaff, J.; Altman, D.G.; Grp, P. Preferred Reporting Items for Systematic Reviews and Meta-Analyses: The PRISMA Statement (Reprinted from Annals of Internal Medicine). *Phys. Ther.* **2009**, *89*, 873–880.
57. Tuena, C.; Serino, S.; Gaston-Bellegarde, A.; Orriols, E.; Makowski, D.; Riva, G.; Piolino, P. How virtual embodiment affects episodic memory functioning: A proof-of-concept study. *Annu. Rev. Cyberther. Telemed.* **2017**, *15*, 98–103.
58. Carassa, A.; Geminiani, G.; Morganti, F.; Varotto, D. Active and passive spatial learning in a complex virtual environment: The effect of effcient exploration. *Cogn. Process.* **2002**, *3*, 65–81.
59. Sandamas, G.; Foreman, N. Drawing maps and remembering landmarks after driving in a virtual small town environment. *J. Maps* **2007**, *3*, 35–45. [CrossRef]
60. Wallet, G.; Sauzéon, H.; Larrue, F.; N'Kaoua, B. Virtual/real transfer in a large-scale environment: Impact of active navigation as a function of the viewpoint displacement effect and recall tasks. *Adv. Hum. Comput. Interact.* **2013**, *2013*, 8. [CrossRef]
61. Meade, M.E.; Meade, J.G.; Sauzéon, H.; Fernandes, M.A. Active Navigation in Virtual Environments Benefits Spatial Memory in Older Adults. *Brain Sci.* **2019**, *9*, 47. [CrossRef]
62. Gaunet, F.; Vidal, M.; Kemeny, A.; Berthoz, A. Active, passive and snapshot exploration in a virtual environment: Influence on scene memory, reorientation and path memory. *Cogn. Brain Res.* **2001**, *11*, 409–420. [CrossRef]
63. Taillade, M.; Sauzéon, H.; Pala, P.A.; Déjos, M.; Larrue, F.; Gross, C.; N'Kaoua, B. Age-Related Wayfinding Differences in Real Large-Scale Environments: Detrimental Motor Control Effects during Spatial Learning Are Mediated by Executive Decline? *PLoS ONE* **2013**, *8*, e67193. [CrossRef]
64. Dalgarno, B.; Bennett, S.; Harper, B. The Importance of Active Exploration, Optical Flow, and Task Alignment for Spatial Learning in Desktop 3D Environments. *Hum. Comput. Interact.* **2010**, *25*, 25–66. [CrossRef]

65. von Stülpnagel, R.; Steffens, M.C. Active route learning in virtual environments: Disentangling movement control from intention, instruction specificity, and navigation control. *Psychol. Res.* **2013**, *77*, 555–574. [CrossRef]
66. Wilson, P.N. Active exploration of a virtual environment does not promote orientation or memory for objects. *Environ. Behav.* **1999**, *31*, 752–763. [CrossRef]
67. Peruch, P.; Vercher, J.; Gauthier, G.M. Acquisition of Spatial Knowledge Through Visual Exploration of Simulated Environments. *Ecol. Psychol.* **1995**, *7*, 1–20. [CrossRef]
68. Sauzéon, H.; N'Kaoua, B.; Arvind Pala, P.; Taillade, M.; Guitton, P. Age and active navigation effects on episodic memory: A virtual reality study. *Br. J. Psychol.* **2016**, *107*, 72–94. [CrossRef]
69. Sauzéon, H.; Pala, P.A.; Larrue, F.; Wallet, G.; Déjos, M.; Zheng, X.; Guitton, P.; N'Kaoua, B. The use of Virtual Reality for episodic memory assessment: Effects of active navigation. *Exp. Psychol.* **2012**, *59*, 99–108. [CrossRef]
70. Plancher, G.; Tirard, A.; Gyselinck, V.; Nicolas, S.; Piolino, P. Using virtual reality to characterize episodic memory profiles in amnestic mild cognitive impairment and Alzheimer's disease: Influence of active and passive encoding. *Neuropsychologia* **2012**, *50*, 592–602. [CrossRef]
71. Plancher, G.; Nicolas, S.; Piolino, P. Apport de la réalité virtuelle en neuropsychologie de la mémoire: Étude dans le vieillissement. *Psychol. Neuropsychiatr. Vieil.* **2008**, *6*, 7–22.
72. Wallet, G.; Sauzéon, H.; Rodrigues, J.; Larrue, F.; N'Kaoua, B. Virtual/real transfer of spatial learning: Impact of activity according to the retention delay. *Stud. Health Technol. Inform.* **2010**, *154*, 145–149.
73. Hahm, J.; Lee, K.; Lim, S.-L.; Kim, S.-Y.; Kim, H.-T.; Lee, J.-H. Effects of active navigation on object recognition in virtual environments. *CyberPsychol. Behav.* **2007**, *10*, 305–308. [CrossRef]
74. Cutmore, T.R.H.; Hine, T.J.; Maberly, K.J.; Langford, N.M.; Hawgood, G. Cognitive and gender factors influencing navigation in a virtual environment. *Int. J. Hum. Comput. Stud.* **2000**, *53*, 223–249. [CrossRef]
75. Sandamas, G.; Foreman, N. Active Versus Passive Acquisition of Spatial Knowledge While Controlling a Vehicle in a Virtual Urban Space in Drivers and Non-Drivers. *SAGE Open* **2015**, *5*, 2158244015595443. [CrossRef]
76. Farrell, M.J.; Arnold, P.; Pettifer, S.; Adams, J.; Graham, T.; MacManamon, M. Transfer of route learning from virtual to real environments. *J. Exp. Psychol. Appl.* **2003**, *9*, 219–227. [CrossRef]
77. Wallet, G.; Sauzéon, H.; Pala, P.A.; Larrue, F.; Zheng, X.; N'Kaoua, B. Virtual/real transfer of spatial knowledge: Benefit from visual fidelity provided in a virtual environment and impact of active navigation. *Cyberpsychol. Behav. Soc. Netw.* **2011**, *14*, 417–423. [CrossRef]
78. Allison, C.; Redhead, E.S. Factors in fl uencing orientation within a nested virtual environment: External cues, active exploration and familiarity. *J. Environ. Psychol.* **2017**, *51*, 158–167. [CrossRef]
79. Palermo, E.; Laut, J.; Nov, O.; Cappa, P.; Porfiri, M. Spatial memory training in a citizen science context. *Comput. Hum. Behav.* **2017**, *73*, 38–46. [CrossRef]
80. Liu, I.; Levy, R.M.; Barton, J.J.S.; Iaria, G. Age and gender differences in various topographical orientation strategies. *Brain Res.* **2011**, *1410*, 112–119. [CrossRef]
81. Pacheco, D.; Verschure, P.F.M.J. Long-term spatial clustering in free recall. *Memory* **2018**, *26*, 798–806. [CrossRef]
82. Pettijohn, K.A.; Radvansky, G.A. Walking through doorways causes forgetting: Active and passive interaction. *J. Cogn. Psychol.* **2018**, *30*, 771–777. [CrossRef]
83. Barry, C.; Burgess, N. Neural Mechanisms of Self-Location. *Curr. Biol.* **2014**, *24*, R330–R339. [CrossRef]
84. Chrastil, E.R.; Warren, W.H. Active and Passive Spatial Learning in Human Navigation: Acquisition of Graph Knowledg. *J. Exp. Psychol. Learn. Mem. Cogn.* **2015**, *41*, 1162–1178. [CrossRef]
85. Greenwood, P.M. The frontal aging hypothesis evaluated. *J. Int. Neuropsychol. Soc.* **2000**, *6*, 705–726. [CrossRef]
86. Charness, G.; Gneezy, U.; Kuhn, M.A. Experimental methods: Between-subject and within-subject design. *J. Econ. Behav. Organ.* **2012**, *81*, 1–8. [CrossRef]
87. Delis, D.C.; Kramer, J.H.; Kaplan, E.; Thompkins, B.A.O. *CVLT: California Verbal Learning Test-Adult Version: Manual*; Psychological Corporation: London, UK, 1987.
88. Madan, C.R.; Singhal, A. Using actions to enhance memory: Effects of enactment, gestures, and exercise on human memory. *Front. Psychol.* **2012**, *3*, 507. [CrossRef]

89. Dijkstra, K.; Kaschak, M.P.; Zwaan, R.A. Body posture facilitates retrieval of autobiographical memories. *Cognition* **2007**, *102*, 139–149. [CrossRef]
90. Guterstam, A.; Bjornsdotter, M.; Bergouignan, L.; Gentile, G.; Li, T.-Q.; Ehrsson, H.H. Decoding illusory self-location from activity in the human hippocampus. *Front. Hum. Neurosci.* **2015**, *9*, 412. [CrossRef]
91. Steffens, M.C.; Von Stülpnagel, R.; Schult, J.C. Memory Recall After 'Learning by Doing' and 'Learning by Viewing': Boundary Conditions of an Enactment Benefit. *Front. Psychol.* **2015**, *6*, 1907. [CrossRef]
92. Potter, M.C. Recognition and memory for briefly presented scenes. *Front. Psychol.* **2012**, *3*, 32. [CrossRef]
93. Migo, E.M.; Mayes, A.R.; Montaldi, D. Measuring recollection and familiarity: Improving the remember/know procedure. *Conscious. Cogn.* **2012**, *21*, 1435–1455. [CrossRef]
94. Nyberg, L.; Persson, J.; Nilsson, L.G. Individual differences in memory enhancement by encoding enactment: Relationships to adult age and biological factors. *Neurosci. Biobehav. Rev.* **2002**, *26*, 835–839. [CrossRef]
95. Zimmer, H.D.; Cohen, R.L. *Memory for Action: A Distinct Form of Episodic Memory?* Oxford University Press: Oxford, UK, 2001.
96. Wechsler, D. *WAIS-R Manual: Wechsler Adult Intelligence Scale-Revised*; Psychological Corporation: London, UK, 1981.
97. Stroop, J.R. Studies of interference in serial verbal reactions. *J. Exp. Psychol.* **1935**, *18*, 643. [CrossRef]
98. Vandenberg, S.G.; Kuse, A.R. Mental rotations, a group test of three-dimensional spatial visualization. *Percept. Mot. Skills* **1978**, *47*, 599–604. [CrossRef]
99. Reitan, R.M. Validity of the Trail Making Test as an indicator of organic brain damage. *Percept. Mot. Skills* **1958**, *8*, 271–276. [CrossRef]
100. García-Betances, R.I.; Arredondo Waldmeyer, M.T.; Fico, G.; Cabrera-Umpiérrez, M.F. A succinct overview of virtual reality technology use in Alzheimer's disease. *Front. Aging Neurosci.* **2015**, *7*, 80.
101. Serino, S.; Pedroli, E.; Tuena, C.; Leo, G.D.; Stramba-Badiale, M.; Goulene, K.; Mariotti, N.G.; Riva, G. A Novel Virtual Reality-Based Training Protocol for the Enhancement of the 'Mental Frame Syncing' in Individuals with Alzheimer' s Disease: A Development-of-Concept Trial. Serino, Silvia et al. "A Novel Virtual Reality-Based Training Protocol for the Enhancement of the "Mental Frame Syncing" in Individuals with Alzheimer's Disease: A Development-of-Concept Trial.". *Front. Aging Neurosci.* **2017**, *9*, 240.
102. Serino, S.; Riva, G. Getting lost in Alzheimer's disease: A break in the mental frame syncing. *Med. Hypotheses* **2013**, *80*, 416–421. [CrossRef]
103. Triberti, S.; Riva, G. Being present in action: A theoretical model about the 'interlocking' between intentions and environmental affordances. *Front. Psychol.* **2016**, *6*, 2052. [CrossRef]
104. Münzer, S.; Zimmer, H.D.; Schwalm, M.; Baus, J.; Aslan, I. Computer-assisted navigation and the acquisition of route and survey knowledge. *J. Environ. Psychol.* **2006**, *26*, 300–308. [CrossRef]
105. Doeller, C.F.; King, J.A.; Burgess, N. Parallel striatal and hippocampal systems for landmarks and boundaries in spatial memory. *Proc. Natl. Acad. Sci. USA* **2008**, *105*, 5915–5920. [CrossRef]
106. Kontaxopoulou, D.; Beratis, I.N.; Fragkiadaki, S.; Pavlou, D.; Yannis, G.; Economou, A.; Papanicolaou, A.C.; Papageorgiou, S.G. Incidental and Intentional Memory: Their Relation with Attention and Executive Functions. *Arch. Clin. Neuropsychol.* **2017**, *32*, 19–532. [CrossRef]
107. Guderian, S.; Dzieciol, A.M.; Gadian, D.G.; Jentschke, S.; Doeller, C.F.; Burgess, N.; Mishkin, M.; Vargha-Khadem, F. Hippocampal Volume Reduction in Humans Predicts Impaired Allocentric Spatial Memory in Virtual-Reality Navigation. *J. Neurosci.* **2015**, *35*, 14123–14131. [CrossRef]
108. Serino, S.; Repetto, C. New Trends in Episodic Memory Assessment: Immersive 360 Ecological Videos. *Front. Psychol.* **2018**, *9*, 1878. [CrossRef]
109. Salthouse, T.A. When does age-related cognitive decline begin? *Neurobiol. Aging* **2009**, *30*, 507–514. [CrossRef]
110. Hedden, T.; Gabrieli, J.D.E. Insights into the ageing mind: A view from cognitive neuroscience. *Nat. Rev. Neurosci.* **2004**, *5*, 87–96. [CrossRef]
111. Kinugawa, K.; Schumm, S.; Pollina, M.; Depre, M.; Jungbluth, C.; Doulazmi, M.; Mariani, J. Aging-related episodic memory decline: Are emotions the key? *Front. Behav. Neurosci.* **2013**, *7*, 2. [CrossRef]
112. Robitsek, R.J.; Fortin, N.J.; Koh, M.T.; Gallagher, M.; Eichenbaum, H. Cognitive Aging: A Common Decline of Episodic Recollection and Spatial Memory in Rats. *J. Neurosci.* **2008**, *28*, 8945–8954. [CrossRef]
113. Wolbers, T.; Dudchenko, P.A.; Wood, E.R. Spatial memory—A unique window into healthy and pathological aging. *Front. Aging Neurosci.* **2014**, *6*, 35. [CrossRef]

114. Colombo, D.; Serino, S.; Tuena, C.; Pedroli, E.; Dakanalis, A.; Cipresso, P.; Riva, G. Egocentric and allocentric spatial reference frames in aging: A systematic review. *Neurosci. Biobehav. Rev.* **2017**, *80*, 605–621. [CrossRef]
115. Alexander, A.S.; Nitz, D.A. Retrosplenial cortex maps the conjunction of internal and external spaces. *Nat. Neurosci.* **2015**, *18*, 1143–1151. [CrossRef]
116. Dubois, B.; Feldman, H.H.; Jacova, C.; DeKosky, S.T.; Barberger-Gateau, P.; Cummings, J.; Delacourte, A.; Galasko, D.; Gauthier, S.; Jicha, G.; et al. Research criteria for the diagnosis of Alzheimer's disease: Revising the NINCDS-ADRDA criteria. *Lancet Neurol.* **2007**, *6*, 734–746. [CrossRef]
117. Nordahl, C.W.; Ranganath, C.; Yonelinas, A.P.; DeCarli, C.; Reed, B.R.; Jagust, W.J. Different mechanisms of episodic memory failure in mild cognitive impairment. *Neuropsychologia* **2005**, *43*, 1688–1697. [CrossRef] [PubMed]
118. Dunn, C.J.; Duffy, S.L.; Hickie, I.B.; Lagopoulos, J.; Lewis, S.J.; Naismith, S.L.; Shine, J.M. Deficits in episodic memory retrieval reveal impaired default mode network connectivity in amnestic mild cognitive impairment. *NeuroImage Clin.* **2014**, *4*, 473–480. [CrossRef] [PubMed]
119. Petersen, R.C.; Doody, R.; Kurz, A.; Mohs, R.C.; Morris, J.C.; Rabins, P.V.; Ritchie, K.; Rossor, M.; Thal, L.; Winblad, B. Current Concepts in Mild Cognitive Impairment. *Arch. Neurol.* **2011**, *58*, 1985–1992. [CrossRef]
120. Hafkemeijer, A.; van der Grond, J.; Rombouts, S.A.R.B. Imaging the default mode network in aging and dementia. *Biochim. Biophys. Acta Mol. Basis Dis.* **2012**, *1822*, 431–441. [CrossRef]
121. Buckner, R.L.; Snyder, A.Z.; Shannon, B.J.; LaRossa, G.; Sachs, R.; Fotenos, A.F.; Sheline, Y.I.; Klunk, W.E.; Mathis, C.A.; Morris, J.C.; et al. Molecular, Structural, and Functional Characterization of Alzheimer's Disease: Evidence for a Relationship between Default Activity, Amyloid, and Memory. *J. Neurosci.* **2005**, *25*, 7709–7717. [CrossRef] [PubMed]
122. Buckner, R.L.; Andrews-Hanna, J.R.; Schacter, D.L. The brain's default network: Anatomy, function, and relevance to disease. *Ann. N. Y. Acad. Sci.* **2008**, *1124*, 1–38. [CrossRef] [PubMed]
123. Serino, S.; Morganti, F.; Di Stefano, F.; Riva, G. Detecting early egocentric and allocentric impairments deficits in Alzheimer's disease: An experimental study with virtual reality. *Front. Aging Neurosci.* **2015**, *7*, 88. [CrossRef]
124. Ruggiero, G.; Iavarone, A.; Iachini, T. Allocentric to egocentric spatial switching: Impairment in amci and Alzheimer's disease patients? *Curr. Alzheimer Res.* **2018**, *15*, 229–236. [CrossRef]
125. Piolino, P.; Desgranges, B.; Belliard, S.; Matuszewski, V.; Lalevée, C.; De La Sayette, V.; Eustache, F. Autobiographical memory and autonoetic consciousness: Triple dissociation in neurodegenerative diseases. *Brain* **2003**, *126*, 2203–2219. [CrossRef]
126. Rauchs, G.; Piolino, P.; Mézenge, F.; Landeau, B.; Lalevée, C.; Pélerin, A.; Viader, F.; De La Sayette, V.; Eustache, F.; Desgranges, B. Autonoetic consciousness in Alzheimer's disease: Neuropsychological and PET findings using an episodic learning and recognition task. *Neurobiol. Aging* **2007**, *28*, 1410–1420. [CrossRef]

6

A Computational Approach for the Assessment of Executive Functions in Patients with Obsessive–Compulsive Disorder

Elisa Pedroli [1,2,*], Filippo La Paglia [3], Pietro Cipresso [1,4], Caterina La Cascia [3], Giuseppe Riva [1,4] and Daniele La Barbera [3]

1. Applied Technology for Neuro-Psychology Lab, IRCCS Istituto Auxologico Italiano, Via Magnasco 2, 20149 Milano, Italy; Pietro.Cipresso@unicatt.it (P.C.); giuseppe.riva@unicatt.it (G.R.)
2. Faculty of Psychology, eCampus University, Via Isimbardi, 10, 22060 Novedrate, Italy
3. Department of Experimental Biomedicine and Clinical Neuroscience, University of Palermo, Piazza Marina, 61, 90133 Palermo, Italy; filippo.lapaglia@unipa.it (F.L.P.); erika.lacascia@unipa.it (C.L.C.); daniele.labarbera@unipa.it (D.L.B.)
4. Psychology Department, Catholic University of Milan, Largo Gemelli 1, 20123 Milan, Italy

* Correspondence: e.pedroli@auxologico.it

Abstract: Previous studies on obsessive–compulsive disorder (OCD) showed impairments in executive domains, particularly in cognitive inhibition. In this perspective, the use of virtual reality showed huge potential in the assessment of executive functions; however, unfortunately, to date, no study on the assessment of these patients took advantage of the use of virtual environments. One of the main problems faced within assessment protocols is the use of a limited number of variables and tools when tailoring a personalized program. The main aim of this study was to provide a heuristic decision tree for the future development of tailored assessment protocols. To this purpose, we conducted a study that involved 58 participants (29 OCD patients and 29 controls) to collect both classic neuropsychological data and precise data based on a validated protocol in virtual reality for the assessment of executive functions, namely, the VMET (virtual multiple errands test). In order to provide clear indications for working on executive functions with these patients, we carried out a cross-validation based on three learning algorithms and computationally defined two decision trees. We found that, by using three neuropsychological tests and two VMET scores, it was possible to discriminate OCD patients from controls, opening a novel scenario for future assessment protocols based on virtual reality and computational techniques.

Keywords: Obsessive–compulsive disorders; virtual reality; multiple errands test; cognitive assessment; executive functions; computational models; decision tree; cross-validation

---

1. Introduction

According to the Diagnostic and Statistical Manual of Mental Disorders, Fifth Edition (DSM-5) [1], patients with obsessive–compulsive disorder (OCD) usually show obsessions and/or compulsions that reduce quality of life because of interference with daily routines, as well as work, social, or family life. This disorder affects about 2% of the population, and the World Health Organization highlighted that OCD is one of the 20 causes of disability in subjects within the 15–44 age range [2]. Moreover, OCD patients show dysfunctions in executive domains, particularly in cognitive inhibition [3], probably caused by a serotoninergic and dopaminergic dysfunction [4]. A deficit in executive functions may give problems when responding to both internal and external requirements, by inhibiting the ability to manage and orient the necessary cognitive resources. Specifically, the term "executive function" indicates a complex domain that includes a large number of cognitive processes and behavioral capabilities such as problem-solving, planning, sequencing, ability to sustain attention, resisting interference, utilizing feedback, cognitive inhibition, multitasking, cognitive flexibility, etc. [5–7]. Despite this abnormality, research on neuropsychological impairments in OCD produced unclear results [8]. Analyzing this specific syndrome, we can find some symptoms strongly related to dysexecutive deficits, such as checking behaviors. It is important to understand which one has a causal role in OCD and which one is a consequence of the syndrome [9]. Some articles showed deficits in planning abilities and nonverbal memory, while other studies reported deficits in cognitive flexibility and inhibition, and others displayed no neuropsychological deficits [10–14]. There are many possible explanations, e.g., differences in the methodology, in the instruments used, or in the characteristics of the samples. Specifically, the diversity of tools used during the assessment phase is related to an unsolved debate: the difference between paper-and-pencil and ecological tests [15]. Classic tasks in a classic setting analyze single aspects of complex domains and request simple responses to single events. Conversely, tasks in naturalistic settings may analyze cognitive functions in a complete way, requiring complex answers and, sometimes, the inhibition of inappropriate or irrelevant actions within several subtasks [6]. Therefore, it is critical to increase the ecological validity of a neuropsychological battery, especially for a complex cognitive domain such as an executive function. The assessment procedure has to become more sensitive to different aspects of patient behavior reflecting real-life situations [16]. However, it is too difficult to create a feasible assessment of executive functions during real-life situations because of implementation problems and the difficulty in involving patients in the procedure [17].

Virtual reality (VR) represents a valid solution to address the problems of classical assessment protocols. VR is a new technology that allows users to actively interact in a computer-generated tridimensional environment that simulates the real world [18]. This technology allows subjects to explore and manage several situations inspired by daily experiences using real correspondent behaviors in a more controlled, safe, and low-cost setting than real-life situations [19]. In the last few years, VR was applied for the assessment and rehabilitation of several psychological diseases such as post-traumatic stress disorder [20–22], anxiety [23,24], and eating disorders [25], as well as for neuropsychological domains such as neglect [26,27], executive functions [28,29], decision-making [30], spatial memory and orientation [31–33], and cognitive rehabilitation of schizophrenia [34].

In the current study, we proposed a computational approach based on classification learning algorithms to discriminate OCD patients from a control group. There were many studies that highlighted the usefulness of a VR-based approach for the assessment of executive functions in OCD patients [35–37]. These patients showed a specific pattern of symptoms that could be easily detected with the use of VR or an integrated assessment. Our purpose was to provide a heuristic decision tree for a more precise but simple diagnosis, giving evidence-based indications for a possible rehabilitation protocol using virtual reality tailored to these patients. The assessment of the OCD disorder was based on a clinical interview, integrated with a questionnaire, as well as neuropsychological assessment in rare cases. This last aspect is important because it may highlight a particular pattern of functioning in OCD patients [38]. We tried providing indications of the most useful assessment tools for the analysis of these specific aspects.

2. Materials and Methods

2.1. Participants

The 58 participants consisted of 29 OCD patients (mean age: 33.07; SD: 9.91), diagnosed by a clinical psychologist or psychiatrist as meeting the DSM-5 [1] criteria for OCD, and 29 healthy and partially matched controls (mean age: 40.48; SD: 15.59). The mean value for years of education (y.o.e.) of patients was 12.03 (SD: 3.2) and that for the healthy control group was 12.03 (SD: 3.2). In the OCD group, there were 14 females and 15 males, and, in the healthy control group, there were 14 females and 15 males. In Table 1, the descriptive statistics of both groups are presented. In Table 2, a comparison between age and y.o.e. and between the cognitive level of control and patient groups is presented. According to the results, the two groups were matched for both age and y.o.e. but not for cognitive level. The general exclusion criteria were as follows: (1) presence of sensory and/or motor limitation; (2) presence of deficit in general cognitive level (Mini Mental State Examination <19); (3) deficit in perception (Street Test <2.25); (4) deficit in language comprehension (Token Test <26.5); (5) anxiety (State Trait Anxiety Inventory - STAI >40); (6) depression (Beck Depression Inventory >16). We did not control the level of OCD symptoms with quantitative methods; however, all patients were currently undergoing treatment and, according to a clinician, in partial remission. Furthermore, OCD patients with comorbidities and healthy controls with any psychiatric diagnosis were excluded. The subjects involved were treated with both drugs and psychotherapy according to the standard. All participants were experienced with the use of personal computers (PCs) and came from the hospital's area. Participants were asked not to drink caffeine or alcohol and not to smoke prior to the experimental test to avoid any effects of these substances on test execution and performance.

Table 1. Descriptive statistics of the two groups. SE—standard error; y.o.e.—years of education; MMSE—Mini Mental State Examination.

	Group	*N*	Mean	SD	SE
Age	1	29	33.07	9.906	1.840
	2	29	40.48	15.588	2.895
y.o.e.	1	29	12.03	3.201	0.594
	2	29	12.03	3.029	0.563
MMSE	1	29	26.56	2.675	0.497
	2	29	28.53	1.028	0.191

Table 2. Independent sample Mann–Whitney U test.

	W	*p*
Age	312.5	0.094
y.o.e.	425.5	0.936
MMSE	194.0	<0.001

2.2. *Ethics Statement*

The study was approved by the scientific review board of the "U.O. di Psichiatria dell'Azienda Universitaria Ospedaliera Policlinico 'Paolo Giaccone' di Palermo", in accordance with the Declaration of Helsinki. All participants gave written informed consent to the experimental procedure according to the rules of the scientific review board. All participant data were stored in encrypted and password protected files, following the criteria to protect personal health information [39].

2.3. *Protocol*

Participants were selected from the outpatient Unit of Psychiatry of Palermo University Hospital. The subject who met the experimental criteria were contacted, and a meeting was scheduled at the University Hospital. The experimental session was held by a specialized psychiatrist of the University of Palermo. At the beginning of the session, the examiner explained the general goals of the clinical protocol and the procedures to be used, and discussed the patient's doubts and concerns. During the experimental session, two parts were planned: the classical neuropsychological assessment and the VR-based assessment. The presentation order was counterbalanced; half of the patients started the assessment with the VR test, and the other half started with the classic neuropsychological battery. Before the VR-based assessment, patients were trained for the use of a joypad within a virtual environment.

2.4. Neuropsychological Battery

To understand the cognitive profile of the participants, a complete neuropsychological battery was administered. A Mini Mental State Evaluation (MMSE) [40] was administered to assess the general cognitive level. To assess verbal memory, the Digit Span (Digit S) Test [41] was used to assess short-term memory, the Short Story Recall Test and the Paired-Associate Learning Test (PALT) [42] were used to assess long-term memory, and the Corsi Span (Corsi S) and the Corsi Block Task (Corsi BT) [41] were used for the assessment of short- and long-term spatial memory. For analysis of the executive domain, several tests were used: the Frontal Assessment Battery (FAB) [43], a general battery to assess frontal lobe functions, the Trail Making Test (TMT, forms A, B, and B-A) [44] for the assessment of selective attention, and the Tower of London (TOL) Test [45] for the assessment of planning abilities. Also, a Phonemic Fluency (PF) Test and a Semantic Fluency (SF) Test [46] were used. All scores of the tests were corrected for age, education level, and gender where appropriate.

2.5. VMET

The assessment protocol was created with NeuroVR (Version 2.0, Istituto Auxologico Italiano, Milan, Italy), a free software where the user can modify a pre-existing virtual environment by selecting contents from a database of objects (both two- and three-dimensional (2D and 3D)) and videos [47], expanded with NeuroVirtual 3D [48]. The scene was visualized in the player using non-immersive displays. The task took place in a virtual supermarket shown on a laptop screen, and the patient had to use a joypad to move around the environment. All users were trained for virtual reality use in another smaller shop, specifically designed for training purposes. In the virtual supermarket, all products were organized in categories such as beverages, fruits and vegetables, breakfast foods, hygiene products, frozen foods, garden products, and animal products.

2.6. VMET Scoring

Before starting the task, the participants received a shopping list, a sheet with the rules, a map of the supermarket, information about the supermarket (opening and closing times, products on sale, etc.), a pen, and a wristwatch. The examiner read and explained all the information relative to the subject in order to guarantee complete understanding. The VMET test was composed of four main tasks. The first involved purchasing six items (e.g., one product on sale). The second involved asking the examiner information about one item to be purchased. The third involved writing the shopping list 5 min after beginning the test. The fourth involved responding to some questions at the end of the virtual session by using the given materials (e.g., the closing time of the virtual supermarket). The rules that the patients had to follow to complete the task were as follows: (1) they had to execute all the proposed tasks; (2) they could execute all tasks in any order; (3) they could not go to a place unless it was a part of a task; (4) they could not pass through the same passage more than once; (5) they could not buy more than two items per category (looking at the chart); (6) they had to take as little time as possible to complete the exercise; (7) they could not talk to the researcher unless this was a part of the task; (8) they had to go to their "shopping cart" 5 min after the beginning of the task and make a list of all their products. After the explanation of the material, the clinician measured the time, stopping it when the participant said they finished the task. During the assessment, the examiner recorded all the participant's behaviors in the virtual environment according to a predefined form. To better understand the patient's work, the following items were recorded [49]: task failures (total and partial), inefficiencies, strategies, rule breaks, and interpretation failures. When a subtask was not totally completed, a task failure occurred, and the scoring range for total errors was from 11 (all 11 subtasks were correctly done) to 33 (all 11 subtasks were incorrectly done). To calculate the scoring for each task, the scale ranged from 1–3 (1 = the task was performed correctly; 2 = the participant performed part of the task; 3 = the participant totally omitted the task). An inefficiency was deemed a behavior that could prevent the correct execution of the tasks, such as not grouping similar tasks when possible. The general scoring range was from eight (several inefficiencies) to 32 (no inefficiencies), and the scoring scale for each inefficiency was from 1–4 (1 = always; 2 = more than once; 3 = once; 4 = never). To analyze the strategies, 13 behaviors that facilitated carrying out the tasks were evaluated, such as accurate planning before starting a specific subtask. The scoring scale for each strategy was from 1–4 (1 = always; 2 = more than once; 3 = once; 4 = never), and the total score ranged from 13 (good strategies) to 52 (no strategies). A rule break occurred when patients violated one or more of the eight rules listed (e.g., talking with the examiner when not necessary). The scoring scale for each rule break was from 1–4 (1 = always; 2 = more than once; 3 = once; 4 = never) and the total score ranged from eight (a large number of rule breaks) to 32 (no rule breaks). Finally, an interpretation failure occurred when the requirements of particular tasks were misunderstood, for example, when a participant thought that the subtasks all had to be done in the order presented on the information sheet. The general score ranged from three (a large number of interpretation failures) to six (no interpretation failures), and the score for each interpretation failure ranged from 1–2 (1 = yes; 2 = no). Furthermore, for every subtask, we analyzed the following variables: (1) sustained attention; (2) maintaining the correct sequence of the task; (3) remembering the instructions; (4) divided attention; (5) correct organization of the materials; (6) self-corrections; (7) absence of perseverations. The general score ranged from seven (no errors) to 14 (a large number of errors), and the score for each interpretation failure ranged from 1–2 (1 = yes; 2 = no). According to the analysis prosed by Cipresso and colleagues [35], we analyzed three subtasks that they recognized as particularly crucial in the OCD patients' performance: (1) "going to the shopping chart after 5 min"; (2) "buying two products instead of just one"; (3) "going into a specific place and asking the examiner what to buy". These tasks represented a break during the normal task execution because they required a different, confusing, or stopping behavior, which required attention and the elaboration of different information at the same time. These tasks represented a "break in time", a "break in choice", and a "break in social rules", respectively.

2.7. Data Analysis

Data were analyzed with the aid of the statistical software STATA MP-Parallel Edition (Release 14.0, StataCorp LP, College Station, Texas) Orange (Version 3.3.5, Universitas Labacensis, Ljubljana and Portorož, Slovenia) with Python (Version 3.4, Python Software Foundation, Beaverton, OR, USA), JASP (Version 0.7.1.4, University of Amsterdam, Nieuwe Achtergracht, Amsterdam, The Netherlands) [50]. Comparisons between patients and controls were done by using a series of independent sample *t*-tests. To classify data, we used the following approaches [51,52]:

- Logistic regression classification algorithm with ridge regularization;
- Random forest classification using an ensemble of decision trees;
- Support vector machine (SVM), to map inputs to higher-dimensional feature spaces that best separated different classes.

Specifications about the algorithms used for computational data analyses can be found in the seminal article recently published by Zhou and colleagues (https://bmcmedinformdecismak.biomedcentral.com/track/pdf/10.1186/s12911-019-0890-0)

3. Results

Table 3 shows the results of OCD patients compared with normative data. The results showed intact cognitive levels in these patients.

Tables 4 and 5 report the sample descriptive statistics for the neuropsychological battery and the VMET scores, respectively. Table 6 indicates the independent sample *t*-tests comparing OCD patients with controls, for both the executive function domain and the other cognitive domains. On the other hand, Table 7 reports the independent sample *t*-tests for the VMET scoring.

Table 3. Neuropsychological battery in obsessive–compulsive disorder (OCD) patients compared to deficit level in normative sample.

Test	Mean	Standard Deviation	Normative Data
MMSE	26.56	2.68	>18
Frontal Assessment Battery (FAB)	14.97	1.4	>13.5
Trail Making Task A (TMTA)	63.07	23.58	<93
Trail Making Task B (TMTB)	191.93	112.04	<282
Trail Making Task B-A (TMTBA)	129.93	100.27	<186
Phonemic Fluency (PF)	27.38	9.42	>16
Semantic Fluency (SF)	33.69	8.43	>24
Tower of London (TOL)	22.72 [a]	5.45	Not available
Digit Span (Digit S)	5.28	1.09	>3.5
Paired-Associate Learning Test (PALT)	10.84	4.04	>6
Corsi Span (Corsi S)	4.51	0.78	>3.5
Short Story	12.62	5.24	>7.5
Corsi Block Task (Corsi BT)	16.09	8.21	>5.5

[a] Normally considered non-pathological level.

Table 4. Classical neuropsychological battery descriptive statistics (Group 1: OCD patients; Group 2: controls).

Test	Group	*N*	Mean	SD	SE
MMSE	1	29	26.565	2.675	0.497
	2	29	28.532	1.028	0.191
FAB	1	29	14.965	1.403	0.261
	2	20	16.274	0.849	0.190
TMTA	1	29	63.069	23.584	4.379
	2	29	37.632	15.624	2.901
TMTB	1	29	191.310	112.041	20.806
	2	29	95.448	46.144	8.569
TMTBA	1	29	129.931	100.269	18.619
	2	29	58.616	45.439	8.438
PF	1	29	27.379	9.420	1.749
	2	29	41.138	11.192	2.078
SF	1	29	33.690	8.431	1.566
	2	29	48.172	10.275	1.908
TOL	1	29	22.724	5.450	1.012
	2	29	28.448	3.582	0.665
Digit S	1	29	5.284	1.087	0.202
	2	29	6.010	0.847	0.157
PALT	1	29	10.845	4.036	0.749
	2	20	13.072	4.759	1.064
Corsi S	1	29	4.508	0.778	0.144
	2	29	6.345	2.660	0.494
Short Story	1	29	12.621	5.242	0.973
	2	29	14.491	4.454	0.827
Corsi BT	1	29	16.091	8.208	1.524
	2	29	21.239	5.843	1.085

Table 5. Virtual multiple errands test (VMET) descriptive analysis.

VMET	Group	*N*	Mean	SD	SE
Errors	1	29	17.276	2.840	0.527
	2	29	13.897	1.633	0.303
Break in time	1	29	13.379	2.821	0.524
	2	29	11.655	2.844	0.528
Break in choice	1	29	9.655	1.951	0.362
	2	29	8.379	0.979	0.182
Break in social rules	1	29	10.517	2.181	0.405
	2	29	8.793	1.544	0.287
Inefficiencies	1	29	22.552	4.733	0.879
	2	29	24.379	6.439	1.196
Rule break	1	29	21.172	3.733	0.693
	2	29	22.897	5.453	1.013
Strategies	1	29	36.414	7.238	1.344
	2	29	31.793	6.298	1.170
Interpretation failures	1	29	5.207	0.940	0.175
	2	29	5.241	0.872	0.162
Time	1	29	649.448	320.076	59.437
	2	29	595.759	266.793	49.542
Sustained attention	1	29	8.345	1.610	0.299
	2	29	7.759	0.830	0.154
Sequence	1	29	8.241	1.640	0.305
	2	29	7.828	0.805	0.149
Instructions	1	29	8.276	1.623	0.301
	2	29	7.517	0.634	0.118
Divided attention	1	29	10.448	2.667	0.495
	2	29	8.276	1.556	0.289
Organization	1	29	10.483	3.158	0.586
	2	29	8.000	1.282	0.238
Self-corrections	1	29	9.241	1.902	0.353
	2	29	7.759	0.786	0.146
Perseverations	1	29	8.724	1.830	0.340
	2	29	7.414	0.682	0.127

Clearly, both the neuropsychological battery and the VMET scores were able to differentiate patients from healthy controls; however, the mean scores of the neuropsychological battery for both patients and healthy controls were situated in the normal range (Table 3). Because of this fact, it is important to define classification models able to identify mutual information among the variables to make predictions based on a limited number of tests in a clinical setting. To pursue this aim, we ran three different learning algorithms for a cross-validation based on logistic regression, random forest, and support vector machine. Two different models were built: one based on classical neuropsychological tests for executive functions (FAB, TMTA, TMTB, TMTBA, TOL, PF, and SF) and the other one by also adding the previously defined VMET scores. Results of the two cross-validations can be seen in Table 8.

Table 6. Independent sample *t*-Test comparing OCD patients vs. controls for neuropsychological battery. df—degrees of freedom.

Test	*t*	df	*p*	Mean Difference	SE Difference	Cohen's *d*
Executive Function Domain↓						
FAB	−4.061	46.36	<0.001	−1.309	0.322	−1.082
TMTA	4.842	48.61	<0.001	25.437	5.253	1.272
TMTB	4.260	37.23	<0.001	95.862	22.501	1.119
TMTBA	3.489	39.04	0.001	71.315	20.442	0.916
PF	−5.065	54.42	<0.001	−13.759	2.717	−1.330
SF	−5.868	53.94	<0.001	−14.483	2.468	−1.541
TOL	−4.726	48.38	<0.001	−5.724	1.211	−1.241
Other Cognitive Domains↓						
MMSE	−3.696	36.10	<0.001	−1.967	0.532	−0.971
Digit S	−2.836	52.84	0.006	−0.726	0.256	−0.745
PALT	−1.712	36.44	0.095	−2.228	1.301	−0.513
Corsi S	−3.568	32.75	0.001	−1.837	0.515	−0.937
Short Story	−1.465	54.58	0.149	−1.871	1.277	−0.385
Corsi BT	−2.752	50.58	0.008	−5.149	1.871	−0.723

Note. For all tests, variances of groups were not assumed equal.

Table 7. Independent sample *t*-test for VMET index.

VMET	*t*	df	*p*	Mean Difference	SE Difference	Cohen's *d*
Errors	**5.555**	**56.00**	**<0.001**	3.379	0.608	1.459
Break in time	2.318	56.00	0.024	1.724	0.744	0.609
Break in choice	3.148	56.00	0.003	1.276	0.405	0.827
Break in social rules	3.474	56.00	<0.001	1.724	0.496	0.912
Inefficiencies	−1.232	56.00	0.223	−1.828	1.484	−0.323
Rule break	−1.405	56.00	0.166	−1.724	1.227	−0.369
Strategies	2.593	56.00	0.012	4.621	1.782	0.681
Interpretation failures	−0.145	56.00	0.885	−0.034	0.238	−0.038
Time	−0.033	56.00	0.974	−2.117	64.666	−0.009
Sustained attention	1.743	56.00	0.087	0.586	0.336	0.458
Sequence	1.220	56.00	0.228	0.414	0.339	0.320
Instructions	2.344	56.00	0.023	0.759	0.324	0.616
Divided attention	3.789	56.00	<0.001	2.172	0.573	0.995
Organization	3.923	56.00	<0.001	2.483	0.633	1.030
Self-corrections	3.879	56.00	<0.001	1.483	0.382	1.019
Perseverations	3.613	56.00	<0.001	1.310	0.363	0.949

Note. For all tests, variances of groups were assumed equal.

Table 8. Classification table. Three learning algorithms were compared, namely, logistic regression (LogReg), random forest, and support vector machine (SVM). In the first analysis (Panel A), the classifications were run referring to the classic neuropsychological test used for executive functions. In the second analysis (Panel B), VMET scores were added to the classic test for the classification learning algorithm [53–55].

Panel A: Classification with classic neuropsychological test for executive functions.					
Features:	*FAB, TMTA, TMTB, TMTBA, TOL, PF, SF*				
Sampling type:	Stratified 10-fold cross-validation				
Target class:	Average over classes				
Method	**AUC**	**CA**	**F1**	**Precision**	**Recall**
LogReg	0.742	0.741	0.746	0.733	0.759
Random forest	0.817	0.810	0.800	0.846	0.759
SVM	0.783	0.776	0.787	0.750	0.828

Table 8. *Cont.*

Panel B: Classification with classic neuropsychological test for executive functions and the VMET.					
Features	*FAB, TMTB, TMTA, TMTBA, TOL, PF, SF, ERRORS, break in time, break in choice, break in social rules, inefficiencies, rule break, strategies, interpretation failures, sustained attention, sequence, instructions, divided attention, organization, self-corrections, perseverations*				
Sampling type	Stratified 10-fold cross-validation				
Target class	Average over classes				
Method	**AUC**	**CA**	**F1**	**Precision**	**Recall**
LogReg	0.700	0.707	0.702	0.714	0.690
Random forest	0.850	0.845	0.852	0.812	0.897
SVM	0.775	0.776	0.772	0.786	0.759

AUC (area under the receiver operating characteristic (ROC) curve) is the area under the classic receiver operating characteristic curve. CA (classification accuracy) represents the proportion of examples correctly classified. F1 represents the weighted harmonic average of precision and recall (see below). Precision represents the proportion of true positives among all instances classified as positive. In our case, this was the proportion of OCD patients correctly identified as patients and not controls. Recall represents the proportion of true positives among the positive instances in our data, i.e., the number of OCD patients diagnosed as patients instead of controls.

Finally, a classification tree for both models was built based on feature selection, choosing entropy as a measure of homogeneity [56–58] for split selection (Figures 1 and 2). Small circles indicate the ratio of classifications reported inside the rectangle in terms of percentage of correctness in recognizing the specific characteristics. The colors indicate classification as one of the two groups: blue for OCD patients, red for control participants.

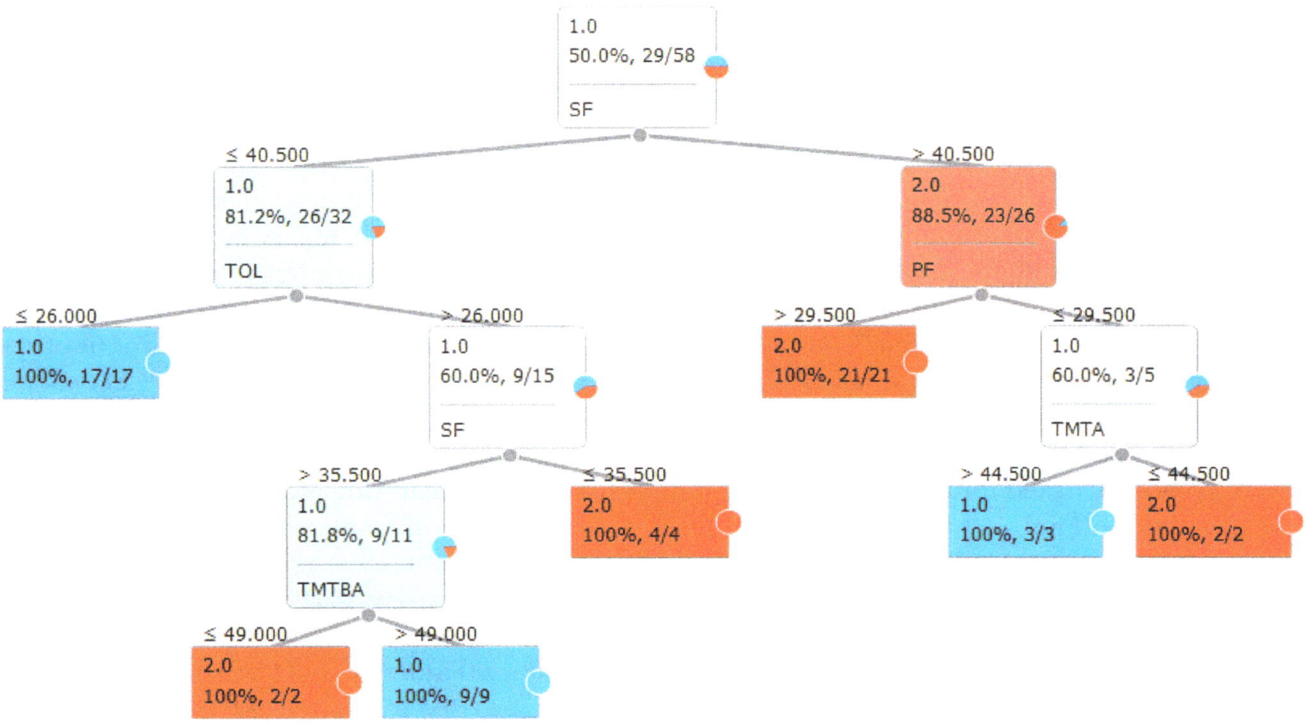

Figure 1. Classification tree using classic neuropsychological test for executive functions.

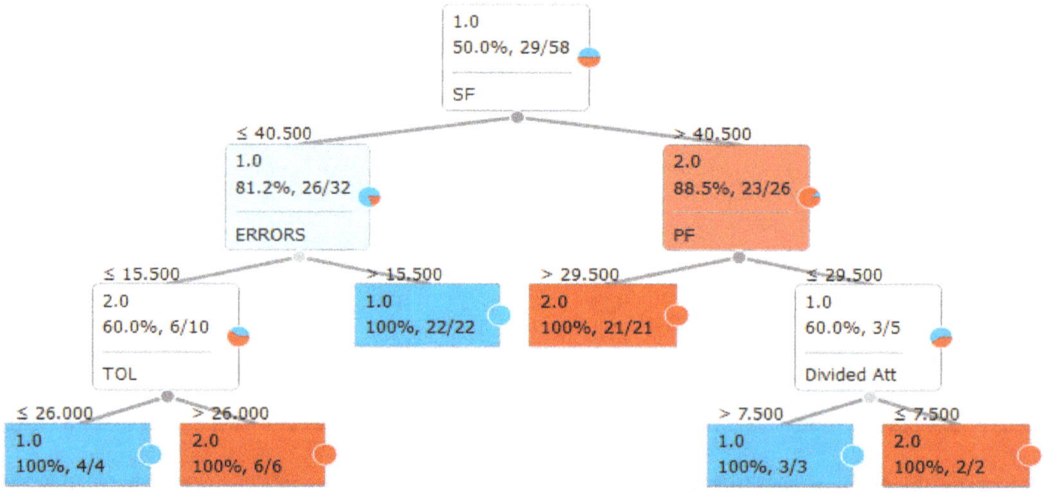

Figure 2. Classification tree using the classic test for executive functions and the virtual multiple errands test (VMET).

4. Discussion

The general aim of this study was twofold. Firstly, we investigated executive functions in OCD patients and controls. To this purpose, we used the virtual version of the multiple errands test and a classic neuropsychological battery. On the other hand, our purpose was to find a method to discriminate the two groups in a better way. Indeed, the goal was scaled on the minimal number of variables possible to pursue an ecological assessment of executive functions with these patients. VMET was demonstrated to be effective in the assessment of several patients, such as for OCD [35], Parkinson's disease [28], and stroke [49]; however, previous studies focused on single scores, such as time, total and partial errors, inefficiencies, and others. In this study, we exploited the multivariate nature of the VMET for the assessment of a particular patient sample (i.e., OCD), where dysfunction is slightly higher than or equal to a normative sample. Thus, this aim shed new light on using multidimensional scaling for understanding the deficits of executive functions.

The results showed a clear difference between OCD patients and the control group, particularly in executive functions, as highlighted in Table 4 for the classic neuropsychological test and Table 5 for most of the VMET scores. However, the complexity of a complete neuropsychological battery with the complete execution of VMET hindered the assessment of these patients. With this limitation in mind, we used computational techniques, which are also used in VR settings [59], to advance our knowledge based on consistent and relevant data from the sample presented. The first strategy was to understand the classification ability within the sample with a supervised machine learning approach. The results showed precision levels between 71.4% and 84.6%, making us confident of the goodness of fit of the model to data. This result is important since, on the one hand, it allowed discriminating OCD patients from healthy subjects (see Table 6, where results are all related to such a domain). On the other hand, at the clinical level, we need to reduce complexity and, consequently, the number of used tests. To this purpose, we opted for a visual classification tree to provide clear indications (based on data) of heuristic choice (Figures 1 and 2). The main and most encouraging result was that, by using both the classic neuropsychological battery and the VMET scores, we obtained a tree based on only five variables (Figure 2), two of which are VMET-based and, not surprisingly, particularly related to OCD patients (errors and divided attention).

Even if the tree based on classic neuropsychological battery (Figure 1) could provide a useful tool for patient evaluation, it does not represent a simple tool to be used for the assessment of executive functions as a whole. On the other hand, the tree based on semantic and phonemic fluency, as well as the TOL and the two VMET scores (Figure 2), can be very useful as a shortened model for the assessment of executive functions in OCD patients.

During the assessment process of OCD, the clinician has many variables to take into account, and deficits of executive function could be one of them. A method which provides clinicians with a simple and complete indication of the best assessment process may have great impact on the clinical process and on rehabilitation.

In clinical neuropsychological assessment, there is always the necessity of integrating different types of information, such as psychometric and ecological data [60,61] in order to better understand the patient's cognitive functioning. VMET is able to play a crucial role in integrating classical neuropsychological tests with ecological settings, especially for executive function assessment in different type of patients.

Making a guided diagnosis for a specific cognitive domain in a specific target of patients is an important goal for both the assessment and the rehabilitation process because it could be able, on one hand, to reduce the time and effort expended by patients and clinicians. On the other hand, a virtual rehabilitation program developed for a targeting assessment would potentially be more personalized and efficient.

This study also had some limitations that could be overcome in future studies. Firstly, the sample size was limited; in a future study, an accurate sample size calculation could be done. Also, adding a clinical control group could be interesting in order to understand the potential of our algorithm for differential diagnosis.

According to our algorithm, the important test for discrimination between OCD patients and controls are fluency, both semantic and phonological, Tower of London, and VMET. This setting would require a minimum amount of time and reduced effort for the clinician during the assessment procedure.

Author Contributions: E.P. wrote the first version of the article. F.L.P. and C.L.C. recruited controls and patients and executed the clinical tests and the experimental protocol. P.C. and E.P. carried out the statistical and computational analyses and wrote the results. G.R. and D.L.B. supervised the scientific and clinical aspects of the study. All authors revised and approved the final version of the manuscript.

References

1. APA. *Diagnostic and Statistical Manual of Mental Disorders-DSM-5*; American Psychiatric Publishing: Arlington, VA, USA, 2013.
2. Garfinkel, P.E.; Goldbloom, D.S. Mental health-getting beyond stigma and categories. *Bull. World Health Organ.* **2000**, *78*, 503. [PubMed]
3. Muller, J.; Roberts, J.E. Memory and attention in Obsessive-Compulsive Disorder: A review. *J. Anxiety Disord.* **2005**, *19*, 1–28. [CrossRef] [PubMed]
4. Morein-Zamir, S.; Craig, K.J.; Ersche, K.D.; Abbott, S.; Muller, U.; Fineberg, N.A.; Bullmore, E.T.; Sahakian, B.J.; Robbins, T.W. Impaired visuospatial associative memory and attention in obsessive compulsive disorder but no evidence for differential dopaminergic modulation. *Psychopharmacology* **2010**, *212*, 357–367. [CrossRef] [PubMed]
5. Burgess, P.W.; Veitch, E.; De Lacy Costello, A.; Shallice, T. The cognitive and neuroanatomical correlates of multitasking. *Neuropsychologia* **2000**, *38*, 848–863. [CrossRef]
6. Chan, R.C.; Shum, D.; Toulopoulou, T.; Chen, E.Y. Assessment of executive functions: Review of instruments and identification of critical issues. *Arch. Clin. Neuropsychol.* **2008**, *23*, 201–216. [CrossRef]
7. Grafman, J.; Litvan, I. Importance of deficits in executive functions. *Lancet* **1999**, *354*, 1921–1923. [CrossRef]
8. Abramovitch, A.; Dar, R.; Schweiger, A.; Hermesh, H. Neuropsychological Impairments and Their Association with Obsessive-Compulsive Symptom Severity in Obsessive-Compulsive Disorder. *Arch. Clin. Neuropsychol.* **2011**, *26*, 364–376. [CrossRef]
9. Lader, M. Current Controversies in the Anxiety Disorders. *BMJ* **1996**, *312*, 984. [CrossRef]
10. Shin, N.Y.; Kang, D.H.; Choi, J.S.; Jung, M.H.; Jang, J.H.; Kwon, J.S. Do organizational strategies mediate nonverbal memory impairment in drug-naïve patients with obsessive-compulsive disorder? *Neuropsychology* **2010**, *24*, 527. [CrossRef]

11. Moritz, S.; Kloss, M.; Von Eckstaedt, F.V.; Jelinek, L. Comparable performance of patients with obsessive–compulsive disorder (OCD) and healthy controls for verbal and nonverbal memory accuracy and confidence: Time to forget the forgetfulness hypothesis of OCD? *Psychiatry Res.* **2009**, *166*, 247–253. [CrossRef]
12. Abramovitch, A.; Abramowitz, J.S.; Mittelman, A. The neuropsychology of adult obsessive–compulsive disorder: A meta-analysis. *Clin. Psychol. Rev.* **2013**, *33*, 1163–1171. [CrossRef] [PubMed]
13. Pauls, D.L.; Abramovitch, A.; Rauch, S.L.; Geller, D.A. Obsessive-compulsive disorder: An integrative genetic and neurobiological perspective. *Nat. Rev. Neurosci.* **2014**, *15*, 410–424. [CrossRef] [PubMed]
14. Penades, R.; Catalan, R.; Rubia, K.; Andres, S.; Salamero, M.; Gasto, C. Impaired response inhibition in obsessive compulsive disorder. *Eur. Psychiatry* **2007**, *22*, 404–410. [CrossRef] [PubMed]
15. Sbordone, R.J.; Purisch, A.D. Hazards of blind analysis of neuropsychological test data in assessing cognitive disability: The role of confounding factors. *Neurorehabilitation* **1996**, *7*, 15–26. [CrossRef]
16. Burgess, N. Spatial memory: How egocentric and allocentric combine. *Trends Cogn. Sci.* **2006**, *10*, 551–557. [CrossRef] [PubMed]
17. Rand, D.; Rukan, S.B.A.; Weiss, P.L.; Katz, N. Validation of the Virtual MET as an assessment tool for executive functions. *Neuropsychol. Rehabil.* **2009**, *19*, 583–602. [CrossRef]
18. Schultheis, M.T.; Himelstein, J.; Rizzo, A.A. Virtual reality and neuropsychology: Upgrading the current tools. *J. Head Trauma Rehabil.* **2002**, *17*, 378–394. [CrossRef]
19. Riva, G. Virtual reality in psychotherapy: Review. *Cyberpsychol. Behav.* **2005**, *8*, 220–230. [CrossRef]
20. Difede, J.; Hoffman, H.G. Virtual reality exposure therapy for World Trade Center post-traumatic stress disorder: A case report. *Cyberpsychol. Behav.* **2002**, *5*, 529–535. [CrossRef]
21. Serino, S.; Triberti, S.; Villani, D.; Cipresso, P.; Gaggioli, A.; Riva, G. Toward a validation of cyber-interventions for stress disorders based on stress inoculation training: A systematic review. *Virtual Real.* **2014**, *18*, 73–87. [CrossRef]
22. Villani, D.; Grassi, A.; Cognetta, C.; Cipresso, P.; Toniolo, D.; Riva, G. The effects of a mobile stress management protocol on nurses working with cancer patients: A preliminary controlled study. *Stud. Health Technol. Inform.* **2012**, *173*, 524–528. [PubMed]
23. Safir, M.P.; Wallach, H.S.; Bar-Zvi, M. Virtual reality cognitive-behavior therapy for public speaking anxiety: One-year follow-up. *Behav. Modif.* **2011**. [CrossRef] [PubMed]
24. Repetto, C.; Gaggioli, A.; Pallavicini, F.; Cipresso, P.; Raspelli, S.; Riva, G. Virtual reality and mobile phones in the treatment of generalized anxiety disorders: A phase-2 clinical trial. *Pers. Ubiquitous Comput.* **2013**, *17*, 253–260. [CrossRef]
25. Serino, S.; Dakanalis, A.; Gaudio, S.; Carrà, G.; Cipresso, P.; Clerici, M.; Riva, G. Out of body, out of space: Impaired reference frame processing in eating disorders. *Psychiatry Res.* **2015**, *230*, 732–734. [CrossRef]
26. Pedroli, E.; Serino, S.; Cipresso, P.; Pallavicini, F.; Riva, G. Assessment and rehabilitation of neglect using virtual reality: A systematic review. *Front. Behav. Neuroscience.* **2015**, *9*, 226. [CrossRef]
27. Cipresso, P.; Pedroli, E.; Serino, S.; Semonella, M.; Tuena, C.; Colombo, D.; Pallavicini, E.; Riva, G. Assessment of Unilateral Spatial Neglect using a free mobile application for Italian clinicians. *Front. Psychol.* **2018**, *9*. [CrossRef]
28. Cipresso, P.; Albani, G.; Serino, S.; Pedroli, E.; Pallavicini, F.; Mauro, A.; Riva, G. Virtual multiple errands test (VMET): A virtual reality-based tool to detect early executive functions deficit in Parkinson's disease. *Frontiers in Behavioral Neuroscience.* **2014**, *8*, 405. [CrossRef]
29. Raspelli, S.; Pallavicini, F.; Carelli, L.; Morganti, F.; Poletti, B.; Corra, B.; Silani, V.; Riva, G. Validation of a Neuro Virtual Reality-based version of the Multiple Errands Test for the assessment of executive functions. *Stud. Health Technol. Inform.* **2010**, *167*, 92–97.
30. La Paglia, F.; La Cascia, C.; Rizzo, R.; Riva, G.; La Barbera, D. Decision Making and Cognitive Behavioral Flexibility in a OCD Sample: A Study in a Virtual Environment. *Stud. Health Technol. Inform.* **2016**, *219*, 53–57.
31. Serino, S.; Pedroli, E.; Keizer, A.; Triberti, S.; Dakanalis, A.; Pallavicini, F.; Chirico, A.; Riva, G. Virtual Reality Body Swapping: A Tool for Modifying the Allocentric Memory of the Body. *Cyberpsychol. Behav. Soc. Netw.* **2016**, *19*, 127–133. [CrossRef]
32. Serino, S.; Mestre, D.; Mallet, P.; Pergandi, J.M.; Cipresso, P.; Riva, G. Do not get lost in translation: The role of egocentric heading in spatial orientation. *Neurosci. Lett.* **2015**, *602*, 84–88. [CrossRef] [PubMed]

33. Ferrucci, R.; Serino, S.; Ruggiero, F.; Repetto, C.; Colombo, D.; Pedroli, E.; Marceglia, S.; Riva, G.; Priori, A. Cerebellar Transcranial Direct Current Stimulation (tDCS), Leaves Virtual Navigation Performance Unchanged. *Front. Neurosci.* **2019**, *13*. [CrossRef] [PubMed]
34. La Paglia, F.; La Cascia, C.; Rizzo, R.; Sideli, L.; Francomano, A.; La Barbera, D. Cognitive rehabilitation of schizophrenia through NeuroVR training. *Stud. Health Technol. Inform.* **2013**, *191*, 158–162. [PubMed]
35. Cipresso, P.; La Paglia, F.; La Cascia, C.; Riva, G.; Albani, G.; La Barbera, D. Break in volition: A virtual reality study in patients with obsessive-compulsive disorder. *Exp. Brain Res.* **2013**, *229*, 443–449. [CrossRef]
36. La Paglia, F.; La Cascia, C.; Rizzo, R.; Cangialosi, F.; Sanna, M.; Riva, G.; La Barbera, D. Cognitive assessment of OCD patients: NeuroVR vs neuropsychological test. *Stud. Health Technol. Inform.* **2014**, *199*, 40–44.
37. Van Bennekom, M.J.; Kasanmoentalib, M.S.; de Koning, P.P.; Denys, D. A virtual reality game to assess obsessive-compulsive disorder. *Cyberpsychol. Behav. Soc. Netw.* **2017**, *20*, 718–722. [CrossRef]
38. Bragdon, L.B.; Gibb, B.E.; Coles, M.E. Does neuropsychological performance in OCD relate to different symptoms? A meta-analysis comparing the symmetry and obsessing dimensions. *Depress. Anxiety* **2018**, *35*, 761–774. [CrossRef]
39. El Emam, K.; Moreau, K.; Jonker, E. How Strong are Passwords Used to Protect Personal Health Information in Clinical Trials? *J. Med. Internet Res.* **2011**, *13*, 13–22. [CrossRef]
40. Magni, E.; Binetti, G.; Bianchetti, A.; Rozzini, R.; Trabucchi, M. Mini-Mental State Examination: A normative study in Italian elderly population. *Eur. J. Neurol.* **1996**, *3*, 198–202. [CrossRef]
41. Monaco, M.; Costa, A.; Caltagirone, C.; Carlesimo, G.A. Forward and backward span for verbal and visuo-spatial data: Standardization and normative data from an Italian adult population. *Neurol. Sci.* **2012**, *34*, 749–754. [CrossRef]
42. Novelli, G.; Papagno, C.; Capitani, E.; Laiacona, M. Tre test clinici di memoria verbale a lungo termine: Taratura su soggetti normali. *Arch. Psicol. Neurol. Psichiatr.* **1986**, *47*, 278–296.
43. Appollonio, I.; Leone, M.; Isella, V.; Piamarta, F.; Consoli, T.; Villa, M.L.; Forapani, E.; Russo, A.; Nichelli, P. The Frontal Assessment Battery (FAB): Normative values in an Italian population sample. *Neurol. Sci.* **2005**, *26*, 108–116. [CrossRef] [PubMed]
44. Amodio, P.; Wenin, H.; Del Piccolo, F.; Mapelli, D.; Montagnese, S.; Pellegrini, A.; Musto, C.; Gatta, A.; Umiltà, C. Variability of trail making test, symbol digit test and line trait test in normal people. A normative study taking into account age-dependent decline and sociobiological variables. *Aging Clin. Exp. Res.* **2002**, *14*, 117–131. [CrossRef]
45. Allamanno, N.; Della Sala, S.; Laiacona, M.; Pasetti, C.; Spinnler, H. Problem solving ability in aging and dementia: Normative data on a non-verbal test. *Ital. J. Neurol. Sci.* **1987**, *8*, 111–119. [CrossRef]
46. Novelli, G.; Papagno, C.; Capitani, E.; Laiacona, M. Tre test clinici di ricerca e produzione lessicale. Taratura su sogetti normali. *Arch. Psicol. Neurol. Psichiatr.* **1986**, *47*, 477–506.
47. Riva, G.; Gaggioli, A.; Grassi, A.; Raspelli, S.; Cipresso, P.; Pallavicini, F.; Vigna, C.; Gagliati, A.; Gasco, S.; Donvito, G. NeuroVR 2-a free virtual reality platform for the assessment and treatment in behavioral health care. *Stud. Health Technol. Inform.* **2011**, *163*, 493–495.
48. Cipresso, P.; Serino, S.; Riva, G. Psychometric assessment and behavioral experiments using a free virtual reality platform and computational science. *BMC Med. Inform. Decis. Mak.* **2016**, *16*(1), 37. [CrossRef]
49. Raspelli, S.; Pallavicini, F.; Carelli, L.; Morganti, F.; Pedroli, E.; Cipresso, P.; Poletti, B.; Corra, B.; Sangalli, D.; Silani, V.; et al. Validating the Neuro VR-based virtual version of the Multiple Errands Test: Preliminary results. *Presence Teleoper. Virtual Environ.* **2012**, *21*, 31–42. [CrossRef]
50. Love, J.; Selker, R.; Marsman, M.; Jamil, T.; Dropmann, D.; Verhagen, A.J.; Wagenmakers, E.J. *JASP (Version 0.7.1.4)[Computer Software]*; JASP Project: Amsterdam, The Netherlands, 2015; Available online: https://jasp-stats.org (accessed on 16 October 2019).
51. Caruana, R.; Niculescu-Mizil, A. An empirical comparison of supervised learning algorithms. In Proceedings of the ACM 23rd International Conference on Machine Learning, Pittsburgh, PA, USA, 25 June 2006.
52. Suthaharan, S. Supervised Learning Algorithms. In *Machine Learning Models and Algorithms for Big Data Classification*; Springer: Berlin, Germany, 2016; pp. 183–206.
53. Wang, S.; Li, D.; Petrick, N.; Sahiner, B.; Linguraru, M.G.; Summers, R.M. Optimizing area under the ROC curve using semi-supervised learning. *Pattern Recognit.* **2015**, *48*, 276–287. [CrossRef]

54. Kotsiantis, S.B.; Zaharakis, I.; Pintelas, P. Supervised Machine Learning: A Review of Classification Techniques. 2007. Available online: https://datajobs.com/data-science-repo/Supervised-Learning-[SB-Kotsiantis].pdfURL (accessed on 16 October 2019).
55. Davis, J.; Goadrich, M. The relationship between Precision-Recall and ROC curves. In Proceedings of the ACM 23rd International Conference on Machine Learning, Pittsburgh, PA, USA, 25 June 2006.
56. Quinlan, J.R. Induction of decision trees. *Mach. Learn.* **1986**, *1*, 81–106. [CrossRef]
57. Wagacha, P.W. Induction of Decision Trees. *Foundations of Learning and Adaptive Systems*. 2003. Available online: https://www.researchgate.net/profile/Peter_Wagacha/publication/283569199_Instance_Based_Learning/links/563f951808ae34e98c4e723a/Instance-Based-Learning.pdfURL (accessed on 16 October 2019).
58. Sheth, N.; Deshpande, A. A Review of Splitting Criteria for Decision Tree Induction. *Fuzzy Syst.* **2015**, *7*, 1–4.
59. Cipresso, P. Modeling behavior dynamics using computational psychometrics within virtual worlds. *Front. Psychol.* **2015**, *6*, 1725. [CrossRef] [PubMed]
60. Macniven, J.A. *Neuropsychological Formulation: A Clinical Casebook*; Springer: Berlin, Germany, 2015.
61. Savage, G. Cognitive Neuropsychological Formulation. In *Neuropsychological Formulation*; Springer: Berlin, Germany, 2016; pp. 221–239.

7

Effectiveness of Psychological Capital Intervention and its Influence on Work-Related Attitudes: Daily Online Self-Learning Method and Randomized Controlled Trial Design

Shu Da, Yue He and Xichao Zhang *

Beijing Key Laboratory of Applied Experimental Psychology, National Demonstration Center for Experimental Psychology Education (Beijing Normal University), Faculty of Psychology, Beijing Normal University, Beijing 100875, China; zhuriyinv@163.com (S.D.); hyue0917@163.com (Y.H.)

* Correspondence: xchzhang@bnu.edu.cn

Abstract: Research on positive psychology intervention is in its infancy; only a few empirical studies have proved the effectiveness and benefits of psychological capital interventions in workplaces. From a practical perspective, a more convenient intervention approach is needed for when organizations have difficulties in finding qualified trainers. This study aims to extend the psychological capital intervention (PCI) model and examine its influence on work-related attitudes. A daily online self-learning approach and a randomized controlled trial design are utilized. A final sample of 104 full-time employees, recruited online, is randomly divided into three groups to fill in self-report questionnaires immediately before (T1), immediately after (T2), and one week after (T3) the intervention. The results indicate that the intervention is effective at improving psychological capital (PsyCap), increasing job satisfaction, and reducing turnover intention. The practical implications for human resource managers conducting a flexible and low-cost PsyCap intervention in organizations are discussed. Limitations related to sample characteristics, short duration effect, small sample size, and small effect size are also emphasized. Due to these non-negligible drawbacks of the study design, this study should only be considered as a pilot study of daily online self-learning PsyCap intervention research.

Keywords: psychological capital intervention; online self-learning; job satisfaction; turnover intention; job embeddedness; cost-effectiveness

---

1. Introduction

In the wake of the influential positive psychology movement, Luthans and Church [1] (p. 59) defined positive organizational behavior (POB) as "the study and application of positively oriented human resource strengths and psychological capacities that can be measured, developed, and effectively managed for performance improvement in today's workplace". Instead of emphasizing relatively stable individual differences such as positive personality traits, POB tries to pay more attention to state-like factors that can be developed through well-designed workplace interventions and targeted managerial policies [2].

It is widely assumed that POB can result in highly valued outcomes that benefit employees and organizations [3]. However, compared to the large number of studies that focus on cross-sectional or longitudinal relationships between POB and outcome variables, empirical research focusing on organizational positive psychology interventions is still in its early stages [4]. In the current situation, we do not have enough evidence to support the supposed benefits of positive psychology interventions in organizations, so it will be difficult for human resource (HR) managers to implement positive psychology practices [5], which reveals the huge gap between the requirements from organizations to promote employees' POB and the tough reality that HR managers do not know how to do so. Therefore, more research on POB interventions is required to not only prove the real value of POBs but also show HR managers how to conduct POB interventions.

Psychological capital (PsyCap), which goes beyond human and social capital, might be one of the most popular POB in both academic and practical fields, and includes four elements: self-efficacy, optimism, hope, and resilience. Many studies have focused on what influences PsyCap and what it leads to [6] but not on PsyCap interventions. Luthans et al. [7] put forward an intervention model, the psychological capital intervention (PCI) model, to operationalize and implement PsyCap interventions. Several intervention studies explore the effectiveness of the PCI model [8–11]. These interventions are typically conducted by training facilitators using face-to-face or online training, lasting one to three consecutive hours, and utilizing a series of group activities, discussions, or individual exercises [7,9,10]. To sum up, previous PsyCap intervention studies have something in common. First, they are mainly based on the PCI model. Second, they provide one to three hours' centralized training and do not clarify trainers' qualifications and styles. Third, they mainly focus on the effectiveness of PsyCap intervention but ignore its influence on other work-related outcomes, except for one study that tests the effect of the intervention on on-the-job performance [9]. Fourth, the participants are all from Western countries.

However, in workplaces, it might be difficult to implement interventions in this way, especially in China. For instance, it is difficult to find a training time suitable for all employees. If employees have emergency work but must attend intervention workshops due to pressure from HR managers, they may be absent-minded or participate halfheartedly, which would counteract the intervention's effect. In addition, if HR managers make employee participation voluntary, it will cost more money for organizations to make all employees get access to the training. Furthermore, small or middle-sized organizations in small or middle-sized cities in China might face difficulties in finding qualified trainers, as the development of psychological talent is uneven in different regions of mainland China.

Therefore, this study aims to extend the PsyCap intervention literature from both a theoretical and a practical perspective in the cultural context of mainland China. First, we add a goal-as-journey metaphor [12] in the hope of supplementing the PCI model. Second, we utilize a daily online self-learning approach to conduct the intervention. Third, based on the conservation of resources (COR) [13,14] theory, we examine the intervention effect on PsyCap and also other work-related attitudes: job satisfaction, turnover intention, and job embeddedness.

1.1. Psychological Capital Development

PsyCap is defined as "an individual's positive psychological state of development and is characterized by: (1) having confidence (self-efficacy) to take on and put in the necessary effort to succeed at challenging tasks; (2) making a positive attribution (optimism) about succeeding now and in the future; (3) persevering toward goals, and when necessary, redirecting paths to goals (hope) in order to succeed; and (4) when beset by problems and adversity, sustaining and bouncing back and even beyond (resiliency) to attain success" [15] (p. 3). It has been argued that these four elements have a synergistic effect and have more influence when combined than separate [7], which indicates that PsyCap, as a core construct, is better than any of its individual components at predicting outcome variables [16].

Moreover, as the concept of PsyCap is derived from the USA and European countries, it is important to illustrate how we can directly apply the PCI model to non-Western countries. From a theoretical perspective, Lomas [17] introduces the idea of positive cross-cultural psychology and argues that most research actually offers a synthesizing perspective on positive psychology, which recognizes universals in the way well-being is sought, constructed, and experienced, but it also allows for extensive variation in the ways these universals are shaped by culture. However, to the best of our knowledge, the literature on cultural differences in PsyCap interventions is still deficient.

From an empirical perspective, although the concept of PsyCap originates from Western countries, it also attracts wide research interest from many other different countries, such as South Africa [18], Ethiopia [19], Russia [20], Korea [21], Malaysia [22], Pakistan [23], China [24–27], and so on, which all support the positive effect of PsyCap. A recent meta-analysis [28] suggests that positive psychology interventions that are conducted in non-Western countries have larger effects than those in Western countries. However, research in the field of positive psychology interventions in non-Western countries is still in its infancy, and researchers urge articles from non-Western countries, even when there is a finding of no effect, as this is likely to reduce the publication bias in positive psychology intervention research [28,29].

Therefore, our study aims to generalize the effectiveness of the PCI model in mainland China in order to enrich the literature on positive psychology interventions in non-Western countries. The theory of the development of the four core constructs of PsyCap has been illustrated in detail in the literature [1,7]. Here, we summarize it briefly.

1.1.1. Developing Efficacy

Bandura's [30] social cognitive theory, especially the content related to efficacy, has been widely accepted. He classified sources of efficacy into four categories: task mastery, modeling or vicarious learning, social persuasion and positive feedback, and physiological or psychological arousal. This became the basic foundation of the PCI model [31]. In the PCI model [7], employees who participate in the intervention will be encouraged to experience and model success through social persuasion and arousal, which will give them a positive emotional experience and confidence to generate plans to achieve their goals. Additionally, combined with hope development, participants can create an imaginary task mastery experience by generating pathways, inventorying resources, and identifying subgoals to enhance and develop their efficacy.

1.1.2. Developing Hope

Positive psychologist Rick Snyder's work [32] is also the foundation of PsyCap development. He identified the basic components of hope as agency, pathways, and goals. In the PCI model, Luthans and colleagues [7] use a three-pronged strategy, embedded in a goal-oriented framework, which included goal design, pathway generation, and overcoming obstacles. First, employees who participate in the intervention will be guided to form personal goals. Then, they will be asked to divide their goals into several steps. After that, they will be encouraged to think about as many different pathways to the goal as possible. They will also consider the obstacles they might face and figure out alternative solutions to overcome them.

In this study, we add a goal-as-journey metaphor as a prime picture to stimulate participants' motivation to put their goals into action. Combining the conceptual metaphor theory [33] and identity-based motivation theory [34], researchers have shown that the journey metaphor implies a feeling of knowing how to achieve a goal and promote identity connection [12].

1.1.3. Developing Resilience

The resilience component in the PCI model [7,35,36] mainly comes from Masten [37], who considered asset factors, risks factors, and influence processes as three major components of resiliency. The most effective strategies to build resilience are based on enhancing assets (e.g., becoming more employable) and proactively avoiding risky, potentially adverse events (e.g., meeting critical deadlines) [37]. In the PCI model, employees who participate in the intervention will be encouraged to write down their reactions to recent feedback at work. Then, they will be guided to form a view of reality and how to react with resilience.

1.1.4. Developing Optimism

Luthans and his colleagues [7] developed the optimism dimension of PsyCap from both an expectancy-value orientation and a positive attributional, explanatory style [38], with realistic optimism being the ideal. They proposed that self-efficacy and hope training can both be used to build optimism [7]. Specifically, employees who participate in PCI will be guided to consider "bad events" as potential challenges or obstacles and then use the methods to develop hope to create alternative pathways to overcome problems.

1.2. Daily Online Self-Learning Method

In order to widely promote PsyCap interventions in China, HR managers should consider more flexible methods of conducting PsyCap interventions. With the development of the Internet, distance education has gradually become more popular. Increasingly, employees have arranged their spare time to allow for self-learning through distance education. Therefore, online self-learning might replace centralized workshops to implement PsyCap intervention in organizations, and intervention time could be divided into several days to allow employees to autonomously choose an appropriate schedule.

In the literature, self-learning modules are defined as self-contained instructional tools that guide learners through a step-by-step process for achieving educational objectives [39]. It contains some basic elements, including clear objectives and directions, materials needed for accomplishing objectives, and post-tests to examine the effectiveness. The instructional materials usually contain text and images that explain what is to be learnt and include examinations for self-assessment after self-learning. Compared with traditional learning methods with teachers, self-learning is a low-cost, nontechnical, and easily and widely disseminated strategy, which is commonly used by students, nurses, and other groups [40–42].

Moreover, traditionally, educators have focused on lecture/discussion teaching methods [43], in which learners are dependent upon instructors and are assumed to have a passive role in learning activities. Lectures assume that all participants are at the same level and learning at the same pace. By contrast, self-learning shows some distinct characteristics. It fosters learners' personal autonomy, allows them to realize self-management, and lets them control the learning process and utilize an independent approach to learning [44].

To conclude, an online-based self-learning intervention approach enjoys the benefits of speed, convenience, cost, and effectiveness, which can be applied to interventions in workplaces to promote employees' PsyCap and further human resource development [8]. Additionally, there have been a number of studies examining the effectiveness of online methods to deliver education, training, and interventions [45]. Therefore, we decided to adopt a daily online self-learning method to implement PsyCap intervention and proposed the following hypothesis:

Hypothesis 1. *The daily online self-learning PsyCap intervention will effectively improve the PsyCap level of employees.*

1.3. Work-Related Attitudes

In this study, we not only pay attention to the effectiveness of an online self-learning method for promoting PsyCap but also assess the influence of PsyCap interventions on work-related attitudes.

According to psychological resource theories such as the conservation of resources (COR) theory [13,14], individuals are motivated to acquire, maintain, and foster the necessary resources, as found in PsyCap, to attain successful performance outcomes. If an individual builds abundant resources including personal, social, economic, etc., he or she will be more capable of overcoming obstacles, enduring severe stress, and seeing accomplishments [46]. PsyCap, as an underlying capacity consisting of four positive psychological resources, is supposed to be beneficial to employees' attitudes and performance [47], both in the workplace and in their personal lives, through the mechanism of improving motivation and cognitive processing.

In addition, plenty of empirical studies have already demonstrated the influence of PsyCap on work-related outcomes, such as satisfaction or commitment [48,49], absenteeism [50], and performance [16]. However, except for Luthans et al. [9], who provided evidence that short training interventions can develop participants' PsyCap and improve on-the-job performance, few intervention studies have attempted to determine whether PsyCap development has a positive influence on employees' work-related attitudes. In this study, we choose job satisfaction, turnover intention, and job embeddedness as outcome indicators of PsyCap intervention, as they are the most common and fundamental work-related attitudes.

1.3.1. Job Satisfaction

Job satisfaction is a multidimensional construct including cognitive and affective perspectives [51]. From the perspective of cognition, job satisfaction is decided by how much an employee's physical and psychological needs are fulfilled by his or her work [52]. From the perspective of affect, job satisfaction is the overall feeling toward different aspects of one's job, including payments, leaders, colleagues, subordinates, environment, content, and so on [53].

With the general expectation of success derived from optimism and the belief in personal abilities derived from efficacy, employees with higher PsyCap show a higher level of job satisfaction, which was also supported by a meta-analysis [54].

1.3.2. Turnover Intention

Employee turnover—employees' voluntary severance of employment ties [55]—has long attracted the attention of scholars and practitioners [56]. March [57] identifies two main factors that affect employees' decision to relinquish their job: movement desirability (or job satisfaction) and ease (or perceived job opportunities). Before actual turnover behavior, employees usually generate initial behavior intentions [58] to indicate their possible choices. Avey, Luthans, and Youssef [59] prove that employees' level of PsyCap has a positive effect on reducing turnover intention as employees with high efficacy are prone to have confidence when facing obstacles (such as high job demands) during work and have higher motivation to overcome difficulties in order to better perform in the organizations; thus, they are more likely to stay within the organization [60].

1.3.3. Job Embeddedness

Mitchell et al. [61] introduce the notion of job embeddedness to elucidate why people stay at an organization or leave. It has been gradually recognized that the motives for leaving and staying are not necessarily opposite to each other [56]. That is, what triggers someone to quit the job (e.g., interpersonal conflicts or low pay) may differ from what makes people want to stay (e.g., opportunities for development or supervisor guidance). Sun et al. [62] prove that, in nurses, high levels of PsyCap are related to higher levels of job embeddedness and performance.

Therefore, we propose the following hypotheses:

Hypothesis 2. *The daily online self-learning PsyCap intervention will effectively promote the job satisfaction of employees.*

Hypothesis 3. *The daily online self-learning PsyCap intervention will effectively reduce the turnover intention of employees.*

Hypothesis 4. *The daily online self-learning PsyCap intervention will effectively promote the job embeddedness of employees.*

2. Materials and Methods

2.1. Participants

Both the recruitment and the intervention in this study were conducted through WeChat, the most popular online social and work connection application in mainland China. The study was open to all who met the following inclusion criteria: 20–60 years old; full-time employees in mainland China; working for five consecutive workdays every week; and ability to access WeChat on a daily basis. Participants were excluded from the study if they had a psychology degree, just in case they were familiar with the procedures of psychology interventions and responded to the surveys in accordance with the purpose of the intervention. We utilized a convenience sampling method, posting the recruitment advertisement on researchers' WeChat. Due to the snowball effect, we recruited 171 participants at time 1 (T1). Due to dropout, 118 participants completed the questionnaire at time 2 (T2), and 110 participants finished the questionnaire at time 3 (T3). After data cleaning, the final sample consisted of 104 participants (Figure 1). The rate of valid data was 60.82%.

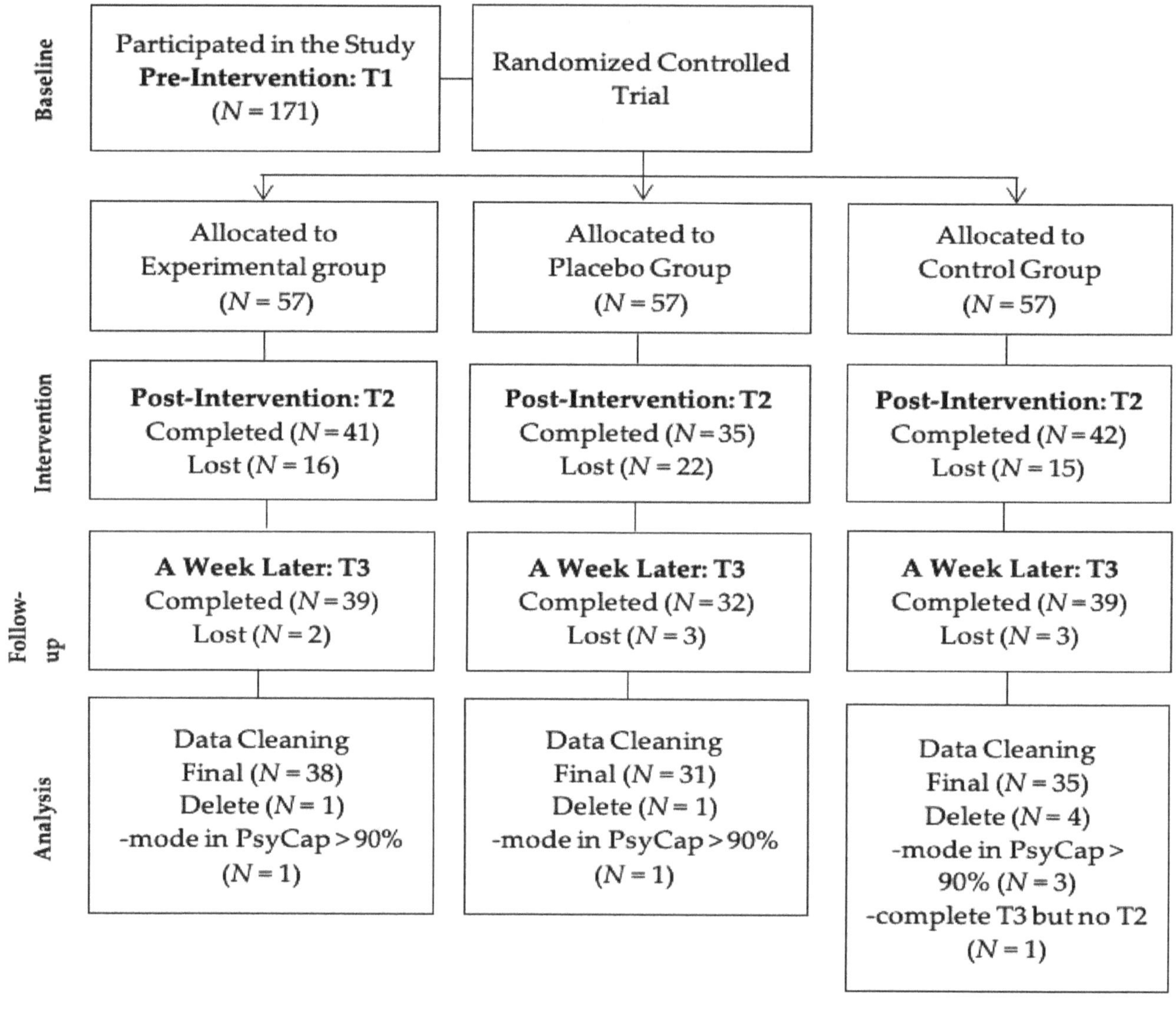

Figure 1. Participants' flowchart.

To check for potential selection bias due to dropout, independent-samples *t* tests and chi-square tests were calculated for the study variables and demographic variables. The results showed that the dropouts—those who did not complete post-intervention and follow-up questionnaires—differed with regard to gender, $\chi^2(1, N = 104) = 7.497$, $p < 0.01$: more men dropped out of the study than women. The means of the study variables (PsyCap, job satisfaction, turnover intention, and job embeddedness) and other demographic variables (age, job tenure, education, and marital status) did not differ significantly.

The final sample included 38 participants in the experimental group, 31 participants in the placebo group, and 35 participants in the control group; 27 of the total participants were men and 77 were women. Most participants (61.5%) were aged between 26 and 35 years, with 31.7% between 36 and 45, 3.8% between 46 and 55, and 2.9% under 25. As for work experience, 47.1% of the participants had five to 10 years of work experience, 38.5% had more than 10 years, and 14.4% had under five years. Regarding education, 57.7% of the participants had a bachelor's degree, 33.7% had a Master's degree, and 8.7% had a high school or associate's degree. Most participants were married (60.6%), while 34.6% were unmarried, 3.8% were divorced, and 1% were remarried. The sample represented a broad range of industries: the three most common were healthcare (20.0%), education (19.0%), and information technology (9.5%). In addition, the three most common job positions in this sample were consultants (12.4%), human resources personnel (11.4%), and managers (11.4%). The complicated composition of the final sample, the small sample size, and the short follow-up appeared to be limitations of our study and are discussed in detail at the end of the study.

2.2. Procedure

All subjects gave their informed consent for inclusion before they participated in the study. The study was conducted in accordance with the Declaration of Helsinki, and the protocol was approved by Institutional Review Board of the Faculty of Psychology, BNU on 19th, December 2019 (201912190084). This study was conducted using a randomized controlled trial (RCT) intervention method.

First, participants voluntarily filled out the informed consent form, baseline questionnaire (T1), and contact information (e-mail address and nickname) online after they viewed the study's advertisement and decided to participate. We made the study purpose, inclusion and exclusion criteria, and rewards very clear in our online recruitment advertisement. It was stated that this was a three-fold survey on occupational psychological health and the lucky participants could get access to a five-day online activity to promote mental health.

Then, after finishing a pretest questionnaire, participants were randomly assigned to one of three WeChat online groups (assigned by e-mail) according to the sequence in which they finished the pretest: experimental group, placebo group, and control group. After creating three WeChat online groups, the researcher again explained the study purpose and procedures to the different groups. Participants in the control group were thanked for participating in a survey on occupational psychological health and told when and how to complete the online questionnaires three times. As to the experimental and placebo groups, the researcher thanked them for their participation in a survey on occupational psychological health and told them that they were the lucky ones, getting an opportunity for a five-day activity to promote mental health. Therefore, it was a single-blind design, as the participants in the placebo group had the same study guidance but a different intervention from the experimental group to ensure that the results were due to the experimental design instead of the organizational process or instruction. Next, interventions were conducted by sending daily online links to reading materials and practice activities to the experimental group and online links to write down self-reflections to the placebo group for five consecutive workdays. The links were sent in the morning, and participants could choose a convenient time to read and complete the content before the next day. Nothing was sent to the control group. On day six, participants in all three groups were sent a posttest questionnaire (T2). One week later, they were sent a follow-up questionnaire (T3). Participants were asked to complete the intervention in a quiet setting, free from interference. It took approximately 20 min to finish the intervention each day. Each participant won 10-yuan rewards every time they completed a survey.

For PsyCap intervention according to the PCI model and journal metaphor, in the links sent to experimental group, participants were asked to read materials or engage in related activities and record their answers to questions (Figure 2).

In order to balance the Hawthorne effect that may exist in an experimental group, we utilized an expressive writing [63] and a self-reflection [64] intervention method for participants in the placebo group. A growing number of studies have found that expressive writing improves a variety of outcomes, ranging from improved immunity and reduced stress [65]. A meta-analysis [66] reveals that emotional disclosure confers lots of benefits, including increased physical and psychological well-being. Therefore, in the links sent to the placebo group, participants were guided to engage in self-reflection and record anything impressive from the work in at least 50 Chinese characters every day.

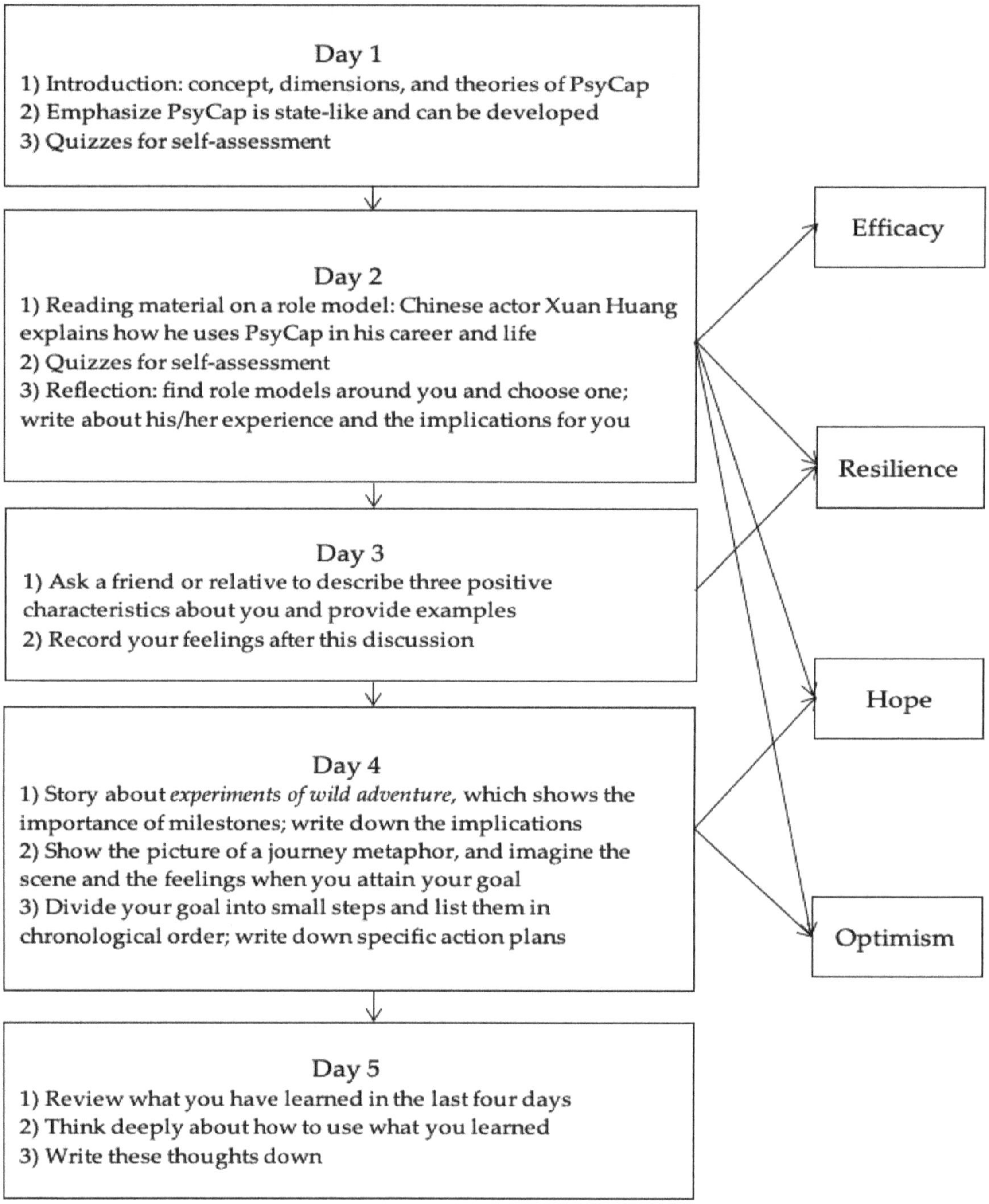

Figure 2. The intervention process.

2.3. Measures

All four study variables (psychological capital, job satisfaction, turnover intention, and job embeddedness) were assessed at all three measurement points (T1, T2, and T3) using the scales outlined below with the exception of demographic variables, which were collected only at T1. All participants created unique nicknames for themselves, which were used to match the three questionnaires. Given that the nicknames might reveal a participant's identity, we stored them in a separate file. All scales showed good internal consistency at all measurement times (see Table 1).

Psychological capital. Psychological capital was measured by the Psychological Capital Questionnaire-24 developed by Luthans, Avolio, and Norman [16], which included four dimensions: efficacy, optimism, hope, and resilience. All 24 items were rated on a six-point Likert scale, ranging from 1 (*completely disagree*) to 6 (*completely agree*).

Job satisfaction was measured by the six-item Overall Job Satisfaction short form developed by Agho, Price, and Mueller [67]. Items such as "I find real enjoyment in my job" and "I am seldom bored with my job" were rated on a five-point Likert scale, ranging from 1 (*completely disagree*) to 5 (*completely agree*).

Turnover intention was measured with a five-item scale used in previous research by Bluedom [68], including items such as "I intend to quit my present job." Respondents indicated their answers on a seven-point Likert scale, ranging from 1 (*completely disagree*) to 7 (*completely agree*).

We used the seven-item version of a global measure of job embeddedness [69]. Items such as "I feel attached to this organization" and "It would be easy for me to leave this organization" were accompanied by responses on a five-point Likert scale, ranging from 1 (*completely disagree*) to 5 (*completely agree*).

Table 1. Correlations and reliability of all study variables.

	1	2	3	4	5	6	7	8	9	10	11	12
1. PC T1	(0.89)											
2. PC T2	0.77 **	(0.91)										
3. PC T3	0.75 **	0.89 **	(0.93)									
4. JS T1	0.61 **	0.51 **	0.53 **	(0.83)								
5. JS T2	0.48 **	0.55 **	0.58 **	0.80 **	(0.89)							
6. JS T3	0.49 **	0.57 **	0.63 **	0.77 **	0.89 **	(0.90)						
7. TI T1	−0.30 **	−0.27 **	−0.31 **	−0.60 **	−0.53 **	−0.57 **	(0.94)					
8. TI T2	−0.30 **	−0.29 **	−0.36 **	−0.59 **	−0.61 **	−0.63 **	0.90 **	(0.93)				
9. TI T3	−0.27 **	−0.28 **	−0.34 **	−0.57 **	−0.59 **	−0.62 **	0.90 **	0.95 **	(0.96)			
10. JE T1	0.21 *	0.20 *	0.26 **	0.51 **	0.58 **	0.55 **	−0.62 **	−0.65 **	−0.64 **	(0.81)		
11. JE T2	0.19	0.24 *	0.27 **	0.49 **	0.60 **	0.59 **	−0.58 **	−0.65 **	−0.66 **	0.87 **	(0.87)	
12. JE T3	0.21 *	0.28 **	0.34 **	0.47 **	0.57 **	0.64 **	−0.62 **	−0.68 **	−0.70 **	0.83 **	0.88 **	(0.83)

Note. T1 = Time 1; T2 = Time 2; T3 = Time 3. PC = Psychological capital; JS = Job Satisfaction; TI = Turnover Intention; JE = Job Embeddedness. Coefficient alphas appear in parentheses along the diagonal. * $p < 0.05$. ** $p < 0.01$.

2.4. Data Analysis

SPSS 18.0 and MPLUS 7.0 were used to analyze the data. Descriptive analyses and tests of baseline homogeneity of three groups were conducted using analysis of variance (ANOVA) and chi-square analysis. Data are available from the corresponding author.

To test the hypotheses, we conducted a mixed between-within ANOVA. The interaction of Group (experimental, placebo, control) × Time (T1, T2, T3) was analyzed to test whether three groups showed different development over time. Moreover, we conducted post hoc analyses to test mean differences between three groups at T1, T2, and T3 with three multivariate analyses of variance (MANOVAs). In addition, analysis of covariance (ANCOVA) was used to support the differences between the groups. Then, pairwise comparisons were conducted to test within-group differences, that is, whether the experimental group showed a significant difference in the study variables at different time points. Partial eta-squared (η_p^2), Cohen's d, and 95% confidence intervals were calculated to examine the effect size. Cohen's d was considered to be a small effect if $d \geq 0.2$, a medium effect if $d \geq 0.5$, and a large effect if $d \geq 0.8$ [70]. Partial eta-squared was interpreted as a small effect if $\eta_p^2 \geq 0.01$, a medium effect if $\eta_p^2 \geq 0.06$, and a large effect if $\eta_p^2 \geq 0.14$ [70].

3. Results

3.1. Preliminary Analysis

The ANOVA indicated that random assignment was truly effective at establishing an initial equivalence between the three groups, as no significant differences were found between their levels of PsyCap ($p = 0.981$). Furthermore, at the baseline, no significant differences were found between groups for job satisfaction ($p = 0.952$); turnover intention ($p = 0.731$); job embeddedness ($p = 0.514$) (Table 2); gender, χ^2 (1, N = 104) = 0.98, $p = 0.612$; age, χ^2 (3, N = 104) = 4.51, $p = 0.608$; job tenure, χ^2 (4, N = 104) = 12.81, $p = 0.118$; education, χ^2 (3, N = 104) = 4.24, $p = 0.644$; or marriage, χ^2 (3, N = 104) = 3.35, $p = 0.764$.

Table 2. Means, standard deviations, and results of the multivariate analyses of variance (MANOVAs) for study variables at pretest (time 1), posttest (time 2), and follow-up (time 3), comparing experimental, placebo, and control groups.

Variable	Group	*M (SD)*			Results of MANOVA					
					Pre (T1)		Post (T2)		Follow-up (T3)	
		Pre (T1)	Post (T2)	Follow-up (T3)	Univariate *F*, *p*-Value	η_p^2	Univariate *F*, *p*-Value	η_p^2	Univariate *F*, *p*-Value	η_p^2
PsyCap	E	4.47 (0.559)	4.66 (0.503)	4.69 (0.513)	0.020, 0.981	0.000	1.673, 0.193	0.032	1.705, 0.187	0.033
	P	4.48 (0.434)	4.52 (0.489)	4.51 (0.473)						
	C	4.49 (0.514)	4.44 (0.554)	4.49 (0.532)						
Job Satisfaction	E	3.29 (0.651)	3.52 (0.632)	3.57 (0.636)	0.048, 0.952	0.001	0.438, 0.646	0.009	0.852, 0.430	0.017
	P	3.34 (0.689)	3.38 (0.812)	3.41 (0.785)						
	C	3.33 (0.795)	3.38 (0.774)	3.35 (0.782)						
Turnover Intention	E	3.65 (1.64)	3.45 (1.51)	3.48 (1.59)	0.314, 0.731	0.006	0.725, 0.487	0.014	0.308, 0.736	0.006
	P	3.69 (1.80)	3.90 (1.63)	3.77 (1.59)						
	C	3.39 (1.69)	3.62 (1.58)	3.52 (1.59)						
Job Embeddedness	E	3.12 (0.471)	3.16 (0.618)	3.15 (0.535)	0.671, 0.514	0.013	0.051, 0.950	0.001	0.172, 0.842	0.003
	P	2.99 (0.899)	3.14 (0.904)	3.15 (0.861)						
	C	3.18 (0.671)	3.20 (0.763)	3.07 (0.609)						

Note. Group: E = Experimental; P = Placebo; C = Control. N (experimental group) = 38; N (placebo group) = 31; N (control group) = 35. df = 2; η_p^2 = partial eta-squared.

3.2. Intervention Effects on PsyCap

To test the first hypothesis, which proposed that the intervention would effectively improve the PsyCap level, we performed a mixed between-within ANOVA. The results revealed a significant interaction effect for groups by time for PsyCap, $F = 3.77$, $df = 3.439$, $p = 0.009$, $\eta_p^2 = 0.069$. As a post hoc analysis, we conducted MANOVA to test whether the three groups differed significantly regarding their means at T1, T2, and T3 for PsyCap. The results indicated no significant differences between the groups (Table 2).

In addition, we conducted ANCOVA for a more rigorous test for mean differences. Specifically, PsyCap data at T2 and T3 were compared among the experimental, placebo, and control groups, controlling for PsyCap at T1. In addition to controlling for the effect of PsyCap at T1, we also included the covariates of age, gender, job tenure, education, and marriage. The results (Table 3) suggested that the group variable was a significant predictor of PsyCap at T2 and T3 ($p < 0.05$), whereas age, gender, job tenure, education, and marriage were not ($p > 0.05$).

Table 3. Analysis of covariance (ANCOVA) controlling for study variables at T1, demographic, and job variables.

Dependent Variable	Variables	*F* Value	*p*-Value	Dependent Variable	Variables	*F* Value	*p*-Value
PsyCap at T2	PsyCap at T1	159.629	<0.001	JS at T2	JS at T1	176.522	<0.001
	Age	0.855	0.357		Age	0.001	0.979
	Gender	0.131	0.719		Gender	0.170	0.681
	Job Tenure	0.144	0.705		Job Tenure	0.221	0.639
	Education	0.589	0.455		Education	0.072	0.790
	Marriage	0.534	0.467		Marriage	0.221	0.639
	Group	4.546	0.013		Group	1.688	0.190
PsyCap at T3	PsyCap at T1	129.698	<0.001	JS at T3	JS T1	140.703	<0.001
	Age	0.028	0.867		Age	0.822	0.367
	Gender	2.132	0.148		Gender	0.018	0.893
	Job Tenure	0.092	0.762		Job Tenure	0.813	0.370
	Education	0.663	0.417		Education	0.298	0.587
	Marriage	0.102	0.750		Marriage	0.095	0.758
	Group	5.018	0.008		Group	3.089	0.050
TI at T2	TI at T1	433.628	<0.001	JE at T2	JE at T1	314.839	<0.001
	Age	0.265	0.608		Age	0.013	0.908
	Gender	2.175	0.144		Gender	0.483	0.489
	Job Tenure	0.125	0.724		Job Tenure	0.398	0.530
	Education	2.470	0.119		Education	0.499	0.482
	Marriage	0.616	0.434		Marriage	0.929	0.338
	Group	5.017	0.008		Group	1.044	0.356
TI at T3	TI at T1	419.907	<0.001	JE at T3	JE at T1	230.827	<0.001
	Age	0.182	0.670		Age	0.037	0.848
	Gender	0.397	0.530		Gender	0.701	0.405
	Job Tenure	0.005	0.943		Job Tenure	0.923	0.339
	Education	1.416	0.237		Education	5.835	0.018
	Marriage	0.044	0.835		Marriage	0.405	0.526
	Group	1.544	0.219		Group	3.028	0.053

Note. T1 = Time 1; T2 = Time 2; T3 = Time 3. JS = Job Satisfaction; TI = Turnover Intention; JE = Job Embeddedness.

We also analyzed whether the means in the experimental group were significantly distinct from T1 to T2 and from T1 to T3, expecting an increase across this time frame. Pairwise comparison showed a significant promotion in PsyCap over time in the experimental group (Figure 3): the means changed significantly from T1 to T2 ($\Delta(T2–T1) = 0.198$, $p = 0.001$, $d = 0.501$, 95% CI [0.044, 0.958]) and from T1 to T3 ($\Delta(T3–T1) = 0.224$, $p = 0.000$, $d = 0.557$, 95% CI [0.098, 1.015]). For the placebo group, pairwise comparison showed no significant distinctions from T1 to T2 ($\Delta(T2–T1) = 0.043$, $p = 1.000$, $d = 0.136$, 95% CI [−0.363, 0.634]) or from T1 to T3 ($\Delta(T3–T1) = 0.03$, $p = 1.000$, $d = 0.098$, 95% CI [−0.4, 0.596]). For the control group, pairwise comparison also showed no significant differences from T1 to T2 ($\Delta(T2–T1) = -0.043$, $p = 1.000$, $d = -0.143$, 95% CI [−0.613, 0.326]) or from T1 to T3 ($\Delta(T3–T1) = 0$, $p = 1.000$, $d = 0$, 95% CI [−0.469, 0.469]). Thus, only the experimental group saw a significant promotion in PsyCap level, which supported Hypothesis 1.

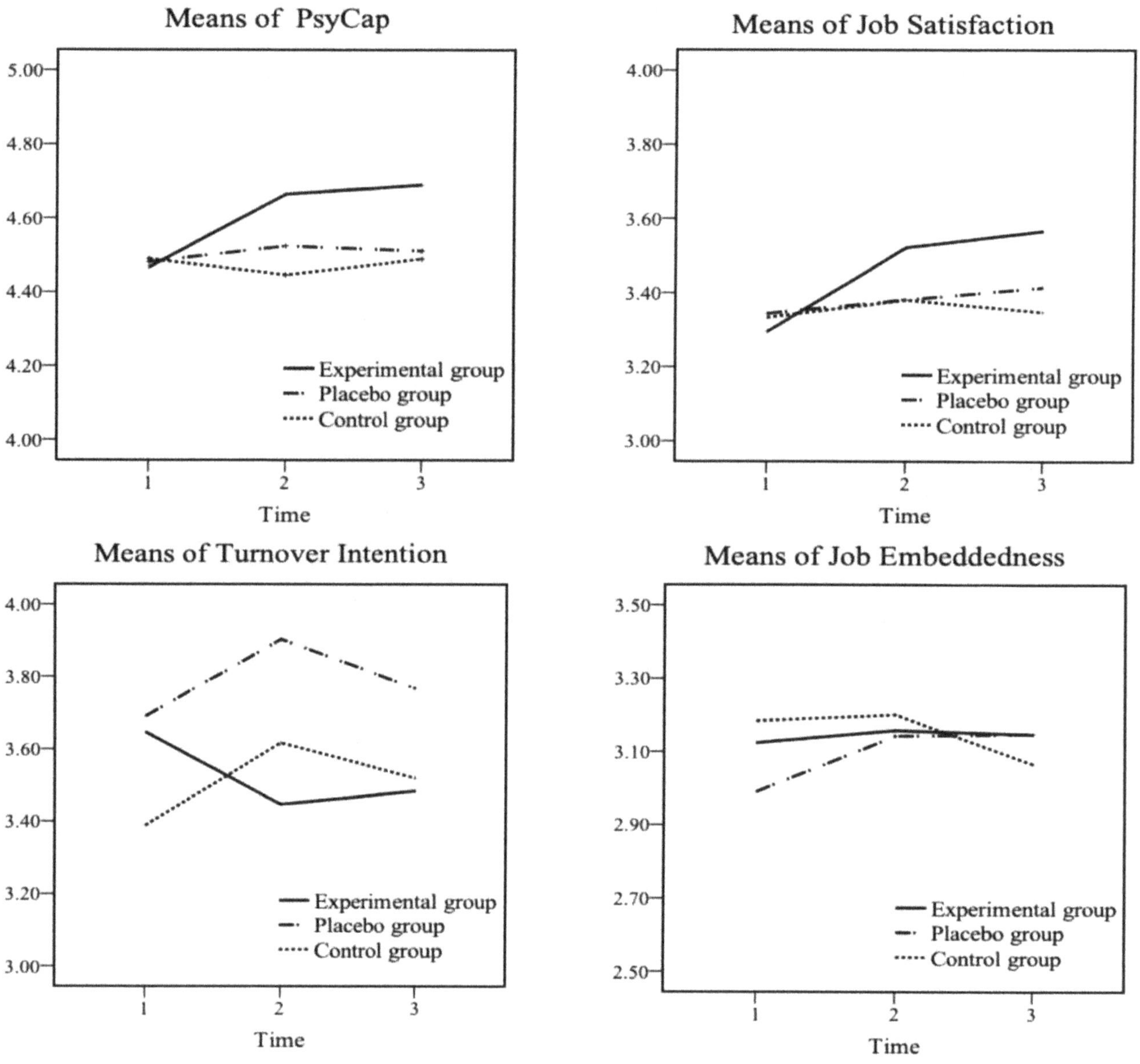

Figure 3. Development of PsyCap and work-related attitudes for the three groups over time.

3.3. Intervention Effects on Work-Related Attitudes

For job satisfaction, the mixed between-within ANOVA showed no significant interaction effect of group by time, $F = 2.015$, $df = 3.643$, $p = 0.101$, $\eta_p^2 = 0.038$. However, the main effect of time was significant, $F = 4.571$, $df = 1.821$, $p = 0.014$, $\eta_p^2 = 0.043$, whereas the main effect of group was not significant, $F = 0.242$, $df = 2$, $p = 0.786$, $\eta_p^2 = 0.005$.

Furthermore, we conducted ANCOVA for a more rigorous test for mean differences of job satisfaction. The results (Table 3) suggested that the group variable was not a significant predictor of job satisfaction at T2 ($p > 0.05$) but was a marginally significant one at T3 ($p = 0.050$), whereas age, gender, job tenure, education, and marriage were not significant at either interval ($p > 0.05$).

In addition, pairwise comparison showed a significant promotion in job satisfaction over time in the experimental group (Figure 3): the means changed significantly from T1 to T2 (Δ(T2–T1) = 0.228, $p = 0.002$, $d = 0.559$, 95% CI (0.1, 1.017)) and from T1 to T3 (Δ(T3–T1) = 0.272, $p = 0.001$, $d = 0.634$, 95% CI (0.173, 1.095)). For the placebo group, pairwise comparison showed no significant differences from T1 to T2 (Δ(T2–T1) = 0.038, $p = 0.642$, $d = 0.092$, 95% CI (−0.406, 0.59)) or between T1 and T3 (Δ(T3–T1) = 0.070, $p = 0.424$, $d = 0.15$, 95% CI (−0.349, 0.648)). For the control group, pairwise comparison showed no significant differences from T1 to T2 (Δ(T2–T1) = 0.048, $p = 0.531$, $d = 0.099$, 95% CI (−0.369, 0.568)) or from T1 to T3 (Δ(T3–T1) = 0.014, $p = 0.082$, $d = 0.037$, 95% CI (−0.431, 0.506)). Thus, the experimental group saw a significant promotion of job satisfaction level, which supported Hypothesis 2.

For turnover intention, the mixed between-within ANOVA showed a marginally significant interaction effect of group by time, $F = 2.476$, $df = 3.607$, $p = 0.052$, $\eta_p^2 = 0.047$. However, neither the main effect of time, $F = 0.842$, $df = 1.804$, $p = 0.422$, $\eta_p^2 = 0.008$, nor the main effect of group, $F = 0.318$, $df = 2$, $p = 0.728$, $\eta_p^2 = 0.006$, was significant.

Nevertheless, the mixed between-within ANOVA revealed a significant interaction effect of group at two time points (T1 and T2), $F = 4.022$, $df = 2$, $p = 0.021$, $\eta_p^2 = 0.074$, which indicated that the effect of the PsyCap intervention on turnover was significant at T2, but the significant effect did not persist to T3. We conducted ANCOVA for a more rigorous test for mean differences of turnover intention; the results shown in Table 3 suggested that the group variable was a significant indicator of turnover intention at T2 ($p < 0.05$) but not at T3 ($p > 0.05$), whereas age, gender, job tenure, education levels, and marriage status were not significant at either interval ($p > 0.05$).

We also analyzed whether the means of turnover intention in the experimental group were significantly changed from T1 to T2, indicating a decrease across this time frame. However, pairwise comparison showed no significant reduction in turnover intention in any of the groups between T1 and T2: the experimental group, Δ(T2–T1) = 0.200, $p = 0.094$, $d = -0.273$, 95% CI (−0.724, 0.179) (Figure 3); the placebo group, Δ(T2–T1) = −0.213, $p = 0.107$, $d = 0.261$, 95% CI (−0.239, 0.761); or control group, Δ(T2–T1) = −0.229, $p = 0.067$, $d = 0.304$, 95% CI (−0.167, 0.776). Although the experimental group did not exhibit a significant reduction in turnover intention level, it appeared that the intervention did prevent participants from increasing turnover intention, which was observed in both the placebo and control groups. Thus, Hypothesis 3 was partially supported.

For job embeddedness, the mixed between-within ANOVA showed a marginally significant interaction effect of group by time, $F = 2.422$, $df = 4$, $p = 0.050$, $\eta_p^2 = 0.046$. However, neither the main effect of time, $F = 1.794$, $df = 2$, $p = 0.169$, $\eta_p^2 = 0.017$, nor main effect of group, $F = 0.067$, $df = 2$, $p = 0.936$, $\eta_p^2 = 0.001$, was significant. Additionally, the ANCOVA results (Table 3) suggested that the group variable was not a significant predictor of job embeddedness at T2 ($p > 0.05$) but was a marginally significant one at T3 ($p = 0.053$), whereas age, gender, job tenure, education, and marriage were not significant at either interval ($p > 0.05$).

In addition, despite expecting an increase over time, pairwise comparison of the means of job embeddedness from T1 to T2 and from T1 to T3 showed no significant promotion in job embeddedness over time in the experimental group (Figure 3): the means did not differ significantly from T1 to T2 (Δ(T2–T1) = 00.034, $p = 0.572$, $d = 0.167$, 95% CI (−0.284, 0.617)) or from T1 to T3 (Δ(T3–T1) = 00.023, $p = 0.712$, $d = 0.109$, 95% CI (−0.341, 0.559)). However, for the placebo group, the pairwise comparison showed significant changes from T1 to T2 (Δ(T2–T1) = 0.152, $p = 0.023$, $d = 0.327$, 95% CI (−0.174, 0.828)) and from T1 to T3 (Δ(T3–T1) = 00.157, $p = 0.027$, $d = 0.305$, 95% CI (−0.196, 0.806)). For the control group, the pairwise comparison showed no significant differences from T1 to T2 (Δ(T2–T1) = 0.016, $p = 0.794$, $d = 0.058$, 95% CI (−0.41, 0.527)) or from T1 to T3 (Δ(T3–T1) = −0.118, $p = 0.075$, $d = -0.281$, 95% CI (−0.752, 0.19)). Thus, the experimental group did not see a significant improvement in job embeddedness. Thus, Hypothesis 4 was not supported.

4. Discussion

The purpose of this study was to extend PsyCap intervention studies from both theoretical and practical perspectives in the cultural context of mainland China, which creatively contributes to the academic literature and, to some degree, organizational practice on PsyCap intervention. Theoretically, we added a goal-as-journey metaphor [12] in the development of the hope dimension. To the best of our knowledge, this is the first attempt to extend the existing content of the PCI model. We believe that it is crucial to generalize the effectiveness of PsyCap interventions [7–10] and at the same time continuously develop previous theories and models. However, it is regrettable that we could not evaluate the effect of adding the journal metaphor into the PCI model. It has been argued by many researchers that the effectiveness of workplace interventions cannot look only at final outcomes [71]. The combination of an outcome evaluation and an evaluation of the process of the intervention is encouraged by researchers [72–74].

Moreover, based on the conservation of resources (COR) theory [13,14], we examined not only the effectiveness of this PsyCap intervention but also its influence on other work-related attitudes: job satisfaction, turnover intention, and job embeddedness. Consistent with both our hypothesis and the results of other studies [8–10], we found that our intervention based on the PCI model significantly enhanced PsyCap. In addition, we found that our intervention significantly improved the job satisfaction level in the experimental group over time, despite the group difference at the three time points not being significant. Moreover, we found that our intervention significantly reduced the turnover intention at time 2, whereas the intervention effect at time 3 was not significant. Specifically, the group difference was significant at time 2, despite the fact that the time difference was not significant. Even though the effect size of PsyCap intervention's influence on job satisfaction and turnover intention was not strong, it still showed a positive tendency in the experimental group, which is worth further exploration.

Contrary to our expectations, we found no significant intervention effects for job embeddedness. However, it is surprising that the time effect for the placebo group was significant, which means that job embeddedness significantly improved in the placebo group from T1 to T3. Although we did not verify our hypothesis on job embeddedness, we proved that job embeddedness and turnover intention are not opposite to each other and may be influenced by different factors in workplaces [56]. The adverse effects of job embeddedness have also been found by other researchers. For example, Nd and Feldman [75] note that employees with high levels of embeddedness are associated with declining social capital development, which is presumably because they have already amassed contacts and felt less need to cultivate new ones. The reason why the intervention effect of PsyCap on job embeddedness was not significant may be related to the different emphases of PsyCap and job embeddedness. Specifically, PsyCap may pay more attention to the difficulties of work and help people to deal with or overcome them, while job embeddedness may pay more attention to the positive sides of work. We consider this a very interesting finding and encourage future studies that examine the relationships between PsyCap and job embeddedness, as well as the influence of PsyCap intervention on this variable and also on some other work-related outcomes.

Practically, a daily online self-learning approach was utilized to conduct the intervention, which provides more possible methods for implementing PsyCap interventions in workplaces. As discussed, ascertaining that a proposed training intervention is effective per se, regardless of the person or method delivering it, is meaningful to the intervention itself and also to practice [10]. A self-learning perspective also challenges the traditional mindset of interventions with trainers. With the development of technology, the Internet can be quite a useful and convenient medium for psychological interventions; it is able to reach a broad audience, flexible and time-efficient, cost-effective, and anonymous [76], which can help organizations and employees overcome different kinds of difficulties, such as getting access to professional trainers, gathering employees together at the same time, increasing more active participation, and so on. Our study encourages future researchers and managers to be creative and flexible when designing targeted and suitable interventions for organizations and employees.

Furthermore, our study enriches the literature of PsyCap interventions in non-Western countries. To the best of our knowledge, this study is one of very few PsyCap intervention studies in Asia or China. According to a previous meta-analysis [29], 78% of the randomized controlled trials on the effectiveness of positive psychology interventions are conducted in Western countries. A systematic review [28] also reveals that research in the field of positive psychology intervention in non-Western countries is still in its infancy, and the low quality of the studies from non-Western countries may explain the larger difference in effect sizes. Therefore, our study utilized a rigid randomized controlled trial design to practice PsyCap intervention in China and may contribute to the field of positive psychology interventions by better comparing the cultural differences between Western and non-Western countries.

4.1. Limitations and Implications for Future Research

Meanwhile, we admit the following limitations of our study. First, our study sample was not confined to one organization. Participants from various occupations were recruited online using a convenience sampling method and then randomly allocated into three groups. Although this makes the sample more representative, this diversity may have produced differences during the intervention, despite no significant difference being found between three groups at T1. Due to differences in organizational culture, the intervention effect may have been contaminated, and the effect of the PsyCap intervention may have been underestimated. This might explain why Hypotheses 2 and 3 were partially supported: employees' job attitudes and behaviors may have been influenced by some organizational elements. Future research should consider conducting the interventions in the same organizations to further test the effect of the PsyCap intervention. In addition, conducting interventions in the same organizations would allow for the addition of some group-level or organization-level outcome variables to verify the intervention effect on both groups and organizations. Furthermore, our use of self-report methods to measure all variables may have led to common method bias; an intervention study confined to one organization could include other measurements, such as objective data, peer assessment, and leader assessment, to reduce such bias.

Second, our study tested all four variables just before (T1), just after (T2), and one week after (T3) the intervention. A one-week follow-up is definitely not strong enough to verify the duration effect of the intervention. When designing the study, as participants are all recruited online, it is difficult to maintain connections with participants for a month or several months, which may lead to a higher rate of dropout. Therefore, we chose a one-week follow-up. However, there is no doubt that one-week follow-up is not sufficient to prove the duration effect of the intervention. Therefore, future research on PsyCap intervention should consider test the duration effect through a longer follow-up, such as one month or three months.

Third, the final sample size was quite small, with about 30 to 40 participants in each group. Based on the limited sample size, it should be stressed that this is at best a pilot study and no valid conclusions can be reached. In addition, more men dropped out of our study than women, which produced a final sample composed mostly of women (68.4%), suggesting gender bias. Future research should attempt to enlarge the sample size and balance the gender distribution. Last but not least, the effect size of some of our significant findings is also small, and it may have resulted from the short duration of the intervention, the small sample size, and so on. Future research could extend the intervention duration to several weeks, as researchers have found that long-term training can lead to a higher effect than short-term training [77].

To conclude, this study has some non-negligible drawbacks to the study design, such as the short follow-up and small sample size, which makes the conclusions of this study unconvincing. Therefore, this study should only be considered as a pilot study [78] of PsyCap intervention, and future research is required to further verify the effectiveness of a daily online self-learning PsyCap intervention and its influence on other work-related variables.

4.2. Practical Implications

Our results are promising for human resources development and management because we demonstrate that a daily self-learning PsyCap intervention over five working days can promote employees' PsyCap level, increase their job satisfaction, and decrease their turnover intention to some degree. Our findings encourage managers to flexibly apply the PCI model to meet the needs of their organizations and employees. Our study also indicates that PsyCap intervention can be provided through daily self-learning materials without professional trainers, which allows employees to receive a PsyCap intervention more conveniently and at lower cost.

5. Conclusions

This study reveals that a daily online self-learning PsyCap intervention is effective at improving PsyCap levels and has positive influences, increasing job satisfaction and decreasing turnover intention. This is another replication and extension of the PCI model and proves the effectiveness of the model on PsyCap and several work-related attitudes.

Author Contributions: Conceptualization, S.D., Y.H., and X.Z.; methodology, S.D., Y.H., and X.Z.; software, S.D.; validation, S.D., Y.H., and X.Z.; formal analysis, Y.H. and X.Z.; investigation, Y.H. and X.Z.; resources, Y.H. and X.Z.; data curation, S.D. and Y.H.; writing—original draft preparation, S.D.; writing—review and editing, S.D., Y.H., and X.Z.; visualization, S.D.; supervision, X.Z.; project administration, X.Z.; funding acquisition, X.Z. All authors have read and agreed to the published version of the manuscript.

Acknowledgments: The authors thank Liuqin Yang for insightful comments on a previous version of this article, Siw Tone Innstrand for the help on manuscript revision, and the two anonymous reviewers and the action editor for their constructive comments during the review process.

References

1. Luthans, F.; Church, A.H. Positive Organizational Behavior: Developing and Managing Psychological Strengths. *Acad. Manag. Exec.* **2002**, *16*, 57–75. [CrossRef]
2. Luthans, F.; Youssef, C.M. Human, Social, and Now Positive Psychological Capital Management: Investing in People for Competitive Advantage. *Organ. Dyn.* **2004**, *33*, 143–160. [CrossRef]
3. Cameron, K.S.; Caza, A. Contributions to the Discipline of Positive Organizational Scholarship. *Am. Behav. Sci.* **2004**, *47*, 731–739. [CrossRef]
4. Meyers, M.C.; Woerkom, M.V.; Bakker, A.B. The Added Value of the Positive: A Literature Review of Positive Psychology Interventions in Organizations. *Eur. J. Work Organ. Psychol.* **2013**, *22*, 618–632. [CrossRef]
5. Cameron, K.S.; Mora, C.; Leutscher, T.; Calarco, M. Effects of Positive Practices on Organizational Effectiveness. *J. Appl. Behav. Sci.* **2011**, *47*, 266–308. [CrossRef]
6. Nolzen, N. The concept of psychological capital: A comprehensive review. *Manag. Rev. Q.* **2018**, *68*, 237–277. [CrossRef]
7. Luthans, F.; Avey, J.B.; Avolio, B.J.; Norman, S.M.; Combs, G.M. Psychological capital development: Toward a micro-intervention. *J. Organ. Behav.* **2006**, *27*, 387–393. [CrossRef]
8. Luthans, F.; Avey, J.B.; Patera, J.L. Experimental Analysis of a Web-Based Training Intervention to Develop Positive Psychological Capital. *Acad. Manag. Learn. Educ.* **2008**, *7*, 209–221. [CrossRef]
9. Luthans, F.; Avey, J.B.; Avolio, B.J.; Peterson, S.J. The Development and Resulting Performance Impact of Positive Psychological Capital. *Hum. Resour. Dev. Q.* **2010**, *21*, 41–67. [CrossRef]
10. Dello Russo, S.; Stoykova, P. Psychological Capital Intervention (PCI): A Replication and Extension. *Hum. Resour. Dev. Q.* **2015**, *26*, 329–347. [CrossRef]
11. Demerouti, E.; van Eeuwijk, E.; Snelder, M.; Wild, U. Assessing the effects of a "personal effectiveness" training on psychological capital, assertiveness and self-awareness using self-other agreement. *Career Dev. Int.* **2011**, *16*, 60–81. [CrossRef]
12. Landau, M.J.; Oyserman, D.; Keefer, L.A.; Smith, G.C. The College Journey and Academic Engagement: How Metaphor Use Enhances Identity-Based Motivation. *J. Personal. Soc. Psychol.* **2014**, *106*, 679–698. [CrossRef] [PubMed]
13. Hobfoll, S.E. Social and psychological resources and adaptation. *Rev. Gen. Psychol.* **2002**, *6*, 307. [CrossRef]
14. Wright, T.A.; Hobfoll, S.E. Commitment, psychological well-being and job performance: An examination of conservation of resources (COR) theory and job burnout. *J. Bus. Manag.* **2004**, *9*, 389–406.
15. Luthans, F.; Youssef, C.M.; Avolio, B.J. *Psychological Capital: Developing the Human Competitive Edge*; Oxford University Press: Oxford, UK, 2007.
16. Luthans, F.; Avolio, B.J.; Avey, J.B.; Norman, S.M. Positive Psychological Capital: Measurement and Relationship with Performance and Satisfaction. *Pers. Psychol.* **2007**, *60*, 541–572. [CrossRef]

17. Lomas, T. Positive cross-cultural psychology: Exploring similarityand difference in constructions and experiences of wellbeing. *Int. J. Wellbeing* **2015**, *5*, 60–77. [CrossRef]
18. Reichard, R.J.; Dollwet, M.; Louw-Potgieter, J. Development of Cross-Cultural Psychological Capital and Its Relationship with Cultural Intelligence and Ethnocentrism. *J. Leadersh. Org. Stud.* **2014**, *21*, 150–164. [CrossRef]
19. Tsegaye, W.K.; Su, Q.; Ouyang, Z. Cognitive adjustment and psychological capital influences on expatriate workers' job performance: An Ethiopian study. *J. Psychol. Afr.* **2019**, *29*, 1–6. [CrossRef]
20. Tatarko, A. Are Individual Value Orientations Related to Socio-Psychological Capital? A Comparative Analysis Data from Three Ethnic Groups in Russia. *Glob. Bus. Issues Ejournal* **2012**. [CrossRef]
21. Jin, C.-H. The effect of psychological capital on start-up intention among young start-up entrepreneurs: A cross-cultural comparison. *Chin. Manag. Stud.* **2017**, *11*, 707–729. [CrossRef]
22. Chua, R.; Ng, Y.L.; Park, M. Mitigating Academic Distress: The Role of Psychological Capital in a Collectivistic Malaysian University Student Sample. *Open Psychol. J.* **2018**, *11*, 171–183. [CrossRef]
23. Nawaz, M.; Bhatti, G.; Ahmad, S.; Ahmed, Z. How Can the Organizational Commitment of Pakistan Railways' Employees Be Improved? The Moderating Role of Psychological Capital. *J. Entrep. Manag. Innov.* **2018**, *14*, 123–142. [CrossRef]
24. Shen, X.; Yang, Y.; Wang, Y.; Liu, L.; Wang, S.; Wang, L. The association between occupational stress and depressive symptoms and the mediating role of psychological capital among Chinese university teachers: A cross-sectional study. *BMC Psychiatry* **2014**, 14. [CrossRef]
25. Li, X.; Kan, D.; Liu, L.; Shi, M.; Wang, Y.; Yang, X.; Wang, J.; Wang, L.; Wu, H. The mediating role of psychological capital on the association between occupational stress and job burnout among bank employees in China. *Int. J. Environ. Res. Public Health* **2015**, *12*, 2984–3001. [CrossRef] [PubMed]
26. Chen, Q.; Kong, Y.; Niu, J.; Gao, W.; Li, J.; Li, M. How Leaders' Psychological Capital Influence Their Followers' Psychological Capital: Social Exchange or Emotional Contagion. *Front. Psychol.* **2019**, 10. [CrossRef] [PubMed]
27. Tian, F.; Shu, Q.; Cui, Q.; Wang, L.-l.; Liu, C.; Wu, H. The Mediating Role of Psychological Capital in the Relationship between Occupational Stress and Fatigue: A Cross-Sectional Study among 1104 Chinese Physicians. *Front. Public Health* **2020**, 8. [CrossRef]
28. Hendriks, T.; Schotanus-Dijkstra, M.; Hassankhan, A.; Graafsma, T.; Bohlmeijer, E.; Jong, J.D. The efficacy of positive psychology interventions from non-Western countries: A systematic review and meta-analysis. *Int. J. Wellbeing* **2018**, *8*, 71–98. [CrossRef]
29. Hendriks, T.; Warren, M.A.; Schotanus-Dijkstra, M.; Hassankhan, A.; Graafsma, T.; Bohlmeijer, E.; Jong, J.D. How WEIRD are positive psychology interventions? A bibliometric analysis of randomized controlled trials on the science of well-being. *J. Posit. Psychol.* **2019**, *14*, 489–501. [CrossRef]
30. Bandura, A. *Self-Efficacy: The Exercise of Control*; W.H. Freeman and Company: New York, NY, USA, 1997.
31. Stajkovic, A.D.; Luthans, F. Social Cognitive Theory and Self-Efficacy: Goin beyond Traditional Motivational and Behavioral Approaches. *Organ. Dyn.* **1998**, *26*, 62–74. [CrossRef]
32. Snyder, C.R. *Handbook of Hope*; Academic Press: San Diego, CA, USA, 2000.
33. Lakoff, G.; Johnson, M. *Metaphors We Live By*; University of Chicago Press: Chicago, IL, USA, 1980.
34. Oyserman, D. Not just any path: Implications of identity-based motivation for disparities in school outcomes. *Econ. Educ. Rev.* **2013**, *33*, 179–190. [CrossRef]
35. Luthans, F.; Vogelgesang, G.R.; Lester, P.B. Developing the Psychological Capital of Resiliency. *Hum. Resour. Dev. Rev.* **2006**, *5*, 25–44. [CrossRef]
36. Luthans, F. The Need for and Meaning of Positive Organizational Behavior. *J. Organ. Behav.* **2002**, *23*, 695–706. [CrossRef]
37. Masten, A.S. Ordinary Magic: Resilience Processes in Development. *Am. Psychol.* **2001**, *56*, 227–238. [CrossRef] [PubMed]
38. Seligman, M.E.P. *Learned Optimism*; Pocket Books: New York, NY, USA, 1998.
39. De Tornyay, R.T.M. *Strategies for Teaching Nursing*, 3rd ed.; Delmar Publishers: Albany, NY, USA, 1987.
40. Khalil, M.K.; Nelson, L.D.; Kibble, J.D. The Use of Self-learning Modules to Facilitate Learning of Basic Science Concepts in an Integrated Medical Curriculum. *Anat. Sci. Educ.* **2010**, *3*, 219–226. [CrossRef]
41. Feldman, M.A.; Case, L. Teaching Child-Care and Safety Skills to Parents with Intellectual Disabilities through Self-learning. *J. Intellect. Dev. Disabil.* **1999**, *24*, 27–44. [CrossRef]

42. Kalbfeld, K. *Evaluating the Effect of a Self-Learning Packet on Change in Nursing Practice*; Southern Connecticut State University: New Haven, CT, USA, 2006.
43. Dougal, J.; Gonterman, R. A Comparison of Three Teaching Methods on Learning and Retention. *J. Nurses Staff Dev.* **1999**, *15*, 205–209. [CrossRef]
44. Candy, P.C. *Self-Direction for Lifelong Learning: A Comprehensive Guide to Theory and Practice*; Jossey-Bass: San Francisco, CA, USA, 1991.
45. Sitzmann, T.; Kraiger, K.; Stewart, D.; Wisher, R. The Comparative Effectiveness of Web-based and Classroom Instruction: A Meta-Analysis. *Pers. Psychol.* **2006**, *59*, 623–664. [CrossRef]
46. Updegraff, J.A.; Taylor, S.E. From Vulnerability to Growth: Positive and Negative Effects of Stressful Life Events. In *Loss and Trauma: General and Close Relationship Perspectives*; Harvey, J., Miller, E., Eds.; Brunner-Routledge: Philadelphia, PA, USA, 2000; pp. 3–28.
47. Peterson, S.J.; Luthans, F.; Avolio, B.J.; Walumbwa, F.O.; Zhang, Z. Psychological Capital and Employee Performance: A Latent Growth Modeling Approach. *Pers. Psychol.* **2011**, *64*, 427–450. [CrossRef]
48. Luthans, F.; Norman, S.M.; Avolio, B.J.; Avey, J.B. The Mediating Role of Psychological Capital in the Supportive Organizational Climate-Employee Performance Relationship. *J. Organ. Behav.* **2008**, *29*, 219–238. [CrossRef]
49. Youssef, C.M.; Luthans, F. Positive Organizational Behavior in the Workplace: The Impact of Hope, Optimism, and Resilience. *J. Manag.* **2007**, *33*, 774–800. [CrossRef]
50. Avey, J.B.; Patera, J.L.; West, B.J. The Implications of Positive Psychological Capital on Employee Absenteeism. *J. Leadersh. Organ. Stud.* **2006**, *13*, 42–60. [CrossRef]
51. Locke, E.A. What is Job Satisfaction? *Organ. Behav. Hum. Perform.* **1969**, *4*, 309–336. [CrossRef]
52. Wolf, M.G. Nedd Gratification Theory: A Theoretical Reformulation of Job Satisfaction/Dissatisfaction and Job Motivation. *J. Appl. Psychol.* **1970**, *54*, 87–94. [CrossRef]
53. Spector, P.E. *Job Satisfaction*; Sage Publications Inc.: New York, NY, USA, 1997.
54. Avey, J.B.; Reichard, R.J.; Luthans, F.; Mhatre, K.H. Meta-Analysis of the Impact of Positive Psychological Capital on Employee Attitudes, Behaviors, and Performance. *Hum. Resour. Dev. Q.* **2011**, *22*, 127–152. [CrossRef]
55. Hom, P.W.; Griffeth, R.W. *Employee Turnover*; South-Western College Publishing: Cincinnati, OH, USA, 1995.
56. Hom, P.W.; Lee, T.W.; Shaw, J.D.; Hausknecht, J.P. One Hundred Years of Employee Turnover Theory and Research. *J. Appl. Psychol.* **2017**, *102*, 530–545. [CrossRef]
57. March, J.G.; Simon, H.A. *Organizations*; Wiley: New York, NY, USA, 1958.
58. Ajzen, I. The Theory of Planned Behavior. *Organ. Behav. Hum. Decis. Process.* **1991**, *50*, 179–211. [CrossRef]
59. Avey, J.B.; Luthans, F.; Youssef, C.M. The Additive Value of Positive Psychological Capital in Predicting Work Attitudes and Behaviors. *J. Manag.* **2010**, *36*, 430–452. [CrossRef]
60. Siu, O.L.; Cheung, F.; Lui, S. Linking Positive Emotions to Work Well-Being and Turnover Intention among Hong Kong Police Officers: The Role of Psychological Capital. *J. Happiness Stud.* **2015**, *16*, 367–380. [CrossRef]
61. Mitchell, T.R.; Holtom, B.C.; Wee, T.W.; Sablyskyi, C.J.; Erez, M. Why People Stay: Using Job Embeddedness to Predict Voluntary Turnonver. *Acad. Manag. J.* **2001**, *44*, 1102–1121. [CrossRef]
62. Sun, T.; Zhao, X.W.; Yang, L.B.; Fan, L.H. The Impact of Psychological Capital on Job Embeddedness and Job Performance among Nurses: A Structural Equation Approach. *J. Adv. Nurs.* **2012**, *68*, 69–79. [CrossRef]
63. Lu, Q.; Dong, L.; Wu, I.H.C.; You, J.; Huang, J.; Hu, Y. The impact of an expressive writing intervention on quality of life among Chinese breast cancer patients undergoing chemotherapy. *Supportive Care Cancer* **2018**, *27*, 165–173. [CrossRef] [PubMed]
64. Dolev-Amit, T.; Rubin, A.; Zilcha-Mano, S. Is Awareness of Strengths Intervention Sufficient to Cultivate Wellbeing and Other Positive Outcomes? *J. Happiness Stud.* **2020**, 1–22. [CrossRef]
65. Smyth, J.M. Written Emotional Expression: Effect Sizes, Outcome Types, and Moderating Variables. *J. Consult. Clin. Psych.* **1998**, *66*, 174–184. [CrossRef]
66. Frattaroli, J. Experimental Disclosure and Its Moderators: A Meta-Analysis. *Psychol. Bull.* **2006**, *132*, 823–865. [CrossRef] [PubMed]
67. Agho, A.O.; Price, J.L.; Mueller, C.W. Discriminant Validity of Measures of Job Satisfaction, Positive Affectivity and Negative Affectivity. *J. Occup. Organ. Psychol.* **1992**, *65*, 185–195. [CrossRef]
68. Bluedom, A.C. A Unified Model of Turnover from Organizations. *Hum. Relat.* **1982**, *35*, 135–153. [CrossRef]

69. Crossley, C.D.; Bennett, R.J.; Jex, S.M.; Burnfield, J.L. Development of a Global Measure of Job Embeddedness and Integration into a Traditional Model of Voluntary Turnover. *J. Appl. Psychol.* **2007**, *92*, 1031–1042. [CrossRef]
70. Cohen, J. *Statistical Power Analysis for the Behavioral Sciences*, 2nd ed.; Erlbaum: Hillsdale, NJ, USA, 1988.
71. Innstrand, S.T.; Christensen, M. Healthy Universities. The development and implementation of a holistic health promotion intervention programme especially adapted for staff working in the higher educational sector: The ARK study. *Promot. Educ.* **2018**, *27*, 68–76. [CrossRef]
72. Nielsen, K.; Randall, R. The importance of employee participation and perceptions of changes in procedures in a teamworking intervention. *Work Stress* **2012**, *26*, 91–111. [CrossRef]
73. Abildgaard, J.S.; Saksvik, P.Ø.; Nielsen, K. How to measure the intervention process? An assessment of qualitative and quantitative approaches to data collection in the process evaluation of organizational interventions. *Front. Psychol.* **2016**, *7*, 1380. [CrossRef]
74. Nielsen, K. Organizational occupational health interventions: What works for whom in which circumstances? *Occup. Med. Oxf.* **2017**, *67*, 410–412. [CrossRef] [PubMed]
75. Ng, T.W.H.; Feldman, D.C. The Effects of Organizational Embeddedness on Development of Social Capital and Human Capital. *J. Appl. Psychol.* **2010**, *95*, 696–712. [CrossRef] [PubMed]
76. Leykin, Y.; Thekdi, S.M.; Shumay, D.; MuÒoz, R.; Riba, M.; Dunn, L. Internet interventions for improving psychological welå being in psycho oncology: Review and recommendations. *Psychè Oncol.* **2012**, *21*. [CrossRef]
77. Walter, N.; Nikoleizig, L.; Alfermann, D. Effects of Self-Talk Training on Competitive Anxiety, Self-Efficacy, Volitional Skills, and Performance: An Intervention Study with Junior Sub-Elite Athletes. *Sports* **2019**, *7*. [CrossRef] [PubMed]
78. Hertzog, M.A. Considerations in determining sample size for pilot studies. *Res. Nurse Health* **2008**, *31*, 180–191. [CrossRef]

8

Working Alliance Inventory for Online Interventions-Short Form (WAI-TECH-SF): The Role of the Therapeutic Alliance between Patient and Online Program in Therapeutic Outcomes

Rocío Herrero [1,2], Mª Dolores Vara [1,2], Marta Miragall [2,3,*], Cristina Botella [2,3], Azucena García-Palacios [2,3], Heleen Riper [4,5], Annet Kleiboer [4] and Rosa Mª Baños [1,2,6]

1 Polibienestar Research Institute, University of Valencia, 46022 Valencia, Spain; ro.herrero.09@gmail.com (R.H.); m.dolores.vara@uv.es (M.D.V.); banos@uv.es (R.M.B.)
2 CIBERObn Physiopathology of Obesity and Nutrition, Instituto de Salud Carlos III, 28029 Madrid, Spain; botella@uji.es (C.B.); azucena@uji.es (A.G.-P.)
3 Department of Basic and Clinical Psychology and Psychobiology, Faculty of Health Sciences, Jaume I University, 12071 Castellon de la Plana, Spain
4 Department of Clinical, Neuro and Developmental Psychology, Vrije Universiteit, 1081-BT Amsterdam, The Netherlands; h.riper@vu.nl (H.R.); a.m.kleiboer@vu.nl (A.K.)
5 Department of Research and Innovation GGZ InGeest, Amsterdam University Medical Center, 1081-HJ Amsterdam, The Netherlands
6 Department of Personality, Evaluation and Psychological Treatment, Faculty of Psychology, University of Valencia, 46010 Valencia, Spain
* Correspondence: miragall@uji.es

Abstract: Background: Therapeutic alliance (TA) between the patient and therapist has been related to positive therapeutic outcomes. Because Internet-based interventions are increasingly being implemented, a tool is needed to measure the TA with Internet-based self-guided programs. The Working Alliance Inventory for online interventions (WAI-TECH-SF) was adapted based on the WAI Short Form (Hatcher & Gillaspy, 2006). The objectives of this study were: (1) to analyse the psychometric properties of the WAI-TECH-SF; (2) to explore the differences in the WAI-TECH-SF scores according to different categories of the sample; and (3) to analyse whether the WAI-TECH-SF can predict therapeutic outcomes and satisfaction with the treatment. Methods: 193 patients diagnosed with depression were included and received blended Cognitive-Behavioural Therapy. Measures of preferences, satisfaction, and credibility about the treatment, TA with the online program, depressive symptoms, and satisfaction with the treatment were administered. Results: An exploratory factor analysis revealed a one-dimensional structure with adequate internal consistency. Linear regression analyses showed that the WAI-TECH-SF predicted changes in depressive symptoms and satisfaction with the treatment. Conclusions: WAI-TECH-SF is a reliable questionnaire to assess the TA between the patient and the online program, which is associated with positive therapeutic outcomes and satisfaction with the treatment.

Keywords: therapeutic alliance; online interventions; therapeutic outcomes; satisfaction with the treatment

---

1. Introduction

Evidence shows that the therapeutic alliance (TA) (also called the working alliance) has a relevant influence on therapeutic outcomes [1]. Several meta-analyses have found that TA is moderately associated with better treatment outcomes in face-to-face therapy [1,2], regardless of the therapeutic framework or patient characteristics, among other aspects [3]. One of the most widely used definitions of TA was proposed by Bordin [4], who considered the alliance to be a general factor with three interrelated components: (a) the degree of mutual trust, collaboration, and acceptance between the therapist and the patient (i.e., the bonds); (b) the agreement between patient and therapist about specific tasks or activities (i.e., the tasks); and (c) the agreement about the therapeutic objectives (i.e., the goals).

Currently, the ways of delivering therapeutic interventions are changing. The need for psychological support is growing, and the dominant model of psychotherapy from past centuries—individual, face-to-face, and long-lasting—is not likely to fulfil this need [5]. New forms of treatment delivery are emerging to face the challenge of providing well-established interventions that can reach a wider population. This situation has promoted the development of interventions that require less therapist involvement, such as Internet-based Interventions (IBIs) [6], either self-guided or hybrid therapeutic approaches (blended treatments) where face-to-face sessions are combined with online therapy [7]. Well-established evidence shows that interventions fully or partially delivered through the Internet (especially those based on Cognitive Behavioural Therapy (CBT)) are effective in treating different psychological disorders [8–10] and can be as effective as face-to-face therapy [11,12]. Therefore, IBIs are attractive and useful strategies to be applied by healthcare professionals in clinical settings [13]. Nevertheless, different questions have arisen about the therapeutic process, such as what happens to the TA when there is no direct contact with a therapist or when this contact is scarce [14].

The research triggered by this question has focused on the development and validation of measures that make it possible to assess the TA in IBIs and study of the role of the TA in predicting the therapeutic outcomes. To measure the TA in therapies supported by technological tools, most studies have used an adapted version of the Working Alliance Inventory (WAI) [15], or its short form (WAI-SF) [16,17]. In general, evidence supports the relevance of the TA in IBIs, because similar TA scores have been found for face-to-face therapy and IBIs [3,14,18–20], as well as similar moderate effect sizes for the relationship between TA and therapeutic outcomes [3,21]. In this regard, Clarke et al. [22] conducted a qualitative and quantitative study to examine the TA in the context of a self-guided intervention, and they found that TA is high even when the intervention does not involve human support. In addition, the study highlighted that a positive TA, in terms of feeling a meaningful connection and working collaboratively, is relevant for engaging with the intervention. In this study, they did not find a relationship between TA and therapeutic outcomes. Nonetheless, a systematic review showed an effect of TA on anxiety and depressive outcomes, pointing out that higher levels of TA were related to better clinical outcomes [23]. Recently, Gómez-Penedo et al. [24] explored the reliability and validity of the WAI-SF in guided IBIs, taking into account the relational aspects involved in this type of intervention (e.g., therapist support, online program). In this validation, the bond subscale was adapted to refer to the acceptance and trust between the patient and the therapist who supported him/her in the online program. Results of the WAI for guided Internet interventions (i.e., WAI-I) showed a two-factor solution ("tasks-goals" and "bonds") with adequate internal consistency and external validity in a sample of patients with mild to moderate depression. Moreover, patients with higher scores on TA were more satisfied with the intervention after the treatment.

The approach used to carry out the adaptation of the WAI questionnaire in previous studies consisted of following Bordin's classic conceptualization [4], considering the three dimensions of TA (bond, tasks, and goals) and making slight modifications in the statements [25,26]. This approach has been questioned by some authors, who suggest that the definition of TA is grounded in the specific characteristics of face-to-face therapy and, therefore, is not necessarily the same in other formats [27,28]. In fact, in the WAI adapted to measure the TA between the patients and the virtual environment, where the word "therapist" was replaced by "virtual environment", the three dimensions proposed by Bordin [4] did not arise in the exploratory factor analysis, and only one general dimension was found [25]. By contrast, Kiluk et al. [29] conducted an adaptation of the 36-item original version of the WAI called WAI-Tech, which was designed to measure the TA between cocaine-dependent patients and the online program, and it showed similar psychometric properties to the original scale (i.e., the WAI). In this adaptation, items were slightly adapted by replacing "therapist" with "online program", and items corresponding to the bond subscale were reworded to preserve comprehension. Results showed lower scores on the bond subscale, and the total scores on WAI-Tech were not associated with the change in therapeutic outcomes. However, findings are limited due to the small sample size and the absence of factor analysis to analyse the psychometric properties in this study.

Thus, the TA developed by the patients in IBIs and, specifically, in blended Cognitive-Behavioural Therapy (CBT) (i.e., combining individual face-to-face sessions with online intervention modules) has not been completely understood. The present study was conducted in the context of a European project called "e-Compared", in which previous findings found that only therapist-rated TA (but not patient-rated TA) was predictive of changes in depression scores during a blended treatment in a sample of 73 patients [30]. Thus, it seems that technology is a third factor in the relationship between patient and therapist, which adds more complexity to this relationship. Hence, the need to measure not only the relationship between the patient and the therapist, but also between the patient and the technology, is undeniably relevant due to the growing emergence of IBIs.

Previous studies have found that individuals have the ability to form a bond and be open with an online application [28]. However, it is still important to develop a reliable questionnaire and explore whether the three-dimensional structure proposed originally for face-to-face therapy is also maintained in the TA with the online program in self-guided IBIs where there is hardly any interaction with a therapist or person supporting the intervention. To do so, an adaptation of the WAI-SF to measure the TA with the online program was carried out. An exploratory factor analysis was conducted in order to avoid determining the psychometric structure a priori, given the controversial structure of TA when technologies are involved (e.g., the structure was uni-dimensional in Miragall et al. [25]; or bi-dimensional in Gómez-Penedo et al. [24]). In addition, other potential variables influencing the TA with the online program were explored, as well as the capacity of the TA with the online program to predict therapeutic outcomes and satisfaction with the treatment. The study was conducted in a sample of depressive patients who were receiving a self-guided IBI in the context of the National Health Systems of different European countries.

Hence, the aims of this study were: (1) to analyse the psychometric structure of the WAI-TECH-SF, a questionnaire designed to assess the TA between the patient and the online program in a self-guided IBI; (2) to explore whether there are differences in WAI-TECH-SF scores based on sex, age-range, level of education, initial severity of depression, preference for any of the treatments offered, and expectations about and credibility of the treatment; and (3) to explore whether higher WAI-TECH-SF scores predict the therapeutic outcomes (i.e., change in depressive symptom scores) and satisfaction with the treatment.

2. Materials and Methods

2.1. Participants

One-hundred and ninety-three patients took part in this study (ages ranging from 19 to 69 years old: $M = 40.44$ years old; $SD = 12.79$; 64.2% women). Patients were recruited as part of the clinical trial conducted in the e-Compared Project (EU-HEALTH.2013 N.603098). The sample was composed of European citizens diagnosed with depression in either primary or specialized care. Regarding their nationalities, 38.2% of the sample were from Germany, 16.2% from Sweden, 12.0% from Spain, 9.8% from France, 8.4% from the Netherlands, 6.3% from the UK, and 2.1% from Switzerland. Patients were excluded if they were under 18 years old, had serious psychiatric comorbidity, or did not have access to a computer or the Internet. All the patients were diagnosed with depression using the MINI. In terms of their symptoms, 10.9% of the sample showed mild symptoms of depression, 33.2% showed moderate symptoms, 36.8% showed moderate–severe symptoms, and 19.2% showed severe depressive symptomatology. In addition, 50.8% of the sample had some suicidal risk, and 61.1% of the sample had a comorbid diagnosis, such as panic disorder, agoraphobia, or social phobia. Regarding their educational level, 56.0% of the sample had a high educational level, 31.6% had a medium educational level, and 12.4% had a low educational level. All participants were informed about the study and gave their informed consent before the beginning of the trial, in accordance with the Declaration of Helsinki. The study was approved by the corresponding ethical committee in each country: (a) France: Comité de protection des personnes, Ile de France V (15033-n° 2015-A00565-44); (b) Germany: Ethik Kommison DGPsychologie, Universitat Trier (MB 102014); (c) The Netherlands: METC VUMC (2015.078); (d) Poland: Komisja ds. Etyki Badan Naukowych (10/2014); (e) Spain: Comision Deontologica/Comite Ético de Investigacion en Humanos de la Universidad de Valencia (H1414775276823); (f) Sweden: Regionala etikprovningsnamnden (2014/428-31); (g) Switzerland: Kantonale Ethikkomission Bern (001/2015); (h) UK: NRES Committee London-Camden and King's Cross (15/LO/0511). All participants received a blended CBT (bCBT) for depression.

2.2. Intervention

All the e-Compared project interventions combined individual CBT delivered through face-to-face sessions and online sessions [31]. The interventions received by patients had some variations across the countries, but followed common guidelines [31]. In this regard, the ratio between the number of face-to-face sessions and the number of online modules varied across countries, but at least 1/3 of the sessions were face-to-face (i.e., between 3 and 10 sessions), and at least 1/3 were online (i.e., between 6 and 10 sessions). As a minimum, the bCBT included modules of psychoeducation, cognitive restructuring, behavioural activation, and relapse prevention. In addition, each country site was able to include additional components, such as mindfulness, coping skills training, or problem solving, but these additional components could not make up more than a quarter of the total intervention. Face-to-face sessions were provided by: (1) licensed CBT therapists in mental health care; (2) CBT therapists in training under the supervision of an experienced licensed CBT therapist in mental health care; (3) a licensed psychologist with a CBT orientation in primary care; or (4) psychologists in training under the supervision of a licensed psychologist with a CBT orientation in primary care. All of them were trained in how to deliver the blended treatment. Each face-to-face session lasted around 20–60 min (i.e., 45–60 min in specialized care and 20–45 min in primary care), while the online session lasted for as long as the patients took to read each session. A summary of the intervention components and the online vs. face-to face ratio are shown in Table 1.

Table 1. Overview of blended treatment applied in each country.

					Mandatory Modules				Additional Modules		
Country	**Platform**	**Duration**	**Online/ Face-to-Face Sessions**	**Session Sequence**	**PE**	**CR**	**BA**	**RP**	**Problem Solving**	**Physical Exercise**	**Other**
Netherlands	Moodbuster	20 weeks	10/10	Alternate	X	X	X	X	X	X	
France	Moodbuster	16 weeks	8/8	Alternate	X	X	X	X	X	X	
Poland	Moodbuster	6–10 weeks	6/6	Alternate	X	X	X	X	X	X	
United Kingdom	Moodbuster	11 weeks	5/6	Alternate	X	X	X	X	X	X	
Switzerland	Deprexis	18 weeks	9/9	Alternate	X	X	X	X	X	X	X
Sweden	Itherapi	12 weeks	8/4	Alternate	X	X	X	X			
Spain	Smiling is fun	10 weeks	8/3	1-4-1-4-1	X	X	X	X			X
Germany	Moodbuster	10–13 weeks	10/5	Alternate	X	X	X	X	X	X	

Notes. PE = Psychoeducation; CR = Cognitive restructuring; BA = Behavioral activation; RP = Relapse prevention.

2.3. Measures

Working Alliance Inventory applied to Internet (WAI-TECH-SF) is an adaptation of the WAI-SF [16] elaborated by the authors. It is a 12-item self-report questionnaire designed to assess the TA with the online program in a self-guided IBI, with responses rated on a seven-point Likert scale, ranging from 1 (never) to 7 (always). The questionnaire was designed to cover the same structure as the original scale, with three dimensions: (1) therapeutic goals (items 1, 2, 8, 10), (2) tasks (items 4, 6, 10, 11), and (3) bonds (items 3, 5, 7, 9). The total score ranges from 12 to 84. The mean and standard deviation for this sample were $M = 57.84$ and $SD = 16.39$. Details about its adaptation appear in the "Procedure" section. The questionnaire was administered at post-assessment.

Patient Health Questionnaire-9 (PHQ-9; [32]) is a nine-item mood module that can be used to screen and diagnose patients with depressive disorders. It is based directly on the criteria for major depressive disorder in the Diagnostic and Statistical Manual of Mental Disorders (4th ed.) [33] and its accuracy for screening to detect major depression has been demonstrated [34]. The nine items are each scored on a 0–3 scale, with the total score ranging from 0–27 and higher scores indicating more severe depression. The means and standard deviations for this sample were M = 15.50 and SD = 4.63 (pre-assessment), and M = 9.05 and SD = 5.35 (post-assessment). The PHQ-9 has been shown to have good psychometric properties [35]. The questionnaire was administered at pre- and post-assessment. In this study, Cronbach's alphas ranged from 0.73 to 0.87.

International Neuropsychiatric Interview (MINI 5.0; [36]) is a structured diagnostic interview based on the Diagnostic and Statistical Manual of Mental Disorders (DSM-IV) and on International Classification of Diseases (ICD-10) criteria. The MINI has been translated into 65 languages and is used for both clinical and research practices. The full MINI. 5.0, with the exception of Anorexia Nervosa, Bulimia Nervosa, and Antisocial Personality Disorder, was used to provide a diagnosis at pre-assessment.

Preference for Treatment Questionnaire (ad-hoc instrument) was used to assess participants' treatment preference from the options of bCBT, TAU, or no preference. Specifically, the following question was asked: "If you had the chance to choose your depression treatment, which one would you prefer to receive?"

Credibility and Expectancy Questionnaire (CEQ; [37]) was used to assess the prior predisposition of patients to the proposed intervention. The scale consists of six items divided into two factors: expectancy (with three questions rated on a 10-point scale, ranging from 1 to 9) and credibility (with one question rated on a 10-point scale and two questions rated on a 1–100% scale). The means and standard deviations for this sample were $M = 17.59$ and $SD = 4.92$ (in a scale ranging from 3 to 27) and $M = 19.32$ and $SD = 5.15$ (on a scale ranging from 3 to 27) for expectancy and credibility, respectively. In this study, Cronbach's alphas were 0.86 for expectancy and 0.72 for credibility.

Client Satisfaction Questionnaire (CSQ-8; [38]) was used to assess patients' satisfaction with the treatment. This questionnaire has been translated into multiple languages, and it is used to measure global patient satisfaction. The questionnaire consists of eight items rated on a four-point scale, with total scores ranging from 8 to 32. The mean and standard deviation for this sample were $M = 25.39$ and $SD = 5.00$. The questionnaire was administered at post-assessment. In this study, Cronbach's alpha was 0.92.

2.4. Procedure

An adaptation of the patient version of the WAI-SF [16] was carried out following the recommendations of Hambleton and Patsula [39]. Thus, the purpose of the WAI-TECH-SF is to measure agreement about goals, tasks, sense of trust, comfort, and bonding between the patient and the "online program". To this end, the sentences on the current scale were kept as similar as possible to the originals, but "my therapist" or therapy was replaced with "online program". Items are displayed in Table 2.

Table 2. Psychometric properties of the WAI-TECH: Descriptive statistics and factorial loadings with a one-factor structure using Maximum Likelihood.

	Skewness Index	Kurtosis Index	M (SD)	λ	h^2
Item 1. As a result of these sessions using the program____ I am clearer as to how I might be able to change.	−0.72	0.19	5.11 (1.40)	0.76	0.58
Item 2. What I am doing with the program____ gives me new ways of looking at my problem.	−0.56	−0.40	4.89 (1.48)	0.88	0.77
Item 3. I believe that I am a good candidate for the program___.	−0.50	−0.36	4.84 (1.46)	0.86	0.74
Item 4. The program___ and I collaborate on setting goals for my therapy.	−0.47	−0.58	4.72 (1.72)	0.87	0.75
Item 5. The program___ and I respect each other.	−0.57	−0.28	4.94 (1.58)	0.84	0.70
Item 6. The program____ and I are working towards mutually agreed upon goals.	−0.64	−0.05	5.04 (1.48)	0.85	0.72
Item 7. I feel that the program____ appreciates me.	−0.35	−0.75	4.44 (1.74)	0.81	0.67
Item 8. The program___ and I agree on what is important for me to work on.	−0.62	−0.25	4.84 (1.61)	0.85	0.73
Item 9. I feel the program_____ cares about me even when I do things that he/she does not approve of.	−0.61	−0.13	4.91 (1.62)	0.89	0.78
Item 10. I feel that the things I do with the program___ will help me to accomplish the changes that I want.	−0.48	−0.34	4.56 (1.54)	0.87	0.76
Item 11. The program___ and I have established a good understanding of the kind of changes that would be good for me.	−0.66	−0.07	4.93 (1.55)	0.91	0.83
Item 12. I believe the way that the program___ and I are working with my problem is correct.	−0.52	−0.43	4.62 (1.65)	0.89	0.79

Notes. λ = Factor loading; h^2 = Communalities.

Once the WAI-TECH-SF had been adapted, it was applied in the context of the e-Compared European project to the participants receiving the bCBT. All the patients in the project were recruited in the National Health Systems of the countries involved, in either primary or specialised care. Their status was assessed with the MINI interview, performed by a clinical psychologist. If patients met the inclusion criteria, they were allocated to one of two conditions: bCBT or Treatment as Usual (TAU) (for more details about the trial, see Kleiboer et al. [31]). All participants filled out the PHQ-9 questionnaire to assess the severity of their depressive symptoms and their preference for the intervention ("blended", "TAU", or "no preference"), and the CEQ scale was used to assess the patients' expectations and credibility with regard to the intervention offered. For the purposes of the current study, only participants allocated to the bCBT condition were taken into account, given that those in the TAU condition did not receive any therapeutic support online. Once patients had finished the intervention, they were assessed again on their depressive symptoms, their satisfaction with the treatment through the CSQ scale, and their TA with the self-guided IBIs using the WAI-TECH-SF.

2.5. Data Analyses

All statistical analyses were performed using the SPSS v.26 (IBM Corp, Armonk, NY, USA). The percentage of missing values in the WAI-TECH-SF, PHQ-9, and CEQ scores ranged from 0% to 1.6%. After testing that the values were missing at random using Little's MCAR test ($p > 0.05$), they were imputed using the Expectation–Maximization Algorithm method [40]. Then, several analyses were carried out. First, to analyse the psychometric properties of the WAI-TECH-SF, skewness and kurtosis were analysed to check the normality of the data [41]. Kaiser-Meyer-Olkin (KMO), and Barlett's Test of Sphericity was used to ensure the suitability of the data for performing an Exploratory Factor Analysis (EFA). Parallel Analysis [42] was applied using a macro for SPSS [43] to determine the number of factors retained in the EFA. Then, to explore the factor structure of the WAI-TECH-SF, an EFA was conducted using a Maximum Likelihood estimation extraction method because the data were normally distributed [41]. Internal consistency of the total score was assessed using Cronbach's alpha coefficient [44].

Second, preliminary analyses were conducted to ensure that relevant assumptions of t-tests, ANOVAs, and simple/multiple regression (i.e., normality, linearity, homoscedasticity, and absence of multicollinearity) were met. Third, independent-samples t-tests and one-way ANOVAs were performed to find out whether there were significant differences in the WAI-TECH-SF scores based on sex, age range (18–34 vs. 35–49 vs. > 50), level of education (low vs. medium vs. high), initial severity on PHQ scores (mild vs. moderate vs. moderate–severe vs. severe), preference for any of the treatments offered (no preference vs. blended vs. TAU), and expectations and credibility towards the treatment. Expectations and credibility scores were categorized as low (Mean–1 Standard deviation), medium (Mean), and high (Mean + 1 Standard deviation). *T*-values are reported as absolute values.

Fourth, two simple linear regression analyses (using the enter method) were carried out to study whether the WAI-TECH-SF scores predicted the changes in PHQ scores and satisfaction with the treatment. PHQ scores were calculated using the differences between post- and pre-assessment scores (Post–Pre). Thus, positive values indicated an increase in depression symptoms, whereas negative values indicated a decrease in depression symptoms.

Finally, a power analysis was conducted to determine whether the present study was adequately powered with our sample size ($N = 193$) (the sample size of this study was initially calculated for testing the hypothesis that bCBT was not inferior to the TAU condition on the primary clinical outcome (i.e., symptoms of depression at 3 months after baseline) (see Kleiboer et al. [31]), but not for the secondary outcomes and analyses). Using G*power v. 3.1.9.743 (Heinrich-Heine-Universität, Düsseldorf, Germany), we calculated power for: (1) an omnibus *F*-test "Fixed effects, one-way"; (2) a *t*-test "Differences between two independent means"; and (3) an omnibus *F*-test "Lineal multiple regression: fixed model, R^2 deviation from zero". An effect size of $f = 0.20$ or $f^2 = 0.12$ was used because there is still limited data in this field and $d = 0.40$ is a standard in Psychology, according to Brysbaert [45]. Results indicated that the current study had 69.38% and 62.68% power for one-way ANOVAs with three and four groups, respectively, 75.49% for the *t*-test, and 99.77% for the regression analyses with one predictor to detect a medium effect size at $p < 0.05$.

3. Results

3.1. Psychometric Properties of WAI-TECH-SF

A random percentage of missing values was found, with Little's MCAR test, $\chi^2(33) = 14.27$, $p = 0.998$, ranging from 0 to 1.6% per item. Consequently, items' missing values were imputed using the Expectation–Maximization Algorithm method [38]. The sample's normality was assumed because skewness values were $<|2|$, and kurtosis values were $<|7|$ [46,47] (see Table 2). The KMO value was (0.96), and the Barlett's Test of Sphericity value, $\chi^2(66) = 2587.26$, $p < 0.001$, showed that it was appropriate to perform a factor analysis. Regarding the number of factors to extract, Parallel Analysis [40] showed that one factor had to be retained because only one factor had an eigenvalue (raw data eigenvalue = 9.08) greater than the eigenvalue at the 95th percentile for randomly generated data (95th percentile eigenvalue = 1.53) [48]. Factorial rotation with one dimension was performed using the Maximum Likelihood extraction method, which showed that one dimension explained 73.49% of the total variance. The factorial solution showed that all the items had minimum factor loadings and communalities above ≥ 0.30 (see Table 2). Cronbach's alpha coefficient for the WAI-TECH-SF was high for the overall scale ($\alpha = 0.97$). We analysed the item–total correlation, and the exclusion of any item increased the alpha value for the overall scale.

3.2. Differences in WAI-TECH-SF Scores According to Socio-Demographic Variables, Initial Severity on PHQ Scores, Preference for the Treatment Offered, and Expectations and Credibility towards the Treatment

Table 3 shows the means and standard deviations of the WAI-TECH-SF scores according to sex, age-range, level of education, initial severity on PHQ scores, preference for any of the treatments offered, and expectations and credibility towards the treatment.

Table 3. Descriptive statistics of WAI-TECH scores in each category.

	Independent-Sample *t*-Tests/ One-Way ANOVAs	N	M	SD
Total sample		193	57.84	16.39
Sex	$t(191) = 0.49$, $p = 0.627$, *Cohen's d* $= 0.07$			
Men		69	57.07	15.03
Women		124	58.27	17.14
Age-range	$F(2,190) = 1.75$, $p = 0.177$, $\eta^2_p = 0.02$			
18–34		70	55.84	17.09
35–49		66	57.12	17.89
>50		57	61.13	13.14
Level of education	$F(2,190) = 3.21$, $p = 0.043$, $\eta^2_p = 0.03$			
Low		24	50.01	15.06
Medium		61	58.72	15.52
High		108	59.08	16.80
Initial severity of depression	$F(3,189) = 0.91$, $p = 0.436$, $\eta^2_p = 0.01$			
Mild		21	59.86	16.16
Moderate		64	56.50	16.38
Moderate-Severe		71	56.66	17.03
Severe		37	61.27	15.27
Preference for any of the treatments offered	$F(2,190) = 1.66$, $p = 0.194$, $\eta^2_p = 0.02$			
No preference		54	57.78	16.09
Blended		107	56.48	16.09
Treatment as usual		32	62.47	17.53
Expectations towards the treatment	$F(2,182) = 1.34$, $p = 0.265$, $\eta^2_p = 0.02$			
Low		34	59.84	15.41
Medium		119	57.92	16.82
High		32	53.47	16.18
Credibility towards the treatment	$F(2,183) = 0.57$, $p = 0.567$, $\eta^2_p = 0.01$			
Low		28	56.38	17.19
Medium		126	57.13	15.65
High		32	60.34	19.13

Independent-sample *t*-tests and one-way ANOVAs showed that there were no significant differences in the WAI-TECH-SF scores based on sex, age-range, initial severity of depression, preferences for any of the treatments offered, expectations about the treatment, and credibility of the treatment. However, there were significant differences in the WAI-TECH-SF scores based on the level of education. Patients with high (vs. low) education levels achieved higher scores on the WAI-TECH-SF, $p = 0.042$.

An Exploratory Multiple Regression Analysis: Socio-Demographic Variables, Initial Severity on PHQ Scores, Preference for the Treatment Offered, and Expectations and Credibility towards the Treatment as Predictors of WAI-TECH-SF Scores

Given the number of potential predictor variables of the WAI-TECH-SF, we also carried out a stepwise linear regression in order to analyse the explained variance by each variable. To do so, age, expectations, and credibility towards the treatment were maintained as continuous variables. Categorical predictor variables (i.e., level of education, initial severity of depression, and preference for any of the treatments offered) were transformed into dummy-coded variables. The reference category was "low" (vs. "medium and high") for level of education, "mild" (vs. moderate, moderate-severe and severe) for initial severity of depression, and "no preference" (vs. blended and treatment as usual) for preference for any of the treatments offered.

Results of this regression analysis showed that two models were significant. The first model included level of education ($\beta = 0.180$, $t = 2.462$, $p = 0.015$) as a positive significant predictor of the WAI-TECH-SF scores. This model was significant, $F(1,181) = 6.059$, $p = 0.015$, explaining 2.7% of the variance.

The second model included level of education ($\beta = 0.205$, $t = 2.798$, $p = 0.006$) and age ($\beta = 0.167$, $t = 2.279$, $p = 0.024$) as positive significant predictors of the WAI-TECH-SF scores. This model was significant, $F(2,181) = 5.696$, $p = 0.004$, explaining 4.9% of the variance.

3.3. Predictive Models: Are Changes in PHQ Scores and Satisfaction with the Treatment Predicted by WAI-TECH-SF Scores?

The model where changes in PHQ pre-post intervention scores were predicted by WAI-TECH-SF scores was statistically significant, $F(1,188) = 14.42$, $p < 0.001$, explaining 6.7% of the variance. Higher scores on the WAI-TECH-SF predicted a greater decrease in depression symptoms.

Similarly, the model in which satisfaction with the treatment was predicted by the WAI-TECH-SF scores was statistically significant, $F(1,187) = 185.53$, $p < 0.001$, explaining 49.7% of the variance. Higher scores on the WAI-TECH-SF predicted higher scores on satisfaction with the treatment (see Table 4).

Table 4. Simple linear regressions of change in PHQ scores and satisfaction with the treatment.

	R	R^2	B	SE	β	t
Change in PHQ scores						
Constant			0.186	1.829		
WAI-TECH	0.268	0.072	−0.115	0.030	−0.268	3.797 ***
Satisfaction with the treatment						
Constant			12.929	0.951		13.601 ***
WAI-TECH	0.707	0.497	0.214	0.016	0.707	13.621 ***

Note. Statistical significance: *** $p < 0.001$. PHQ-9 = Patient Health Questionnaire-9; WAI-TECH-SF = Working Alliance Inventory applied to Internet–Short Form. R = Multiple Correlation Coefficient; R^2 = Coefficient of determination; R^2 Change = Coefficient of determination Change; B = Unstandardized coefficient; SE = Standard Error; β = Beta coefficient; t = t statistic (estimated coefficient divided by its own SE).

4. Discussion

The objectives of this study were: (1) to explore the psychometric structure of a questionnaire (i.e., the WAI-TECH-SF) designed to assess the TA with an online program in a self-guided IBI and CBT program in a sample of depressive patients in the context of the National Health Systems of different European countries; (2) to analyse whether there were differences in the WAI-TECH-SF scores based on several socio-demographic variables, initial symptoms of depression, preference for any of the treatments offered, and expectations and credibility towards the treatment; and (3) to study the capacity of the WAI-TECH-SF scores to predict the therapeutic outcomes (i.e., changes in depressive symptoms) and satisfaction with the treatment.

With regard to the psychometric properties of the WAI-TECH-SF, a unidimensional structure emerged in the EFA that accounted for 73.49% of the explained variance. All the factors had high factor loadings, and the overall scale had excellent internal consistency. This unidimensionality is in line with the structure found in the validation of the WAI applied to virtual and augmented reality (WAI-VAR, [25]). However, this structure is inconsistent with the three-dimensional structure of Bordin's [4] theory and the original validation of the WAI-SF carried out by Hatcher and Gallispy [16] to measure TA in the face-to-face context, distinguishing three separate factors: tasks, goals, and bonds. Nevertheless, the structure of this questionnaire is controversial because a bi-factorial structure has also been found in other validations of the WAI, such as in Gómez-Penedo et al. [24], who found that in the TA with the therapist in IBIs, "goals and tasks" loaded in the same factor, whereas "bond" loaded in a separate factor. According to our findings, a three-dimensional structure cannot be assumed a priori in the context of IBIs. More specifically, in the case of the TA with an online program during a self-guided IBI, the theoretical distinction between task, goals, and bond with the online program was not psychometrically significant, and a single factor could explain the majority of the explained variance of the TA between the patient and the online program. However, these results should be interpreted with caution because IBIs are continuously evolving, and a more personalized treatment that uses algorithms to provide personalized feedback or set individualized goals or tasks depending on the emotional state or unique needs of each patient throughout the treatment could generate a more differentiated factorial structure of the WAI-TECH-SF.

Another possible explanation for the structure of the WAI-TECH-SF is related to the fact that the TA with the online programs is highly complex, and merely replacing the words is not sufficient to capture the subtle differences in these different kinds of TA. In other words, perhaps the dimensions of the questionnaire should be completely reframed [28]. In this regard, Henson, Peck, and Torous [49] developed the Digital-WAI (D-WAI), a six-item self-report questionnaire based on Bordin's three dimensions, but aligned with the purpose of smartphone-based interventions (e.g., "bond" is aimed at measuring the capacity of the app to offer support and guide them through challenges). More recently, Miloff et al. [50] adopted this approach of developing novel items and validated the Virtual Therapist Alliance Scale (VTAS), which assesses the three components of the TA with virtual therapists in an automated exposure treatment format for patients with fear of spiders. Two factors emerged in the exploratory factor analysis ("task, goal, and copresence" and "bond and empathy") that had small and non-significant correlations with therapeutic outcomes at post-treatment, but moderate and significant correlations at follow-up.

Regarding the differences in the WAI-TECH-SF scores according to different characteristics of the sample, overall, no differences were found. That is, the TA with the self-guided IBI was achieved by the patients independently of their sex, their age, the severity of their depression before starting the intervention, their preferences for doing the intervention in the assigned condition, or the expectations and credibility towards the treatment. The average score on the WAI-TECH-SF was around 58 (on a scale ranging from 12 to 84). Nevertheless, patients with a higher level of education scored higher on TA with the online program than patients with a low level of education. This finding was also corroborated by the exploratory multiple regression analysis, in which all the different characteristics of the sample were introduced as potential predictors of the WAI-TECH-SF scores. Results showed that level of education, but also the age, were positive significant predictors of the TA with the self-guided IBI, explaining 4.9% of the variance. Regarding level of education, this higher TA could be related to the fact that more positive therapeutic outcomes in IBIs are also predicted by having a higher level of education [51]. Moreover, these findings may be associated with the lower preferences for IBIs expressed by people with a lower level of education [52], or the related barriers to the use of a less-known technology (e.g., low trust and lack of confidence in the capacity of IBIs to actually help).

The lower preference for technology adoption has also been related to age (e.g., because of their lower proficiency). Moret-Tatay et al. [53] found that older adults showed lower scores in mobile device and computer proficiency than younger adults. Consequently, adapted computer systems for older people have been designed to reduce the barriers that this population encounter. Mitzer et al. [54] found that the use of an adapted computer system for older people at the mid- and long-term was predicted by the earlier use of the system, the higher cognitive abilities (i.e., executive functioning), and computer efficacy. Hence, future studies should assess technology proficiency and cognitive abilities before starting a self-guided IBI in order to avoid the problems associated with the level of education and age, such as the adherence to the therapy. Nevertheless, older patients achieved higher TA in our study. One possible explanation for this finding is that the lower technology proficiency typically found in the population could have been compensated by the greater involvement in the therapy.

Regarding the capacity of the TA with the self-guided IBI to predict therapeutic outcomes, the findings highlight the importance of considering the WAI-TECH-SF scores to predict the change in depressive symptoms and satisfaction with the intervention. The TA with the online program explained 6.7% of the change in depressive symptoms, and 49.7% of the satisfaction with the treatment. Consequently, the relationship between "patient-online program TA" and therapeutic outcomes is also in line with the positive relationship found between the "patient-therapist TA" and the therapeutic outcomes in face-to-face therapy [1,2] and IBIs [3,21]. However, to our knowledge, this is the first study to confirm the relationship between "patient and online program TA" and therapeutic outcomes. By contrast, Kiluk et al. [29] did not find that the total scores on the long form of the WAI-Tech were associated with the change in therapeutic outcomes. Hence, so far, only the present study and Miragall et al. [25] found a significant relationship between the TA with the technology (i.e., the TA between the patient and virtual and augmented reality) and therapeutic outcomes. Therefore, this finding supports the need to work directly on the TA when it is poor because it has important consequences for therapeutic outcomes. Future studies should include algorithms to detect low TA scores after each session, in order to adjust the goals, tasks, and bond between the patient and the online program during an IBI.

This study has some limitations. First, the WAI-TECH-SF was only administered at the end of the treatment, which did not allow us to explore whether the "patient and online program TA" preceded the symptoms and satisfaction throughout the therapeutic sessions. Thus, having these measures during the treatment would allow us to establish the causal effect of TA on the therapeutic outcomes. Future studies should administer the WAI-TECH-SF in earlier therapeutic sessions (e.g., third session) in order to examine the TA through the therapy. Second, the study sample was only composed of depressive patients. Therefore, future studies should replicate this study in a sample of patients with several diagnoses (e.g., anxiety, post-traumatic stress disorder) in order to confirm whether the same psychometric structure is found, and to detect its capacity to predict therapeutic changes in other mental disorders. Third, the adherence or number of sessions performed by the patients was not registered. Thus, future studies should analyse whether the TA affects adherence and, in turn, the therapeutic outcomes. Fourth, the statistical analyses of TA were only conducted with the patients that accepted to fill in the questionnaire after the self-guided IBI was finished. However, the normal distribution (e.g., skewness = −0.56; kurtosis = −0.83) and the wide range of variability of the WAI-TECH-SF scores (i.e., from 12 to 84) allowed us to draw reliable conclusions. The importance shown by the TA with the technology points out the question regarding the impact of TA at early stages of the treatment, and the role that it can play in predicting efficacy and preventing dropouts.

Finally, the importance of having self-guided IBI that promotes an adequate TA between the patient and the online program should be noted, especially when resources are scarce. Several situations, such as the COVID-19 pandemic, could prevent individuals from accessing the traditional face-to-face therapy. Consequently, CBT delivered through telehealth services are undeniably crucial in order to provide timely psychological support, especially in vulnerable populations [55].

5. Conclusions

In conclusion, this study reveals that patients with major depression can develop TA with an online program during a self-guided IBI in the context of primary care. Thus, patients can feel that the program is "taking care" of them, in terms of allowing them to achieve therapeutic goals, proposing appropriate tasks to achieve these goals, and making them feel "embraced" and "cared for" by the program. According to our exploratory factor analysis, the WAI-TECH-SF is a reliable questionnaire to measure this construct, but it would be advisable to calculate an overall score for the total scale, rather than using the traditional theoretical three-dimensional "task-goals-bonds" structure of TA. Moreover, it would be beneficial to explore the IBI preferences of the patients with lower education levels before starting the intervention, in order to ensure that their level of education does not interfere with their capacity to develop TA with the online program. Finally, this study highlights the importance of considering the "patient and online program TA" because the WAI-TECH-SF score was a significant predictor variable of both the change in depressive symptoms and satisfaction at the end of the treatment. Further research is needed to more deeply understand the TA achieved in the "patient-technology-therapist" triangulation in blended treatments.

Author Contributions: Conceptualization, R.H., C.B., A.G.-P., H.R., A.K., and R.M.B.; methodology, R.H. and A.K.; software, R.H. and A.K.; formal analysis, R.H., M.D.V. and M.M., resources, C.B., A.G.-P., H.R., and R.M.B.; data curation, R.H., M.D.V. and M.M.; writing—original draft preparation, R.H., M.D.V. and M.M.; writing—review and editing, all authors; supervision, C.B., A.G.-P., H.R., A.K. and R.M.B.; funding acquisition, C.B., A.G.-P., H.R., A.K. and R.M.B. All authors have read and agreed to the published version of the manuscript.

Acknowledgments: We would like to thank CIBERObn, an initiative of ISCIII (ISC III CB06 03/0052).

References

1. Cameron, S.K.; Rodgers, J.; Dagnan, D. The relationship between the therapeutic alliance and clinical outcomes in cognitive behaviour therapy for adults with depression: A meta-analytic review. *Clin. Psychol. Psychother.* **2018**, *25*, 446–456. [CrossRef] [PubMed]
2. Horvath, A.O.; Del Re, A.C.; Flückiger, C.; Symonds, D. Alliance in individual psychotherapy. *Psychotherapy* **2011**, *48*, 9–16. [CrossRef] [PubMed]
3. Flückiger, C.; Del Re, A.C.; Wampold, B.E.; Horvath, A.O. The alliance in adult psychotherapy: A meta-analytic synthesis. *Psychotherapy* **2018**, *55*, 316–340. [CrossRef] [PubMed]
4. Bordin, E.S. The generalizability of the psychoanalytic concept of the working alliance. *Psychol. Psychother.* **1979**, *16*, 252–260. [CrossRef]
5. Kazdin, A.E.; Blase, S.L. Rebooting Psychotherapy Research and Practice to Reduce the Burden of Mental Illness. *Perspect. Psychol. Sci.* **2011**, *6*, 21–37. [CrossRef] [PubMed]
6. Mohr, D.C.; Tomasino, K.N.; Lattie, E.G.; Palac, H.L.; Kwasny, M.J.; Weingardt, K.; Karr, C.J.; Kaiser, S.M.; Rossom, R.C.; Bardsley, L.R.; et al. IntelliCare: An eclectic, skills-based app suite for the treatment of depression and anxiety. *J. Med. Internet Res.* **2017**, *19*, e10. [CrossRef]
7. Erbe, D.; Eichert, H.C.; Riper, H.; Ebert, D.D. Blending face-to-face and Internet-based interventions for the treatment of mental disorders in adults: Systematic review. *J. Med. Internet Res.* **2017**, *19*, e306. [CrossRef]
8. Richards, D.; Richardson, T. Computer-based psychological treatments for depression: A systematic review and meta-analysis. *Clin. Psychol. Rev.* **2012**, *32*, 329–342. [CrossRef]
9. Schröder, J.; Berger, T.; Westermann, S.; Klein, J.P.; Moritz, S. Internet interventions for depression: New developments. *Dialogues Clin. Neurosci.* **2016**, *18*, 203–212.
10. Sztein, D.; Koransky, C.; Fegan, L.; Himelhoch, S. Efficacy of cognitive behavioural therapy delivered over the Internet for depressive symptoms: A systematic review and meta-analysis. *J. Telemed. Telecare* **2018**, *24*, 527–539. [CrossRef]
11. Andersson, G.; Cuijpers, P.; Carlbring, P.; Riper, H.; Hedman, E. Guided internet-based vs. face-to-face cognitive behavior therapy for psychiatric and somatic disorders: A systematic review and meta-analysis. *World Psychiatry* **2014**, *13*, 288–295. [CrossRef] [PubMed]

12. Wagner, B.; Horn, A.B.; Maercker, A. Internet-based versus face-to-face cognitive-behavioral intervention for depression: A randomized controlled non-inferiority trial. *J. Affect. Disord.* **2014**, *152–154*, 113–121. [CrossRef] [PubMed]
13. Topooco, N.; Riper, H.; Araya, R.; Berking, M.; Brunne, M.; Chevreul, K.; Cieslak, R.; Ebert, D.D.; Etchemendy, E.; Herrero, R.; et al. On behalf of the E-COMPARED consortium. Attitudes towards digital treatment for depression: A European stakeholder survey. *Internet Interv.* **2017**, *8*, 1–9. [CrossRef] [PubMed]
14. Kooistra, L.; Ruwaard, J.; Wiersma, J.; van Oppen, P.; Riper, H. Working alliance in blended versus face-to-face cognitive behavioral treatment for patients with depression in specialized mental health care. *J. Clin. Med.* **2020**, *9*, 347. [CrossRef]
15. Horvath, A.O.; Greenberg, L.S. Development and validation of the Working Alliance Inventory. *J. Couns. Psychol.* **1989**, *36*, 223–233. [CrossRef]
16. Hatcher, R.L.; Gillaspy, J.A. Development and validation of a revised short version of the working alliance inventory. *Psychother. Res.* **2007**, *16*, 12–25. [CrossRef]
17. Tracey, T.J.; Kokotovic, A.M. Factor structure of the Working Alliance Inventory. *Psychol. Assess.* **1989**, *1*, 207–210. [CrossRef]
18. Jasper, K.; Weise, C.; Conrad, I.; Andersson, G.; Hiller, W.; Kleinstauber, M. The working alliance in a randomized controlled trial comparing internet-based self-help and face-to-face cognitive behavior therapy for chronic tinnitus. *Internet Interv.* **2014**, *1*, 49–57. [CrossRef]
19. Knaevelsrud, C.; Maercker, A. Internet-based treatment for PTSD reduces distress and facilitates the development of a strong therapeutic alliance: A randomized controlled clinical trial. *BMC Psychiatry* **2007**, *7*, 13. [CrossRef]
20. Preschl, B.; Maercker, A.; Wagner, B. The working alliance in a randomized controlled trial comparing online with face-to-face cognitive-behavioral therapy for depression. *BMC Psychiatry* **2011**, *11*, 189. [CrossRef]
21. Probst, G.H.; Berger, T.; Flückiger, C. The alliance-outcome relation in internet-based interventions for psychological disorders: A correlational meta-analysis. *Verhaltenstherapie* **2019**, 1–12. [CrossRef]
22. Clarke, J.; Proudfoot, J.; Whitton, A.; Birch, M.R.; Boyd, M.; Parker, G.; Manicavasagar, V.; Hadzi-Pavlovic, D.; Fogarty, A. Therapeutic alliance with a fully automated mobile phone and web-based intervention: Secondary analysis of a randomized controlled trial. *JMIR Ment. Health* **2016**, *3*, e10. [CrossRef] [PubMed]
23. Pihlaja, S.; Stenberg, J.H.; Joutsenniemi, K.; Mehik, H.; Ritola, V.; Joffe, G. Therapeutic alliance in guided internet therapy programs for depression and anxiety disorders–a systematic review. *Internet Interv.* **2018**, *11*, 1–10. [CrossRef] [PubMed]
24. Gómez-Penedo, J.M.; Babl, A.M.; Holtforth, M.G.; Hohagen, F.; Krieger, T.; Lutz, W.; Meyer, B.; Moritz, S.; Klein, J.P.; Berger, T. The association of therapeutic alliance with long-term outcome in a guided Internet Intervention for depression: Secondary analysis from a randomized control trial. *J. Med. Internet Res.* **2020**, *22*, e15824. [CrossRef] [PubMed]
25. Miragall, M.; Baños, R.M.; Cebolla, A.; Botella, C. Working alliance inventory applied to virtual and augmented reality (WAI-VAR): Psychometrics and therapeutic outcomes. *Front Psychol.* **2015**, *6*, 1531. [CrossRef]
26. Heim, E.; Roetger, A.; Lorenz, N.; Maercker, A. Working alliance with an avatar: How far can we go with internet interventions? *Internet Interv.* **2018**, *11*, 41–46. [CrossRef]
27. Berger, T.; Boettcher, J.; Caspar, F. Internet-based guided self-help for several anxiety disorders: A randomized controlled trial comparing a tailored with a standardized disorder-specific approach. *Psychotherapy* **2014**, *51*, 207–219. [CrossRef]
28. Berry, K.; Salter, A.; Morris, R.; James, S.; Bucci, S. Assessing therapeutic alliance in the context of mHealth interventions for mental health problems: Development of the mobile Agnew relationship measure (mARM) questionnaire. *J. Med. Internet Res.* **2018**, *20*, e90. [CrossRef]
29. Kiluk, B.D.; Serafini, K.; Frankforter, T.; Nich, C.; Carroll, K.M. Only connect: The working alliance in computer-based cognitive behavioral therapy. *Behav. Res.* **2014**, *63*, 139–146. [CrossRef]
30. Vernmark, K.; Hesser, H.; Topooco, N.; Berger, T.; Riper, H.; Luuk, L.; Backlund, L.; Carlbring, P.; Andersson, G. Working alliance as a predictor of change in depression during blended cognitive behaviour therapy. *Cogn. Behav.* **2019**, *48*, 285–299. [CrossRef]

31. Kleiboer, A.; Smit, J.; Bosmans, J.; Ruwaard, J.; Andersson, G.; Topooco, N.; Berger, T.; Krieger, T.; Botella, C.; Baños, R.; et al. European COMPARative Effectiveness research on blended Depression treatment versus treatment-as-usual (E-COMPARED): Study protocol for a randomized controlled, non-inferiority trial in eight European countries. *Trials* **2016**, *17*, 387. [CrossRef] [PubMed]
32. Kroenke, K.; Spitzer, R.L.; Williams, J.B. The PHQ-9: Validity of a brief depression severity measure. *J. Gen. Intern. Med.* **2001**, *16*, 606–613. [CrossRef] [PubMed]
33. American Psychiatric Association. *Diagnostic and Statistical Manual of Mental Disorders*, DSM IV-4th ed.; American Psychiatric Association: Washington, DC, USA, 1994.
34. Levis, B.; Benedetti, A.; Thombs, B.D. Accuracy of Patient Health Questionnaire-9 (PHQ-9) for screening to detect major depression: Individual participant data meta-analysis. *BMJ* **2019**, *365*. [CrossRef]
35. Wittkampf, K.A.; Naeije, L.; Schene, A.H.; Huyser, J.; van Weert, H.C. Diagnostic accuracy of the mood module of the Patient Health Questionnaire: A systematic review. *Gen. Hosp. Psychiatry* **2007**, *29*, 388–395. [CrossRef] [PubMed]
36. Sheehan, D.V.; Lecrubier, Y.; Sheehan, K.H.; Amorim, P.; Janavs, J.; Weiller, E.; Dunbar, G.C. The Mini-International Neuropsychiatric Interview (M.I.N.I.): The development and validation of a structured diagnostic psychiatric interview for DSM-IV and ICD-10. *J. Clin. Psychiatry* **1998**, *59*, 22–33.
37. Devilly, G.J.; Borkovec, T.D. Psychometric properties of the credibility/expectancy questionnaire. *J. Behav. Exp. Psychiatry* **2000**, *31*, 73–86. [CrossRef]
38. Nguyen, T.D.; Attkisson, C.C.; Stegner, B.L. Assessment of patient satisfaction: Development and refinement of a service evaluation questionnaire. *Eval. Program Plan.* **1983**, *6*, 299–314. [CrossRef]
39. Hambleton, R.K.; Patsula, L. Increasing the validity of adapted tests: Myths to be avoided and guidelines for improving test adaptation practices. *J. Appl. Test. Technol.* **1999**, *1*, 1–12.
40. Schafer, J.L. Analysis of Incomplete Multivariate Data. In *Monographs on Statistics and Applied Probability*; Chapman & Hall: London, UK, 1997; Volume 72.
41. Fabrigar, L.R.; Wegener, D.T.; MacCallum, R.C.; Strahan, E.J. Evaluating the use of exploratory factor analysis in psychological research. *Psychol. Methods* **1999**, *4*, 272–299. [CrossRef]
42. Horn, J.L. A rationale and test for the number of factors in factor analysis. *Psychometrika* **1965**, *30*, 179–185. [CrossRef]
43. O'Connor, B.P. SPSS and SAS programs for determining the number of components using parallel analysis and Velicer's MAP test. *Behav. Res. Methods Instrum. Comput.* **2000**, *32*, 396–402. [CrossRef] [PubMed]
44. Cronbach, L.J. Coefficient alpha and the internal structure of tests. *Psychometrika* **1951**, *16*, 297–334. [CrossRef]
45. Brysbaert, M. How many participants do we have to include in properly powered experiments? A tutorial of power analysis with reference tables. *J. Cogn.* **2019**, *2*, 1–38. [CrossRef] [PubMed]
46. West, S.G.; Finch, J.F.; Curran, P.J. Structural Equation Models with Non Normal Variables: Problems and Remedies. In *Structural Equation Modeling: Concepts, Issues, and Applications*, 1st ed.; Hoyle, R.H., Ed.; Sage Publications: Thousand Oaks, CA, USA, 1995; pp. 56–75.
47. Russell, D.W. In search of underlying dimensions: The use (and abuse) of factor analysis in Personality and Social Psychology Bulletin. *Pers. Soc. Psychol. Bull.* **2002**, *28*, 1629–1646. [CrossRef]
48. Fabrigar, L.R.; Wegener, D.T. *Exploratory Factor Analysis*; Oxford University Press: New York, NY, USA, 2012.
49. Henson, P.; Peck, P.; Torous, J. Considering the therapeutic alliance in digital mental health interventions. *Harv. Rev. Psychiatry* **2019**, *27*, 268–273. [CrossRef] [PubMed]
50. Miloff, A.; Carlbring, P.; Hamilton, W.; Andersson, G.; Reuterskiöld, L.; Lindner, P. Measuring alliance toward embodied virtual therapists in the era of automated treatments with the virtual therapist alliance scale (VTAS): Development and psychometric evaluation. *J. Med. Internet Res.* **2020**, *22*, e16660. [CrossRef]
51. Warmerdam, L.; Van Straten, A.; Twisk, J.; Cuijpers, P. Predicting outcome of Internet-based treatment for depressive symptoms. *Psychother. Res.* **2013**, *23*, 559–567. [CrossRef]
52. Batterham, P.J.; Calear, A.L. Preferences for internet-based mental health interventions in an adult online sample: Findings from an online community survey. *JMIR Ment. Health* **2017**, *4*, e26. [CrossRef]
53. Moret-Tatay, C.; Beneyto-Arrojo, M.J.; Gutierrez, E.; Boot, W.R.; Charness, N. A spanish adaptation of the computer and mobile device proficiency questionnaires (CPQ and MDPQ) for older adults. *Front Psychol.* **2019**, *10*, 1165. [CrossRef]

9

Brief Psychological Intervention Through Mobile App and Conference Calls for the Prevention of Depression in Non-Professional Caregivers

Patricia Otero [1,*], Isabel Hita [2], Ángela J. Torres [3] and Fernando L. Vázquez [2]

1 Department of Psychology, University of A Coruña, 15071 A Coruña, Spain
2 Department of Clinical Psychology and Psychobiology, University of Santiago de Compostela, 15782 Santiago de Compostela, Spain; isabel.hita@usc.es (I.H.); fernandolino.vazquez@usc.es (F.L.V.)
3 Department of Psychiatry, Radiology and Public Health, University of Santiago de Compostela, 15782 Santiago de Compostela, Spain; angelajuana.torres@usc.es
* Correspondence: patricia.otero.otero@udc.es

Abstract: Despite its potential, no intervention aimed at non-professional caregivers administered through a smartphone app has been proven to prevent depression. The objective of this pilot study was to evaluate the efficacy and feasibility of an indicated depression-prevention intervention for non-professional caregivers administered through an app with the addition of conference-call contact. The intervention was administered to 31 caregivers (Mean age = 54.0 years, 93.5% women). An independent evaluation determined the incidence of depression, depressive symptoms, risk of developing depression, and the variables in the theoretical model (positive environmental reinforcement, negative automatic thoughts) at the pre-intervention and post-intervention, as well as the one- and three-month follow-ups. The incidence of depression at 3 months of follow-up was 6.5%. There was a significant reduction in depressive symptoms ($p < 0.001$) and in the risk of developing depression ($p < 0.001$) at the post-intervention and at the one- and three-month follow-ups. The model's variables improved significantly after the intervention and were associated with post-intervention depressive symptoms. The intervention was more effective in caregivers who had a lower level of depressive symptoms at the pre-intervention. Adherence and satisfaction with the intervention were high. The results encourage future research using a randomized controlled clinical trial.

Keywords: depression; nonprofessional caregiver; prevention; cognitive; behavioral; telephone; app

1. Introduction

Caregivers for dependent family members perform a job that requires them to meet many demands and cope with difficult situations, oftentimes over a long period of time [1], such as looking for a diagnosis, learning to care for their family member, financial matters [2], decreased environmental reinforcement [3], insomnia or low-quality sleep [4,5], or a decrease in capabilities of the family member [6]. Therefore, caregivers' quality of life is affected [7–9], and these risk factors can increase their vulnerability to mental health disorders, especially depression [10]. In fact, a systematic review and meta-analysis on ten studies with a total of 790 caregivers [11] found a relative risk ranging from 2.80 to 38.68 for suffering from a depressive disorder in caregivers compared to non-caregivers. Specifically, previous research has found that 8.9% of caregivers meet the criteria for an episode of major depression [12], which is nearly fivefold higher than the 1.8% prevalence of major depression in the general population [13]. These figures are quite important because major depression is highly disabling and constitutes the third-leading cause of years lived with disabilities [14]. In addition, it is recurrent in 27% to 42% of people who experienced one major depressive episode and symptoms are chronic in 12% to 16% of those who have developed clinical depression [15–17]. Likewise, it entails enormous socioeconomic costs, resulting in billions of dollars annually [18]. Furthermore, in the case of caregivers, it can interfere with the proper performance of their tasks in caring for the dependent person [19].

Therefore, given the prevalence and serious repercussions of depression, its prevention among the caregiver population is critical. Among preventive strategies, indicated prevention interventions are particularly interesting. These are interventions aimed at individuals with subclinical symptoms who do not meet the diagnostic criteria for a major depressive episode [20]. The goal is to reduce the progression of these symptoms and to prevent their worsening into major depression [21].

There are only three previous studies on the indicated prevention of depression in non-professional caregivers providing care for dependent family members. The first evaluated the efficacy of a five-session problem-solving intervention using a group face-to-face format (about five participants per group) compared to a usual-care control group. It found a lower incidence of depression (4.5% vs. 13.1%) and fewer depressive symptoms (d = 1.54) after the intervention [22] and at the 12-month [23] and eight-year follow-up [24]. The second evaluated the efficacy of a five-session cognitive-behavioral face-to-face group intervention (about five participants per group) compared to a usual-care control group. It found a lower incidence of depression (1.1% vs. 12.2%) and fewer depressive symptoms (d = 1.05) after the intervention [25] and at the 12-month follow-up [26]. The therapeutic changes found were clinically significant [27]. However, these interventions were conducted using a traditional face-to-face format, which could compromise their accessibility. Caregivers often have barriers that make it difficult for them to attend face-to-face interventions, including lack of time, a lack of a substitute caregiver in their absence, a shortage of mental health services, travel and cost concerns, and fear of stigmatization.

The use of communication technologies available to practically all caregivers, such as the telephone, reduces these barriers. The telephone offers travel savings, anonymity, lower cost, and accessibility to the most remote communities [28], in addition to solving specific barriers in the caregiver population, such as lack of time and difficulties in finding a substitute caregiver. Therefore, in the third study of indicated depression prevention aimed at caregivers, Vázquez et al. (2020) [29], took a cognitive-behavioral depression-indicated prevention intervention that had previously been tested in a face-to-face format and adapted it into a five-session conference call format. The study also examined the efficacy of its components using a dismantling strategy. They found that the incidence of depression was lower in the group that received either the complete conference call intervention or the behavioral activation component only, compared to the control group (1.5% and 1.4% vs. 8.8%), and depressive symptoms were significantly lower in both intervention groups compared to the control group (d = 1.16 and d = 1.29), with no differences between them.

Although these results were very promising, the prevention intervention for depression could be optimized by utilizing a smartphone app. Currently, it is estimated that more than five billion people worldwide have mobile devices and more than half of these connections are smartphones. Furthermore, 80% of adults in Spain own a smartphone or use apps [30]. The smartphone app allows the caregiver greater mobility and accessibility by allowing access wherever and whenever they want 24 h a day. It increases the flexibility of program participation and can be adapted to caregivers' personal routines without wait times, having to make appointments, or attend sessions at a fixed time. Users can also review the materials as many times as they want and interact and receive feedback immediately [31,32].

However, given its novelty, there are only two previous studies evaluating apps for the treatment of depression [33,34], and neither of them are aimed at preventing depression or are aimed at caregivers of dependent family members. In particular, Arean et al. (2016) [33] found no significant difference at the post-intervention time point and the one-month follow-up between a cognitive training intervention, another problem-based intervention, and an attention control group in which participants received therapeutically inactive information on health. At the three-month follow-up, participants in both interventions showed higher remission rates compared to controls (50% and 49% vs. 32%), but only those with moderate depressive symptoms who participated in the problem-solving group showed fewer depressive symptoms than the control group ($d = 0.76$). In addition, Ly et al. (2014) [34] found no post-intervention differences between a program based on behavioral activation and another based on mindfulness. At the six-month follow-up, the behavioral activation intervention was more effective for patients with greater initial severity of depression ($d = 0.47$), while the mindfulness intervention was more effective for patients with lower severity ($d = 0.98$).

However, lack of adherence is one of the main limitations of interventions that do not use a face-to-face format. Dropout rates for interventions using apps were high, reaching 31.6%, and the level of compliance with tasks between sessions is unknown [33]. These problems are critical, because when evaluating the efficacy of interventions, high dropout rates can lead to bias and limit the generalizability of the results [35]. Furthermore, task completion is a significant predictor of therapy outcomes in depression prevention interventions among the caregiver population [36]. One way to reduce drop-out rates in interventions that are not conducted in an in-person format would be to establish telephone contact [31]. In addition, using the positive and corrective feedback technique, which consists of reinforcing the correct performance of a behavior and providing instructions to change behaviors that have been conducted incorrectly [37], could increase the effectiveness of interventions and strengthen caregivers' commitment to completing the homework tasks.

The objective of this study was to evaluate the efficacy and feasibility of an indicated depression-prevention intervention for non-professional caregivers with depressive symptoms administered through a smartphone app together with positive and corrective feedback through a telephone conference call.

2. Materials and Methods

2.1. Participants

A pretest–posttest design with a 1- and 3-month follow-up without a comparison group was used. Participants were recruited from the population of officially recognized (by the Administration) non-professional caregivers providing care for people in situations of dependency in the Autonomous Community of Galicia. To obtain a sample with similar characteristics to that of a future large-scale randomized controlled trial, the sample was selected by random stratified sampling following the following steps: (1) we contacted 11 regional and national associations related to caregivers via email and telephone, explained the purpose of the pilot study and obtained their cooperation; (2) every association made a list of all the non-professional caregivers they had, assigning a sequential number to each participant (e.g., 1, 2, 3, ...); (3) a random number generator was used to select the sample, taking 10 participants per association (i.e., 110 random numbers were generated). The staff of every association contacted the randomly selected caregivers personally and put them in contact with the research team, who explained to them the purpose of the study and answered all their questions.

To participate in the study, they had to meet the following criteria: (a) be a non-professional caregiver for a family member in a dependent situation; (b) the dependent family member was officially recognized by the competent public bodies in Spain; (c) have a smartphone; (d) be at risk for depression, defined as a score equal to or greater than 16 on the Center for Epidemiologic Studies Depression Scale (CES-D; [38]; Spanish version [39]); (e) not meet the DSM-5 diagnostic criteria for a major depressive episode (American Psychiatric Association [40]); and (f) agree to participate in all evaluations. Exclusion criteria were: (a) having received psychological or psychopharmacological treatment in the last two months prior to study entry; (b) presenting with other disorders that could act as confounding variables (e.g., symptoms due to substance use); (c) presenting with serious mental health or medical disorders that require immediate intervention (e.g., suicidal ideation) or that make the study impossible (e.g., significant cognitive impairment, severe visual deficit); (d) the dependent family member had a very poor prognosis for the next 6 months; and (e) the caregiver anticipated a change of address or institutionalization of the dependent family member.

Of the 110 caregivers contacted, 101 agreed to take the eligibility assessment. Of these, a total of 33 (32.7%) met the eligibility criteria and were invited to participate in the study, and 2 (6.1%) of these refused to participate due to personal issues and difficulty handling the smartphone (93.9% participated in the pilot study). The final sample consisted of 31 caregivers (93.5% women with a mean age of 54.0 years); no dropout occurred. There were no differences between participants and those who refuse participation on sex ($p = 1.000$, Fisher exact test), age ($U = 24.00$; $z = -0.529$; $p = 0.597$), marital status ($p = 0.216$, Fisher–Freeman–Halton test), social class ($p = 0.557$, Fisher–Freeman–Halton test), monthly household income ($p = 0.097$, Fisher–Freeman–Halton test), level of education ($p = 1.000$, Fisher–Freeman–Halton test), primary activity ($p = 0.432$, Fisher–Freeman–Halton test), care recipient sex ($p = 0.489$, Fisher exact test), care recipient age ($U = 16.50$; $z = -1.094$; $p = 0.274$), relationship to caregiver ($p = 0.424$, Fisher–Freeman–Halton test), care recipient diagnosis ($p = 0.318$, Fisher–Freeman–Halton test), daily hours of care ($U = 20.50$; $z = -0.814$; $p = 0.416$), care duration ($U = 11.50$; $z = -1.477$; $p = 0.140$), depressive symptoms ($U = 20.50$; $z = -0.796$; $p = 0.426$), positive environmental reinforcement ($U = 29.50$; $z = -0.114$; $p = 0.909$), or negative automatic thoughts ($U = 29.00$; $z = -0.151$; $p = 0.880$).

Participation was voluntary and no financial or other incentives were provided. The confidentiality of the participants was guaranteed and all gave their informed consent. The investigation was conducted following the principles of the Declaration of Helsinki and was approved by the Bioethics Committee of the University of Santiago de Compostela (Code number 07/09/2016).

2.2. Instruments

The participants were evaluated at the pre- and post-intervention time points and the 1- and 3-month follow-ups. Data was collected through self-administered instruments through the smartphone app by the participants, and by a structured clinical interview administered via telephone by two independent evaluators. These interviewers were previously trained specifically for this study by two experts with more than 25 years of experience in evaluation and were unaware of the purpose of the study and the administered intervention.

This study used an ad hoc questionnaire to evaluate the sociodemographic variables and the care situation. The Structured Clinical Interview for DSM-5—Clinician Version (SCID-5-CV; [41]) was used to evaluate episodes of major depression, which offers good test-retest reliability for psychiatric patients (kappa index > 0.80 for all disorders). CES-D was administered to assess depressive symptoms ([38]; Spanish version [39]), with an internal consistency of 0.89. In order to assess the variables in the theoretical model in which the intervention was based, we used the Environmental Reward Observation Scale (EROS; [42]; Spanish version [43]), which evaluates positive reinforcement with an internal consistency of 0.86, and the Automatic Thoughts Questionnaire (ATQ; [44]; Spanish version [45]) which assess the frequency of negative automatic thoughts with an internal consistency of 0.96. The Client Satisfaction Questionnaire (CSQ-8; [46]; Spanish version [47]) was used to assess satisfaction with the intervention, with an internal consistency of 0.80.

Finally, to assess the acceptability of the interventions, data on attendance at sessions, and completion of assignments between sessions were collected through an ad hoc record worksheet prepared for this study.

2.3. Intervention

Before the study, a cognitive-behavioral intervention for indicated prevention of depression was adapted for application via a smartphone app. Previous studies had demonstrated that this intervention was effective in reducing the incidence of depression and depressive symptoms in the population of caregivers at short- and long-term when administered in a face-to-face group format [24,25] and in a conference call format [29]. This intervention is based on the Multifactorial Integrative Model of

Depression developed by Lewinsohn et al. [48]. The adaptations consisted of modifying the content for presentation on smartphone screens (summarization and simplification of the content and changes to the format), designing the app interface, developing a daily reminder system that sent notifications to the mobile phone, and recording of between sessions homework tasks. The app-based intervention consisted of five modules that participants downloaded on their mobile and were programmed to be completed one per week. Module 1 explained the concept of depression and the need for active coping with depressive symptoms, and participants were trained in an activation control strategy (controlled breathing technique), self-reinforcement, and daily mood monitoring. Module 2 focused on how pleasant activities affect mood, and participants made plans to introduce them into their day-to-day activities. Module 3 addressed how thoughts affect mood, and participants were trained in techniques to manage negative thoughts. Module 4 explained how social contacts affect mood, and participants were trained in assertive communication and how to increase social contacts. In Module 5, participants reviewed everything they had learned and preventing relapse was addressed (see Table 1). The app, called Happy, was developed by independent programmers using the Apache Cordova framework, thus achieving a hybrid application, which is internally based on HTML, Javascript and CSS. For its development, an agile development methodology was followed. It was available for both Android and iOS in one language (Spanish) at the Google Play Store and the Apple App Store respectively, and operative for Android devices 4.4 or greater and for iOS 9 or greater. After the installation in the participant's device, a user and password login previously facilitated by the research team was mandatory to access the app. The app offered participants the previously mentioned battery of questionnaires and, after being completed by the user, a notification with a summary of the results was sent. If the user met the eligibility criteria, they were invited to participate in the intervention by the research team. Every week, the app allowed access to the contents of the corresponding module, sending a message informing the participants that they could access the next module. Upon completion of the module, between-session tasks were assigned, and the app sent a daily notification to users reminding them to complete and record their intersessional homework tasks. The stored data was hosted on an internal server in a MySQL database protected under username/password, and which can only be accessed from an authorized host (only the research team, complying with all security and confidentiality guarantees).

Table 1. Contents of the brief intervention program.

Module	Content
Module 1	Presentation of group members Purpose of the program Information about depression and active coping of symptoms Mood rating Training in diaphragmatic breathing Self-reinforcement Homework: Mood rating, practice breathing control technique, self-reinforcement
Module 2	Explanation of the relationship between pleasant activities and mood Guidelines and strategies to increase pleasant activities Planning pleasant activities Behavioral contract Homework: Mood rating, practice breathing control technique, self-reinforcement, perform the planned pleasant activities
Module 3	Explanation of the relationship between thoughts and mood Thought management techniques (direct approach, priming, distraction) Planning pleasant activities Behavioral contract Homework: Mood rating, practice breathing control technique, self-reinforcement, perform the planned pleasant activities, practice the thought management techniques

Table 1. *Cont.*

Module	Content
Module 3	Explanation of the relationship between thoughts and mood Thought management techniques (direct approach, priming, distraction) Planning pleasant activities Behavioral contract Homework: Mood rating, practice breathing control technique, self-reinforcement, perform the planned pleasant activities, practice the thought management techniques
Module 4	Explanation of the relationship between social contact and mood Guidelines and strategies to increase and improve social relationships Planning pleasant and social activities Homework: Mood rating, practice breathing control technique, self-reinforcement, perform the planned pleasant activities, practice the thought management techniques, make social contacts
Module 5	Review of what was learned. Maintaining progress Relapse prevention Farewell and closure

In addition, a five-session intervention was manualized to establish telephone contact lasting approximately 30 min (1 session/week) with the participants in a group format (5–6 participants) using a conference call system. In these sessions, the group's rules were explained and positive or corrective feedback was administered following the guidelines of Miltenberger (2012) [37]. The positive feedback consisted of providing information on how to correctly perform the homework tasks and providing reinforcement, and corrective feedback consisted of identifying the tasks that were not completed properly, suggesting relevant changes to improve performance.

The conference call intervention was administered by a psychologist and a doctor of psychology previously trained by experts with more than 25 years of experience in cognitive-behavioral therapies applied in different formats (e.g., individual, group) and through different means (e.g., face-to-face, telephone, online). The sessions were recorded, and adherence to the protocol was evaluated, yielding a protocol adherence of 92%. There were no significant differences between therapists in the results of the intervention.

2.4. Statistical Analysis

The quantitative data were analyzed by intention-to-treat. The missing values were imputed using the Last Observation Carried Forward Method. The McNemar test for paired data was used to analyze the incidence of depression and the risk of depression. Depressive symptoms were analyzed using repeated measures analysis of variance (ANOVA) and post hoc pairwise tests with Bonferroni correction. Student's t-test for paired data was used to analyze the changes in depressive symptoms between the pre- and post-intervention time points and between pre-intervention and follow-ups, and changes in reinforcement and negative automatic thoughts at the pre- and post-intervention time points. The effect size was calculated using Cohen's d (small = 0.2, medium = 0.5 and large = 0.8; [49]). Pearson's correlation was used to analyze the association between positive environmental reinforcement, negative thoughts, and depressive symptoms at the post-intervention time point. Multiple linear regression analyses were performed to analyze variables that were predictive of a reduction in depressive symptoms, following the recommendations of Domenéch and Navarro (2006) [50]. Frequency analyses and descriptive statistics of sessions attended, tasks performed, and CSQ-8 scores were performed to analyze adherence and satisfaction with the intervention. The analyses were conducted using statistical package SPSS for Windows (version 22.0, IBMCorp., Armonk, NY, USA).

3. Results

3.1. Characteristics of the Sample

Table 2 presents the most relevant sociodemographic, care situation and clinical characteristics of the caregivers who participated in the study. The 93.5% of caregivers were women and the mean age of them was 54.0 years (range 41–71; Standard Deviation [*SD*] = 9.4). Of the caregivers, 93.5% lived with a partner; 58.1% declared that they belonged to a low/lower-middle social class; 58.1% had a monthly household income of between 1000 and 1999 Euros; 54.8% had a high school or university-level education; and 51.6% were not active members of the workforce (they were unemployed, did not work outside the home, or were retired).

Table 2. Sociodemographic, care situation and clinical characteristics for the sample.

Sociodemographic Variables	*n* = 31	%
Sex		
Men	2	6.5
Women	29	93.5
Age		
M	54	
SD	9.4	
Range	41–71	
Marital status		
With partner	29	93.5
No partner (single, separated, divorced, widowed)	2	6.5
Social class		
Low/lower middle	18	58.1
Middle/upper middle	13	41.9
Monthly household income		
Up to €999	7	22.6
Between 1000 and 1999 euros	18	58.1
€2000 or more	6	19.3
Level of education		
Up to primary school education	14	45.2
Secondary/University	17	54.8
Primary activity		
Active worker	15	48.4
Unemployed/retired/housework	16	51.6
Care situation variables		
Care recipient sex		
Male	16	51.6
Female	15	48.4
Care recipient age		
M	54	
SD	28.1	
Range	5–93	
Relationship to caregiver		
Son/daughter	12	38.7
Father/mother	9	29
Other family members	10	32.3
Care recipient diagnosis		
Mental/neurological disorders/brain damage	15	48.4
Diseases of the skeletomuscular/connective tissue/cardiovascular/respiratory systems	7	22.6
Chromosomal/congenital/perinatal abnormalities	5	16.1
Others	4	12.9
Daily hours of care		
M	15.7	
SD	7.6	

Table 2. *Cont.*

Sociodemographic Variables	n = 31	%
Care duration (years)		
M	15.9	
SD	11.9	
Clinical variables		
CES-D Score		
M	26.8	
SD	8.6	
EROS Score		
M	24.1	
SD	4.1	
ATQ Score		
M	70.7	
SD	19.9	

M = Mean; SD = Standard Deviation; CES-D: Centre for Epidemiologic Studies Depression Scale; EROS: The Environmental Reward Observation Scale; ATQ: Automatic Thoughts Questionnaire.

In 51.6% of the cases, the family members receiving care were men, with a mean age of 54.0 years (*SD* = 28.1), ranging from 5 to 93 years. Most caregivers provided care to a family member, with the largest percentage being parents providing care for a child (38.7%). The most common type of illness observed among family members receiving care were mental health disorders, neurological diseases, and brain damage (48.4%). The time spent caring for the loved one was intensive and continuous. In this sample, caregivers devoted an average of 15.7 h a day to caring for their family member and had done so for an average of 15.9 years.

The mean depressive symptoms score was 26.8 (*SD* = 8.6). The mean positive environmental reinforcement score was 24.1 (*SD* = 4.1). The mean score for automatic negative thoughts was 70.7 (*SD* = 19.9).

3.2. Incidence of Depression

No participant developed an episode of major depression at the post-intervention time point or the one-month follow-up. Only two participants (6.5%) developed an episode of major depression at the three-month follow-up. Of them, one was diagnosed with an episode of major depression according to the DSM-5 diagnostic criteria, and one received an imputed value indicating depression.

Furthermore, there were no significant differences in the incidence of depression between the pre-intervention and post-intervention time points or between the pre-intervention time point and the one- and three-month follow-ups.

3.3. Depressive Symptomatology

Figure 1 shows the progression of depressive symptom scores at the pre-intervention time point (Mean [*M*] = 26.8), post-intervention time point (*M* = 15.3), and one- and three-month follow-ups (*M* = 17.2 and *M* = 15.5, respectively). The repeated-measures ANOVA showed that changes in depressive symptom scores were statistically significant: $F(3, 90) = 24.434$, $p < 0.001$, $\eta^2 = 0.449$. Compared to the pre-intervention time point, depressive symptoms were significantly lower at the post-intervention time point and at the one- and three-month follow-ups, with large effect sizes (Cohen's *d* between 0.91 and 1.37; see Table 3).

The mean score was reduced to 15.5 points, slightly below the threshold for risk of developing clinical depression, which is considered to be a score of 16 or more. Although this is consistent with other depression-prevention interventions [52], the mean score at the three-month follow-up was higher than that found using the same intervention delivered in face-to-face and conference call format [26,51]. On the other hand, it led to a significantly lower percentage of participants being at risk of developing depression, a figure that went from 100% at the pre-intervention time point to 45.2% at the post-intervention time point, though this is not as low as when the intervention is delivered face-to-face (29.5%) [25] and group conference call (18%) [51]. One possible explanation for these findings may be that the baseline level of depressive symptoms was greater in this study ($M = 26.8$) than for the studies examining the face-to-face format ($M = 23.7$) [26] and the conference-call telephone format ($M = 22.4$) [51]. In addition, administering the intervention through an app could also have some impact. While the face-to-face intervention or conference call-only format is more interactive, the smartphone app format of the intervention depends to a great extent on the caregiver's self-determination and autonomy to read the texts with full attention and interpret them appropriately. Depending on their profile, certain caregivers may benefit more from the program if more human contact is added to the intervention program (such as reviewing the content read on the app during conference calls or increasing the duration of conference call sessions).

Regarding the variables in the theoretical model based on which the intervention was developed, a significant increase in positive environmental reinforcement was found after the intervention with a large effect size ($d = 1.01$), along with a significant decrease in negative thoughts with a medium effect size ($d = 0.62$). These results are consistent with the formulation of the multifactorial integrative model of depression developed by Lewinsohn et al. (1985) [48]. Furthermore, the correlations found between post-intervention positive environmental reinforcement, negative thoughts, and depressive symptoms suggest that there is a relationship between the variables in the theoretical model and depressive symptoms, consistent with the proposed model by Lewinsohn et al. (1985) [48]. However, these results should be taken with caution because the variable associations are not synonymous with causality. The changes in the variables from the theoretical model achieved with the intervention could have had an effect on depressive symptoms, but it is also possible that the change in depressive symptoms affected the variables from the theoretical model (positive environmental reinforcement and negative thoughts).

Those caregivers who had fewer depressive symptoms at the pre-intervention time point had better results after the intervention. One possible explanation is that the therapeutic change is more achievable when depressive symptoms are in their initial phase. Therefore, it is of utmost importance to administer preventive interventions in populations with the initial signs of depressive symptoms to prevent future depression.

Furthermore, adherence to the intervention was high. In this sample, 93.5% of caregivers attended all weekly conference call sessions. It is possible that telephone administration of the intervention, the short duration of the weekly telephone calls (only 30 min), the duration of the intervention (only five weeks), and adjusting to times that were convenient for them facilitated caregivers' attendance at these sessions. Caregivers performed an average of 14.2 homework tasks out of the 18 assigned during the intervention. Notifications to record tasks sent from the app itself to the caregiver's smartphone may have motivated and reminded the caregivers to complete and record the tasks. Lastly, satisfaction with the intervention was high, with a mean of 28.1 out of a maximum of 32 on the CSQ-8. Thus, participants rated the quality of the program very positively and indicated that it helped them better manage the difficulties that they experienced on a day-to-day basis.

This study has important implications for research and clinical practice. This is the first study on a psychological intervention for the indicated prevention of depression aimed at non-professional caregivers and administered through a smartphone app. Its innovative format and conference call delivery increases the accessibility of interventions and gives therapists new tools to reach more patients, following the recommendations of the National Institute of Mental Health Psychosocial

Intervention Development Workgroup (2002) [53] and the New Freedom Commission on Mental Health (2003) [54]. It allows caregivers to receive a psychological intervention program at the most convenient time and place for them. Its duration is short (only five weeks), and the non-face-to-face and group format of the conference calls makes the intervention more cost-efficient, enabling reduced waiting lists and lowering the cost to the healthcare system. In addition, this intervention could prevent the personal suffering associated with depression. If its long-term efficacy is demonstrated in a randomized controlled trial as in the previous face-to-face interventions [26], an intervention of just five modules (via application) could prevent (or at least delay) the onset of depression for 12 months. Later, if depressive symptoms of the caregiver increase, we recommend the caregiver to review the contents learned or conduct reinforcement sessions to refresh the learned skills. If a caregiver develops a major depressive episode, they could resort to appropriate individual treatment in the healthcare system, allowing a clinical step-by-step care [32].

However, the present study has some limitations, mainly its lack of a control group and the corresponding randomization of the participants to the treatment conditions, as well as its small sample size. Likewise, it should be noted that a three-month follow-up could be too soon to draw definitive conclusions on the prevention of depression. Therefore, additional extended follow-ups are recommended. Lastly, although the smartphone app intervention format offers many advantages thanks to its accessibility, we do not know under what conditions the participants interact with the app. We did not have information about how much attention they paid to the texts, if there were distractions while interacting with the app, or how they interpreted the contents of the program. Certain caregivers, depending on their profile, may benefit more from a program with the addition of more human contact.

Despite the limitations, and consistent with the methodological recommendations made by Muñoz et al. (1996) [55] for studies on the prevention of depression, this study included aspects that made it a rigorous scientific study, such as the following: defining the population for which the intervention was designed (inclusion and exclusion criteria; defining the symptoms or objective condition); using specific, replicable, and manualized interventions; assessing therapists' adherence to the protocol; using reliable and valid outcome measures; conducting multimodal evaluations; and blinding evaluation of results.

5. Conclusions

The results of the intervention considered here indicate a reduction in the incidence of depression and depressive symptoms, as well as a significant improvement of positive environmental reinforcement and negative automatic thoughts. Moreover, the high adherence and satisfaction with the intervention shows its acceptability and feasibility. The strengths of this intervention include its brief and innovative format via smartphone app and conference call, increasing its accessibility, flexibility and cost-efficiency, appealing to caregivers and therapists. This innovation could change the way in which psychological interventions are administered and reach a greater number of users, benefiting both caregivers from the present and the future. Taking into account the previously mentioned limitations (a lack of control group and a small sample size), these findings encourage future research of a randomized controlled trial with a larger sample size, and long-term follow-up to confirm the results of this study.

Author Contributions: Conceptualization, F.L.V., P.O., and Á.J.T.; methodology, P.O., F.L.V. and I.H.; validation, P.O., I.H., and F.L.V.; formal analysis, P.O., I.H.; investigation, P.O. and I.H.; writing—original draft preparation, P.O., I.H., and F.L.V.; writing—review and editing, P.O., F.L.V., I.H. and Á.J.T.; supervision, F.L.V. and Á.J.T.; project administration, F.L.V. and Á.J.T.; funding acquisition, F.L.V. and Á.J.T. All authors have read and agreed to the published version of the manuscript.

Acknowledgments: We want to thank the support of non-profit associations related to non-professional family caregivers of the Autonomous Region of Galicia, and the Ministry of Education, University and Professional Training and the Ministry of Economy, Employment and Industry, and the ESF Galicia 2014–2020 operational program (Xunta de Galicia).

References

1. Triantafillou, J.; Naiditch, M.; Repkova, K.; Stiehr, K.; Carretero, S.; Emilsson, T.; Di Santo, P.; Bednarik, R.; Brichtova, L.; Ceruzzi, F.; et al. *Informal Care in the Long-Term Care System: European Overview Paper*; Interlinks: Athens, Vienna, 2010.
2. Palacios-Ceña, D.; Famoso-Pérez, P.; Salom-Moreno, J.; Carrasco-Garrido, P.; Pérez-Corrales, J.; Paras-Bravo, P.; Güeita-Rodriguez, J. "Living an Obstacle Course": A qualitative study examining the experiences of caregivers of children with Rett syndrome. *Int. J. Environ. Res. Public Health* **2019**, *16*, 41. [CrossRef]
3. Vázquez, F.L.; López, L.; Blanco, V.; Otero, P.; Torres, A.J.; Ferraces, M.J. The impact of decreased environmental reward in predicting depression severity in caregivers. *An. Psychol.* **2019**, *35*, 357–363.
4. Simón, M.A.; Bueno, A.; Otero, P.; Blanco, V.; Vázquez, F.L. Caregiver burden and sleep quality in dependent people's family caregivers. *J. Clin. Med.* **2019**, *8*, 1072. [CrossRef] [PubMed]
5. Simón, M.A.; Bueno, A.; Otero, P.; Blanco, V.; Vázquez, F.L. Insomnia in female family caregivers of totally dependent patients with dementia: An exploratory study. *Behav. Psychol.* **2019**, *27*, 107–119.
6. Meuser, T.M.; Marwit, S.J. A comprehensive, stage-sensitive model of grief in dementia caregiving. *Gerontologist* **2001**, *41*, 658–670. [CrossRef] [PubMed]
7. Madruga, M.; Gozalo, M.; Prieto, J.; Adsuar, J.C.; Gusi, N. Psychological symptomatology in informal caregivers of persons with dementia: Influences on health-related quality of life. *Int. J. Environ. Res. Public Health* **2020**, *17*, 1078. [CrossRef] [PubMed]
8. Perpiñá-Galvañ, J.; Orts-Beneito, N.; Fernández-Alcántara, M.; García-Sanjuán, S.; García-Caro, M.P.; Cabañero-Martínez, M.J. Level of burden and health-related quality of life in caregivers of palliative care patients. *Int. J. Environ. Res. Public Health* **2019**, *16*, 4806. [CrossRef]
9. Vázquez, F.L.; Otero, P.; Simón, M.A.; Bueno, A.M.; Blanco, V. Psychometric properties of the Spanish version of the Caregiver Burden Inventory. *Int. J. Environ. Res. Public Health* **2019**, *16*, 217. [CrossRef]
10. Schulz, R.; O'Brien, A.T.; Bookwala, J.; Fleissner, K. Psychiatric and physical morbidity effects of dementia caregiving: Prevalence, correlates, and causes. *Gerontologist* **1995**, *35*, 771–791. [CrossRef]
11. Cuijpers, P. Depressive disorders in caregivers of dementia patients: A systematic review. *Aging Ment. Health* **2005**, *9*, 325–330. [CrossRef]
12. Torres, Á.; Blanco, V.; Vázquez, F.L.; Díaz, O.; Otero, P.; Hermida, E. Prevalence of major depressive episodes in non-professional caregivers. *Psychiatry Res.* **2015**, *226*, 333–339. [CrossRef] [PubMed]
13. Ayuso-Mateos, J.L.; Vázquez-Barquero, J.L.; Dowrick, C.; Lehtinen, V.; Dalgard, O.S.; Casey, P.; Wilkinson, C.; Lasa, L.; Page, H.; Dunn, G.; et al. Depressive disorders in Europe: Prevalence figures from the ODIN study. *Br. J. Psychiatry* **2001**, *179*, 308–316. [CrossRef] [PubMed]
14. GBD 2017 Disease and Injury Incidence and Prevalence Collaborators. Global, regional, and national incidence, prevalence, and years lived with disability for 354 diseases and injuries for 195 countries and territories, 1990–2017: A systematic analysis for the Global Burden of Disease Study 2017. *Lancet* **2018**, *392*, 1789–1858. [CrossRef]
15. Hardeveld, F.; Spijker, J.; De Graaf, R.; Nolen, W.A.; Beekman, A.T.F. Recurrence of major depressive disorder and its predictors in the general population: Results from the Netherlands Mental Health Survey and Incidence Study (NEMESIS). *Psychol. Med.* **2013**, *43*, 39–48. [CrossRef]
16. Hoertel, N.; Blanco, C.; Oquendo, M.A.; Wall, M.M.; Olfson, M.; Falissard, B.; Franco, S.; Peyre, H.; Lemogne, C.; Limosin, F. A comprehensive model of predictors of persistence and recurrence in adults with major depression: Results from a national 3-year prospective study. *J. Psychiatr. Res.* **2017**, *95*, 19–27. [CrossRef]
17. ten Have, M.; de Graaf, R.; van Dorsselaer, S.; Tuithof, M.; Kleinjan, M.; Penninx, B.W.J.H. Recurrence and chronicity of major depressive disorder and their risk indicators in a population cohort. *Acta Psychiatr. Scand.* **2018**, *137*, 503–515. [CrossRef]
18. Greenberg, P.E.; Fournier, A.A.; Sisitsky, T.; Pike, C.T.; Kessler, R.C. The economic burden of adults with major depressive disorder in the United States (2005 and 2010). *J. Clin. Psychiatry* **2015**, *76*, 155–162. [CrossRef]
19. Williamson, G.M.; Shaffer, D.R. Relationship quality and potentially harmful behaviors by spousal caregivers: How we were then, how we are now. *Psychol. Aging* **2001**, *16*, 217–226. [CrossRef]
20. Institute of Medicine. *Reducing Risks for Mental Disorders: Frontiers for Preventive Intervention Research*; National Academic Press: Washington, DC, USA, 1994.

21. Muñoz, R.F.; Beardslee, W.R.; Leykin, Y. Major depression can be prevented. *Am. Psychol.* **2012**, *67*, 285–295. [CrossRef]
22. Vázquez, F.L.; Otero, P.; Torres, A.; Hermida, E.; Blanco, V.; Díaz, O. A brief problem-solving indicated-prevention intervention for prevention of depression in nonprofessional caregivers. *Psicothema* **2013**, *25*, 87–92.
23. Otero, P.; Smit, F.; Cuijpers, P.; Torres, A.; Blanco, V.; Vázquez, F.L. Long-term efficacy of indicated prevention of depression in non-professional caregivers: Randomized controlled trial. *Psychol. Med.* **2015**, *45*, 1401–1412. [CrossRef] [PubMed]
24. López, L.; Smit, F.; Cuijpers, P.; Otero, P.; Blanco, V.; Torres, Á.; Vázquez, F.L. Problem-solving intervention to prevent depression in non-professional caregivers: A randomized controlled trial with 8 years of follow-up. *Psychol. Med.* **2020**, *50*, 1002–1009. [CrossRef] [PubMed]
25. Vázquez, F.L.; Hermida, E.; Torres, A.; Otero, P.; Blanco, V.; Díaz, O. Eficacia de una intervención preventiva cognitivo conductual en cuidadoras con síntomas depresivos elevados. [Efficacy of a brief cognitive-behavioral intervention in female caregivers with high depressive symptoms]. *Behav. Psychol.* **2014**, *22*, 79–96.
26. Vázquez, F.L.; Torres, Á.; Blanco, V.; Otero, P.; Díaz, O.; Ferraces, M.J. Long-term follow-up of a randomized clinical trial assessing the efficacy of a brief cognitive-behavioral depression prevention intervention for caregivers with elevated depressive symptoms. *Am. J. Geriatr. Psychiatry* **2016**, *24*, 421–432. [CrossRef] [PubMed]
27. Blanco, V.; Otero, P.; López, L.; Torres, Á.; Vázquez, F.L. Predictores del cambio clínicamente significativo en una intervención de prevención de la depresión. [Clinically significant predictors of change in an intervention for the prevention of depression]. *Rev. Iberoam. Psicol. Salud.* **2017**, *8*, 9–20. [CrossRef]
28. Reese, R.J.; Conoley, C.W.; Brossart, D.F. The attractiveness of telephone counseling: An empirical investigation of client perceptions. *J. Couns. Dev.* **2006**, *84*, 54–60. [CrossRef]
29. Vázquez, F.L.; López, L.; Torres, Á.J.; Otero, P.; Blanco, V.; Díaz, O.; Páramo, M. Analysis of the components of a cognitive-behavioral intervention for the prevention of depression administered via conference call to nonprofessional caregivers: A randomized controlled trial. *Int. J. Environ. Res. Public Health* **2020**, *17*, 2067. [CrossRef]
30. Taylor, K.; Silver, L. *Smartphone Ownership is Growing Rapidly around the World, but not Always Equally*; Pew Research Center: Washington, DC, USA, 2019.
31. Andersson, G.; Cuijpers, P. Internet-based and other computerized psychological treatments for adult depression: A meta-analysis. *Cogn. Behav. Ther.* **2009**, *38*, 196–205. [CrossRef]
32. Nicholas, J.; Ringland, K.E.; Graham, A.K.; Knapp, A.A.; Lattie, E.G.; Kwasny, M.J.; Mohr, D.C. Stepping up: Predictors of 'stepping' within an iCBT stepped-care intervention for depression. *Int. J. Environ. Res. Public Health* **2019**, *16*, 4689. [CrossRef]
33. Arean, P.A.; Hallgren, K.A.; Jordan, J.T.; Gazzaley, A.; Atkins, D.C.; Heagerty, P.J.; Anguera, J.A. The use and effectiveness of mobile Apps for depression: Results from a fully remote clinical trial. *J. Med. Internet Res.* **2016**, *18*, e330. [CrossRef]
34. Ly, K.H.; Trüschel, A.; Jarl, L.; Magnusson, S.; Windahl, T.; Johansson, R.; Carlbring, P.; Andersson, G. Behavioural activation versus mindfulness-based guided self-help treatment administered through a smartphone application: A randomised controlled trial. *BMJ Open* **2014**, *4*, e003440. [CrossRef] [PubMed]
35. Swift, J.K.; Greenberg, R.P. Premature discontinuation in adult psychotherapy: A meta-analysis. *J. Consult. Clin. Psychol.* **2012**, *80*, 547–559. [CrossRef] [PubMed]
36. Otero, P.; Vázquez, F.L.; Hermida, E.; Díaz, O.; Torres, Á. Relationship of cognitive behavioral therapy effects and homework in an indicated prevention of depression intervention for non-professional caregivers. *Psychol. Rep.* **2015**, *116*, 841–854. [CrossRef] [PubMed]
37. Miltenberger, R.G. *Behavior Modification: Principles and Procedures*, 5th ed.; Wadsworth/Thomson Learning: Belmont, MA, USA, 2012.
38. Radloff, L.S. The CES-D Scale: A self-report depression scale for research in the general population. *Appl. Psychol. Meas.* **1977**, *1*, 385–401. [CrossRef]
39. Vázquez, F.L.; Blanco, V.; López, M. An adaptation of the Center for Epidemiologic Studies Depression Scale for use in non-psychiatric Spanish populations. *Psychiatry Res.* **2007**, *149*, 247–252. [CrossRef]
40. American Psychiatric Association. *Diagnostic and Statistical Manual of Mental Disorders*; American Psychiatric Association: Washington, DC, USA, 2013.

41. First, M.B.; Williams, J.B.W.; Karg, R.S.; Spitzer, R.L. *Structured Clinical Interview for DSM-5® Disorders—Clinician Version (SCID-5-CV)*; American Psychiatric Association Publishing: Arlington, VA, USA, 2015.
42. Armento, M.E.A.; Hopko, D.R. The Environmental Reward Observation Scale (EROS): Development, validity, and reliability. *Behav. Ther.* **2007**, *38*, 107–119. [CrossRef]
43. Barraca, J.; Pérez-Álvarez, M. Adaptación española del Environmental Reward Observation Scale (EROS) [Spanish adaptation of Environmental Reward Observation Scale (EROS)]. *Ansiedad Estrés* **2010**, *16*, 95–107.
44. Hollon, S.D.; Kendall, P.C. Cognitive self-statements in depression: Development of an automatic thoughts questionnaire. *Cognit. Ther. Res.* **1980**, *4*, 383–395. [CrossRef]
45. Otero, P.; Vázquez, F.L.; Blanco, V.; Torres, Á. Propiedades psicométricas del Cuestionario de Pensamientos Automáticos (ATQ) en la población de cuidadores familiares [Psychometric properties of the Automatic Thoughts Questionnaire (ATQ) in family caregivers]. *Behav. Psychol.* **2017**, *25*, 387–403.
46. Larsen, D.L.; Attkisson, C.C.; Hargreaves, W.A.; Nguyen, T.D. Assessment of client/patient satisfaction: Development of a general scale. *Eval. Program Plan.* **1979**, *2*, 197–207. [CrossRef]
47. Vázquez, F.L.; Torres, Á.; Otero, P.; Blanco, V.; Attkisson, C.C. Psychometric properties of the Castilian Spanish version of the Client Satisfaction Questionnaire (CSQ-8). *Curr. Psychol.* **2019**, *38*, 829–835. [CrossRef]
48. Lewinsohn, P.M.; Hoberman, H.; Teri, L.; Hautzinger, M. An integrative theory of depression. In *Theoretical Issues in Behaviour Therapy*; Reiss, S., Bootzin, R.R., Eds.; Academic Press: New York, NY, USA, 1985; pp. 313–359.
49. Cohen, J. *Statistical Power Analysis for the Behavioural Sciences*, 2nd ed.; Lawrence Erlbaum Associates, Inc.: Hillsdale, NJ, USA, 1988.
50. Domenéch, J.M.; Navarro, J.B. *Regresión Lineal Múltiple con Predictores Cuantitativos y Categóricos [Multiple Regression with Quantitative and Cathegorical Predictors]*; Signo: Barcelona, Spain, 2006.
51. Vázquez, F.L.; Otero, P.; López, L.; Blanco, V.; Torres, A.; Díaz, O. La prevención de la depresión en cuidadores a través de multiconferencia telefónica [Prevention of depression in caregivers through conference calls]. *Clin. Salud.* **2018**, *29*, 14–20. [CrossRef]
52. Muñoz, R.F.; Cuijpers, P.; Smit, F.; Barrera, A.Z.; Leykin, Y. Prevention of major depression. *Annu. Rev. Clin. Psychol.* **2010**, *6*, 181–212. [CrossRef] [PubMed]
53. Hollon, S.D.; Muñoz, R.F.; Barlow, D.H.; Beardslee, W.R.; Bell, C.C.; Bernal, G.; Clarke, G.N.; Franciosi, L.P.; Kazdin, A.E.; Kohn, L.; et al. Psychosocial intervention development for the prevention and treatment of depression: Promoting innovation and increasing access. *Biol. Psychiatry* **2002**, *52*, 610–630. [CrossRef]
54. New Freedom Commission on Mental Health. *Achieving the Promise: Transforming Mental Health Care in America*; DHHS: Rockville, MD, USA, 2003.
55. Muñoz, R.F.; Mrazek, P.J.; Haggerty, R.J. Institute of Medicine report on prevention of mental disorders: Summary and commentary. *Am. Psychol.* **1996**, *51*, 1116–1122. [CrossRef] [PubMed]

10

Working Alliance in Blended Versus Face-to-Face Cognitive Behavioral Treatment for Patients with Depression in Specialized Mental Health Care

Lisa Kooistra [1,2,*], Jeroen Ruwaard [2,3,†], Jenneke Wiersma [2], Patricia van Oppen [2,3] and Heleen Riper [1,2,3]

1 Department of Clinical, Neuro-and Developmental Psychology and the Amsterdam Public Health Research Institute, Vrije Universiteit Amsterdam, van der Boechorststraat 7, 1081 BT Amsterdam, The Netherlands; m.m.riper@vu.nl
2 Department of Research and Innovation, GGZ inGeest Specialized Mental Health Care, Oldenaller 1, 1081 HJ Amsterdam, The Netherlands; jennekewiersma@gmail.com (J.W.); p.vanoppen@ggzingeest.nl (P.v.O.)
3 Department of Psychiatry and the Amsterdam Public Health Research Institute, GGZ inGeest/Amsterdam UMC, Vrije Universiteit, de Boelelaan 1117, 1081 HV Amsterdam, The Netherlands
* Correspondence: l.kooistra@ggzingeest.nl
† Died July 2019.

Abstract: This study investigates working alliance in blended cognitive behavioral therapy (bCBT) for depressed adults in specialized mental health care. Patients were randomly allocated to bCBT ($n = 47$) or face-to-face CBT ($n = 45$). After 10 weeks of treatment, both patients and therapists in the two groups rated the therapeutic alliance on the Working Alliance Inventory Short-Form Revised (WAI-SR; Task, Bond, Goal, and composite scores). No between-group differences were found in relation to either patient or therapist alliance ratings, which were high in both groups. In the full sample, a moderate positive association was found between patient and therapist ratings on Task ($\varrho = 0.41$, 95% CI 0.20; 0.59), but no significant associations emerged on other components or composite scores. At 30 weeks, within-and between-group associations between alliance and changes in depression severity (QIDS, Quick Inventory of Depressive Symptomatology) were analyzed with linear mixed models. The analyses revealed an association between depression over time, patient-rated alliance, and group ($p < 0.001$). In face-to-face CBT, but not in bCBT, lower depression scores were associated with higher alliance ratings. The online component in bCBT may have led patients to evaluate the working alliance differently from patients receiving face-to-face CBT only.

Keywords: major depressive disorder; blended cognitive behavioral treatment; specialized mental health care; working alliance; randomized controlled trial

---

1. Introduction

Although major depressive disorder (MDD) is a common and severely disabling illness [1], many individuals with MDD have limited access to mental health care and trained therapists [2–4]. This has prompted development of interventions requiring less therapist involvement, such as self-help interventions [5,6], and online psychotherapy [7,8]. Various studies have shown that online interventions, most often based on cognitive behavioral therapy, are effective in treating common mental disorders [9–13]—especially when patients receive professional guidance, for example, via secured e-mail exchange or an online treatment platform [5,9,14,15]. The past few years have seen growing interest in hybrid treatment approaches, which either combine or integrate face-to-face and online therapy [16]. As this is a relatively new form of treatment, evidence on effectiveness is still scarce. Initial evaluations suggest that blended treatment can be effective in decreasing depression severity [17–24].

The consequent modifications in the amounts and forms of contact between therapists and patients in online and blended interventions, as compared with face-to-face treatments, have led some therapists to worry that therapeutic alliance might be negatively impacted [18] and that this could weaken treatment outcomes. This is relevant, as therapeutic alliance is considered an important common factor in psychotherapy [25]. A stronger alliance between therapists and patients has been shown to be moderately associated with better treatment outcomes in face-to-face treatment [26–28], with meta-analyses reporting overall weighted averages of $r = 0.28$ (95% CI 0.26; 0.30) in psychotherapy for mental disorders [28] and $r = 0.26$ (95% CI 0.19; 0.32) in cognitive behavioral therapy (CBT) for depression [29]. However, such associations might be moderated by other factors. For example, assessment of alliance in a later phase of treatment may detect stronger associations between alliance and treatment effect than early assessment [28,29], and the alliance–outcome association has been found weaker for therapist-rated alliance than patient-rated alliance [29]. Associations might also be positively impacted if patient and therapist ratings of working alliance more strongly concur [30], or if patients have had fewer prior depressive episodes [31].

For blended depression treatments, available evidence on therapeutic alliance is still limited. Initial evaluations showed patient-rated alliance in online interventions to be high and comparable to ratings in face-to-face treatment [32,33]. While the therapeutic alliance in guided online interventions is often assumed to be less salient to outcome [9], Flückiger and colleagues [28] have suggested that the overall alliance–outcome association in online therapy is comparable to the association in face-to-face treatment ($r = 0.28$, 95% CI 0.21, 0.34, $p < 0.001$), with higher alliance accompanying better treatment outcomes. A recent review has suggested that the association between alliance and outcome in online interventions may be stronger in terms of agreement on goals and tasks than in terms of the affective bond between patients and their therapists, partly because patients could have lower or different expectations of the bond that can be formed online [32]. In a recent Swedish study ($n = 73$), patients and therapists provided high alliance ratings for blended CBT [34]. The working alliance as rated by therapists, but not as rated by patients, was found predictive of changes in depression severity during treatment. Among the possible explanations for this finding, the authors suggest that therapists in blended cognitive behavioral therapy (bCBT) might have provided more accurate evaluations of working alliance than patients, because patients would have based their alliance ratings on both the online (self-help) material and the face-to-face contacts, whereas therapists would have rated the interaction with the patient in face-to-face contacts only.

The present study expands on existing knowledge by examining working alliance in a randomized controlled trial (RCT), with comparison of blended cognitive behavioral therapy (bCBT) to face-to-face CBT in patients with major depressive disorder (MDD) requiring specialist mental health care. Information on the working alliance was gathered from both patients and therapists, in order to gain insight into the dyadic nature of this relationship [30]. Data was collected in an RCT focusing on the cost-effectiveness of bCBT versus face-to-face CBT [24,35]. The blended intervention integrated face-to-face and online CBT into a single treatment protocol [20,24,35], replacing half of the face-to-face sessions by online sessions. This paper addresses three research questions: (1) Is there a difference between bCBT and face-to-face CBT in terms of patient and therapist ratings of working alliance? (2) Is there an association between working alliance and change in depressive symptoms? and (3) If so, does that association differ between bCBT and face-to-face CBT?

2. Materials and Methods

2.1. Study Design

Data were collected between August 2014 and May 2017 within a pilot randomized controlled trial ($n = 102$), that compared bCBT with face-to-face CBT in six outpatient specialized mental healthcare clinics. The total RCT sample consisted of 102 participants aged 19–62. A detailed overview of the design and procedures of the trial can be found elsewhere [35]. The trial was registered at the Netherlands Trial Register (number NTR4650) and was approved by the Medical Ethics Committee of the Vrije Universiteit Medical Center (VUmc) (registration number 2014.191).

2.2. Participants

Patients for the trial were recruited during the intake procedure before the start of their specialized depression treatment. All patients had a primary diagnosis of MDD, based on the Mini-international Neuropsychiatric Interview Plus (MINI-plus, [36,37]), and had adequate proficiency in the Dutch language, a valid e-mail address, and a computer with Internet access. Patients with a high risk for suicide, a psychotic disorder, a bipolar disorder, or substance dependence were excluded from study participation. No exclusion criteria were applied regarding treatment histories, other comorbidity, or parallel pharmacological treatments. The current study included patients for whom patient-rated or therapist-rated alliance at week 10 was available ($n = 92$; bCBT $n = 45$, CBT $n = 47$).

2.3. Procedures

Patients were asked to provide written informed consent in order to participate in the study. Demographic data, treatment preference, and diagnostic profiles were assessed prior to random allocation and start of treatment (baseline). Working alliance was assessed ten weeks after the start of treatment. At this time point, both groups ideally would have received ten face-to-face sessions. The bCBT group was expected to have received nine additional online sessions and eight online therapist feedback messages. Patients completed weekly assessments on their depression severity during their treatment. Assessments at baseline and after ten weeks of treatment consisted of online self-report questionnaires and a diagnostic interview, administered by trained assessors who were blinded to treatment allocation.

2.4. Random Allocation

Random allocation (1:1 ratio) was performed by an independent researcher, based on a computer-generated random number table. Random allocation was stratified per treatment center. Patients began treatment approximately three weeks after random allocation (SD 2.0, range 0 to 14).

2.5. Interventions

Depression treatment in both study arms was based on CBT manuals [38,39], which advise therapists to provide 15 to 20 weekly CBT sessions and to include psycho-education, behavioral activation, cognitive restructuring, and relapse prevention. The face-to-face CBT without the online sessions was provided at the outpatient clinics. Therapists were advised to plan weekly sessions but were allowed to deviate from the treatment manual when necessary. Duration of treatment could vary per patient, but was expected to last approximately 20 weeks.

Blended CBT consisted of ten face-to-face sessions at the clinic and nine online sessions. Face-to-face and online sessions were alternated. Therapists had received training in the use of the bCBT manual. The aim was to schedule one face-to-face, one online session, and one online feedback message per week during a ten-week period, beginning with a face-to-face session. Patients planned the sessions together with their therapist. Each session focused on a specific domain of the CBT protocol, such as psycho-education, activity scheduling, and identification of dysfunctional assumptions. The content of the online sessions corresponded with that of the previous face-to-face session. Sessions were provided in a fixed order, but therapists were allowed to repeat an online session. In order to access the web-based part of treatment, patients and therapists logged into a personal account on a secure website (www.minddistrict.com). The online sessions consisted of text, short videos, images, patient vignettes, and homework exercises. Patients also had access to a daily mood diary, weekly monitoring of depression severity (QIDS-SR, Quick Inventory of Depressive Symptomatology,

Self-Report version) [40], and a messaging function to contact their therapists. Therapists provided a written therapeutic feedback message to each completed online session. Feedback was asynchronous and was provided within three working days after patients had completed the online session. After reading their therapist's feedback, patients gained access to the next online session. More detailed information on the form and content of bCBT can be found elsewhere [20,35].

2.6. Therapists

A total of 33 therapists participated in the trial, 5 of whom only provided face-to-face CBT, 12 only provided bCBT only, and the remaining 16 therapists treated patients in both treatment arms. On average, therapists treated three patients (SD 2.5, range 1 to 10). All therapists had at least a master's degree in psychology, were specialized in cognitive behavioral treatment, and had a minimum of two years of relevant work experience.

2.7. Measures

In assessing therapeutic alliance, this study focused on Bordin's definition of working alliance [41], which refers to the *bond* between patient and therapist as well as agreement about the *goals* and *tasks* in treatment. Patients and therapists were asked separately to assess their working alliance with the abbreviated Dutch version of the Working Alliance Inventory Short-form Revised (WAI-SR) questionnaire [42–44]. Both questionnaire versions were scored on a five-point Likert scale, ranging from "never" to "always". Items are grouped to measure the three components of working alliance: agreement on Goals, agreement on Tasks, and the quality of the Bond between therapist and patient [41]; a composite (average) score is also calculated as a global assessment of working alliance. Examples of items are "We are working towards mutually agreed upon goals" for the Goal component; "I believe the way we are working with my problem is correct" for the Task component; and "We respect each other" for the Bond component. The client version (WAI-SR-C) consists of 12 items [45], the therapist version (WAI-SR-T) of 10 items. For descriptive purposes, patient and therapist ratings were transformed to a 0 to 5 range for each component. In the current study, both versions of the WAI displayed good internal consistency. Cronbach's alpha for the patient version was 0.91 (95% CI 0.89; 0.94) for the composite score (all items), 0.86 (95% CI 0.82; 0.91) for the Goal component, 0.90 (95% CI 0.86; 0.93) for the Task component, and 0.82 (95% CI 0.77; 0.87) for the Bond component. For the therapist version, Cronbach's alpha was 0.88 (95% CI 0.84; 0.91) for the composite score, 0.81 (95% CI 0.74; 0.87) for the Goal component, 0.81 (95% CI 0.74; 0.87) for the Task component, and 0.79 (95% CI 0.71; 0.85) for the Bond component.

Change in self-reported depression severity was assessed with the Dutch translation of the 16-item short version of the Inventory of Depressive Symptomatology (QIDS-SR) [40]. Patients were requested to complete the QIDS on a weekly basis during treatment. The questionnaire covers all nine components of the DSM-IV-TR (Diagnostic and Statistical Manual of Mental Disorders, fourth edition, text-revision) depression diagnosis. Total scores range between 1 and 27. In the current study, the Cronbach's alpha at baseline was 0.78 (95% CI 0.71; 0.84).

Before random allocation, demographic information, including age, gender, employment status, and income, was collected with an online self-report questionnaire at baseline. One further item was added to inquire whether patients would prefer receiving bCBT or face-to-face CBT. Diagnosis of depression and psychiatric comorbidity were obtained using the Mini-international Neuropsychiatric Interview Plus (MINI-plus, [36,37]). Information on face-to-face treatment uptake (number of sessions completed) was retrieved from patient records. Information on the number of feedback messages received and online sessions completed by patients was obtained from logfiles from the online treatment environment.

2.8. Statistical Analyses

The current study was based on a data subset from a larger trial ($n = 102$) [24,35], and was therefore not powered a priori. The study sample ($N = 92$) was large enough to detect a correlation of r ~ 0.3 and a group difference of d ~ 0.6 at a power of 80% and a significance level of $p = 0.05$.

Multivariable logistic regression analysis including age, gender, partner status, baseline depression severity, comorbidity, treatment group, a priori treatment preference, and total number of face-to-face sessions received was performed to examine possible differences between patients that did and did not provide working alliance ratings.

Between-group differences in patient and therapist ratings of the separate work alliance components were examined using Welch Two-Sample t-test ($p < 0.05$), with patient and therapist ratings as the dependent variable and treatment group as the independent variable.

The degree of consensus between patients and therapists was examined by calculating correlations between patient and therapist ratings. Shapiro–Wilk tests, at alpha = 0.05 [46], revealed non-normal distributions for all separate components, except for the patient ratings on the Task component. We therefore assessed Spearman's rho (for all component pairs. Correlations were estimated using the psych package (version 1.8.4) [47] in R software (Macintosh; Intel Mac OS X v3.5.1) [48]. The relationship between change in depression severity over time, treatment group, and patient- and therapist-rated working alliance was assessed in separate linear mixed-effect models (LMM) with restricted maximum likelihood (REML). The LMM approach was chosen in order to account for missing QIDS data and the correlation between follow-up time points. Because the Goal, Task, and Bond components were moderately to highly intercorrelated (range Task~Bond = 0.41 to Task~Goal = 0.70), only the composite scores were used to examine the association between general working alliance and outcome. The models thus employed QIDS depression severity scores as the independent variable and time (in weeks), treatment group, and the WAI composite scores as dependent variables. Composite scores were centered. The models also included a random effect for individuals over time, which allowed for estimation of individual intercepts and slopes [49,50]. The Holm–Bonferroni correction [51] was applied to account for multiple testing. In the manuscript, noncorrected nonsignificant p-values are reported for descriptive purposes. The mixed models were estimated using the lmer function from the lme4 package (version 1.1–17) [52] in R software (Macintosh; Intel Mac OS X, v3.5.1) [48].

3. Results

3.1. Patients

From the full trial sample of 102 patients (bCBT $n = 53$, CBT $n = 49$), data on working alliance was available for 92 patients (bCBT $n = 45$, CBT $n = 47$). Both the patient and therapist ratings had been obtained for 71 of them (bCBT $n = 38$, CBT $n = 33$), whereas solely therapist ratings were obtained for 19 patients (bCBT $n = 8$, CBT $n = 11$) and patient ratings for 2 patients (bCBT $n = 1$, CBT $n = 1$). Information on baseline demographic and clinical characteristics of patients included in this study ($N = 92$) is presented in Table 1.

Table 1. Sample characteristics at baseline.

	bCBT *n* = 47	CBT *n* = 45	Total *n* = 92
Demographic			
Gender, female (*n*, %)	30 (63.8)	25 (55.6)	43 (59.8)
Age (mean, SD)	39.5 (11.4)	37.7 (10.5)	38.6 (11.0)
In a relationship (*n*, %)	26 (55.3)	27 (60.0)	53 (57.6)
Education (*n*, %)			
Low	6 (12.8)	1 (2.2)	7 (7.6)
Middle	24 (51.1)	31 (68.9)	55 (59.8)
High	17 (36.2)	13 (28.9)	30 (32.6)
Employed (*n*, %)	27 (57.5)	26 (57.8)	53 (57.6)
Nationality, Dutch (n, %)	42 (89.4)	44 (97.8)	68 (93.5)
Clinical			
Treatment preference, bCBT (*n*, %)	30 (63.8)	30 (66.7)	60 (65.2)
Co-morbid disorder(s) (*n*, %)	31 (66.0)	30 (66.7)	61 (66.3)
QIDS-SR (mean, SD)	16.6 (4.9)	15.9 (4.1)	16.3 (4.6)
Antidepressant medication (*n*, %)	32 (68.0)	27 (60.0)	59 (64.1)

Notes: bCBT: blended cognitive behavioral therapy; CBT: cognitive behavioral treatment (face-to-face only); QIDS-SR: Quick Inventory of Depressive Symptomatology, Self-Report version; SD: Standard deviation.

3.2. *Study Dropout*

Gender, age, relationship status, employment, treatment preference, comorbidity, depression severity, and treatment group were not significantly related to missing working alliance ratings ($p > 0.5$). Patients who received fewer face-to-face sessions during the first ten weeks of treatment had higher odds of not providing information on working alliance ($\beta = -0.849$, OR = 0.43, 95% CI: 0.23; 0.64, $p < 0.001$). In addition, there was a high overlap between study dropout and treatment dropout; six out of nine patients who did not provide data also did not receive any face-to-face sessions.

3.3. *Treatment Received*

Table 2 provides an overview of treatment received before and after the alliance ratings (ten weeks after start of treatment). Before rating therapeutic alliance, patients in the bCBT group had received an average of 7.1 (SD 2.1) face-to-face sessions and 7.9 (SD 2.4) online sessions; those in the face-to-face CBT group had received a mean of 6.6 (SD 2.2) sessions by week 10. Average per-patient therapist time, including time spent on online feedback, during the first ten weeks of treatment was 636 min (SD 187) in bCBT and 395 min (SD 132) in face-to-face CBT. This difference was statistically significant—95% CI −308.7; −173.5, $t\ (90) = -7.08$, Holm-corrected $p < 0.001$. Over the full study period, therapist time between the two groups did not significantly differ (bCBT 944 min SD 274 versus CBT 844 min SD 348, $p = 0.130$). Overall, the face-to-face CBT group received more sessions at the clinic than the bCBT group—14.1 sessions (SD 5.8) versus 11.1 sessions (SD 3.5); mean difference 3.0, 95% CI 1.0; 5.0, $t\ (71.23) = 2.99$, $p = 0.004$, Holm-corrected $p = 0.008$).

Table 2. Treatment received in the two study groups.

	bCBT n = 47	CBT n = 45	Total n = 92
Treatment received before assessment of working alliance: mean (SD)			
Face-to-face sessions	7.1 (2.1)	6.6 (2.2)	6.7 (2.2)
Online sessions	7.9 (2.4)	-	-
Online feedback messages	6.9 (2.5)	-	-
Therapist time in minutes	636 (187)	395 (132)	518 (203)
Treatment received after assessment of working alliance: mean (SD)			
Face-to-face sessions	4.0 (2.7)	7.5 (4.8)	5.7 (4.3)
Online sessions	2.7 (2.8)	-	-
Online feedback messages	2.4 (2.6)	-	-
Therapist time in minutes	308 (208)	449 (289)	377 (258)
Treatment received during the full study period: mean (SD)			
Face-to-face sessions	11.1 (3.5)	14.1 (5.8)	12.5 (5.0)
Online sessions	10.3 (2.9)	-	-
Online feedback messages	9.3 (3.5)	-	-
Therapist time in minutes	944 (274)	844 (348)	895 (315)

Notes: bCBT: blended cognitive behavioral therapy; CBT: cognitive behavioral treatment (face-to-face only).

Comparing the total amount of treatment received in both groups with the planned amount of sessions based on the bCBT and CBT treatment protocols, we found that the bCBT group received on average 111% of the planned sessions (averaging one additional face-to-face session and one additional online session) and the CBT group received 70% to 94% (14 out of 15 to 20 planned sessions).

3.4. Working Alliance

After applying a Holm–Bonferroni correction [51] to account for multiple testing, we found no statistically significant differences between treatment groups on either the patient-rated or the therapist-rated composite scores, and also not on the separate Task, Goal, and Bond components of working alliance. Results are shown in Table 3.

Table 3. Patient- and therapist-rated working alliance in the two treatment groups.

	Patients				Therapists			
Outcome [1]	bCBT $n = 39$	CBT $n = 34$	Total $n = 73$	Mean difference (95% CI) bCBT vs. CBT	bCBT $n = 46$	CBT $n = 44$	Total $n = 90$	Mean difference (95% CI) bCBT vs. CBT
Goal	16.3 (3.1)	16.1 (3.2)	16.2 (3.1)	0.25 (−1.22; 1.71)	12.4 (1.9)	11.7 (1.8)	12.1 (1.9)	0.73 (0.04; 1.50) [a]
Scaled	4.1 (0.8)	4.0 (0.8)	4.1 (0.8)		4.1 (0.6)	3.9 (0.6)	4.0 (0.6)	
Task	12.4 (4.1)	11.9 (4.2)	12.2 (4.1)	0.47 (−1.45; 2.40)	12.1 (2.0)	11.2 (1.6)	11.7 (1.9)	0.93 (0.17; 1.68) [b]
Scaled	3.1 (1.0)	3.0 (1.1)	3.0 (1.0)		4.0 (0.7)	3.7 (0.5)	3.9 (0.6)	
Bond	15.6 (3.3)	14.7 (3.6)	15.2 (3.4)	0.97 (−0.64; 2.57)	17.9 (1.9)	17.6 (2.1)	17.7 (2.0)	0.28 (−0.52; 1.17)
Scaled	3.9 (0.8)	3.7 (0.9)	3.8 (0.9)		4.6 (0.5)	4.4 (0.5)	4.4 (0.5)	
Composite	3.7 (0.7)	3.6 (0.8)	3.6 (0.8)	0.14 (−0.22; 0.50)	4.2 (0.5)	4.0 (0.4)	4.1 (0.5)	0.20 (0.00; 0.40) [c]

Notes: [1] Data are presented as mean (standard deviation). bCBT: blended cognitive behavioral therapy; CBT: cognitive behavioral treatment (face-to-face only). [a] uncorrected: $p = 0.063$, Holm-corrected: $p = 0.144$; [b] uncorrected: $p = 0.016$, Holm-corrected: $p = 0.063$; [c] uncorrected: $p = 0.048$, Holm-corrected: $p = 0.424$.

Linear regression analyses showed no significant differences between treatment groups in the associations between patient and therapist evaluations of Task and Goal. In terms of the Bond and the composite scores, positive therapist evaluations appeared to have stronger associations with more positive patient evaluations in the bCBT group, but these were not significant after correction for multiple testing (Bond: 95% CI 0.16; 1.72, $p = 0.019$, Holm-corrected $p = 0.077$; composite: 95% CI −0.0; 1.49; $p = 0.053$, Holm-corrected: $p = 0.160$).

Controlling for therapist time invested in treatment in explorative linear regression analyses led to similar outcomes as described above in the uncontrolled analyses, showing nonsignificant between-group differences in patient-rated alliance, therapist-rated alliance, and associations between patient and therapist evaluations ($p > 0.05$).

In the full sample, patient and therapist composite scores were not significantly related, nor were ratings with regard to the Goal and Bond components. On the Task component, a significant moderate correlation of $\varrho = 0.41$ was found (95% CI: 0.20; 0.59, $p < 0.001$, Holm-corrected $p = 0.001$). In order to gain further insight into the level of agreement between patients and therapists, a difference score was calculated by subtracting the (recoded) therapist composite score from the patient composite score (range 0 to 5). Results showed that 43 out of 71 patients (61%) gave lower ratings than their therapists (mean −1.1, range −2.2 to −0.3); 14 patients (20%) gave similar ratings (mean −0.1, range −0.2 to 0.2), and 11 patients (16%) gave more positive evaluations (mean 0.7, range 0.3 to 4.0).

Explorative linear regression models assessing the relationship between therapist time and the therapist and patient ratings revealed only a significant positive association between therapist time and therapists' ratings of the Task component. This relationship remained significant after controlling for treatment condition (t (85) = 2.84, $p = 0.006$, Holm-corrected $p = 0.023$).

3.5. Working Alliance and Depression Severity

On average, patients completed 22.7 (SD 8.6, range 1 to 42) QIDS measurements. In the week before the assessment of working alliance at ten weeks, the mean QIDS depression severity score was 13.3 (SD 6.2, range 1 to 27), indicating moderately severe depression. Visual inspection of change in depression severity over time suggested a curvilinear pattern. Therefore, linear and quadratic trends were tested in a polynomial model. Adding the polynomial terms to the model led to a better model fit ($p < 0.001$). For patient-rated working alliance (composite score), there was a significant three-way interaction between both the linear and quadratic trends, treatment group and alliance—linear: $b = 0.61$ (95% CI 0.34; 0.88), t (169.50) = 4.25, Holm-corrected $p < 0.001$, quadratic: $b = -0.03$ (95% CI −0.04; −0.02), t (1028) = −5.34, Holm-corrected $p < 0.001$. In Figure 1, the association is visualized by rounding centered alliance scores to low (−1, $n = 21$, range 2.0 to 3.0), medium (0, $n = 32$, range 3.1 to 3.9), and high alliance (1, $n = 21$, range 4.0 to 5.0). Combined with weekly QIDS data, there were 320, 543, and 255 data points available in the respective categories. Density of data points is displayed along the x-axes of the three graphs. The direction of the regression lines after 20 weeks should be interpreted cautiously, because fewer data points were available after that time point.

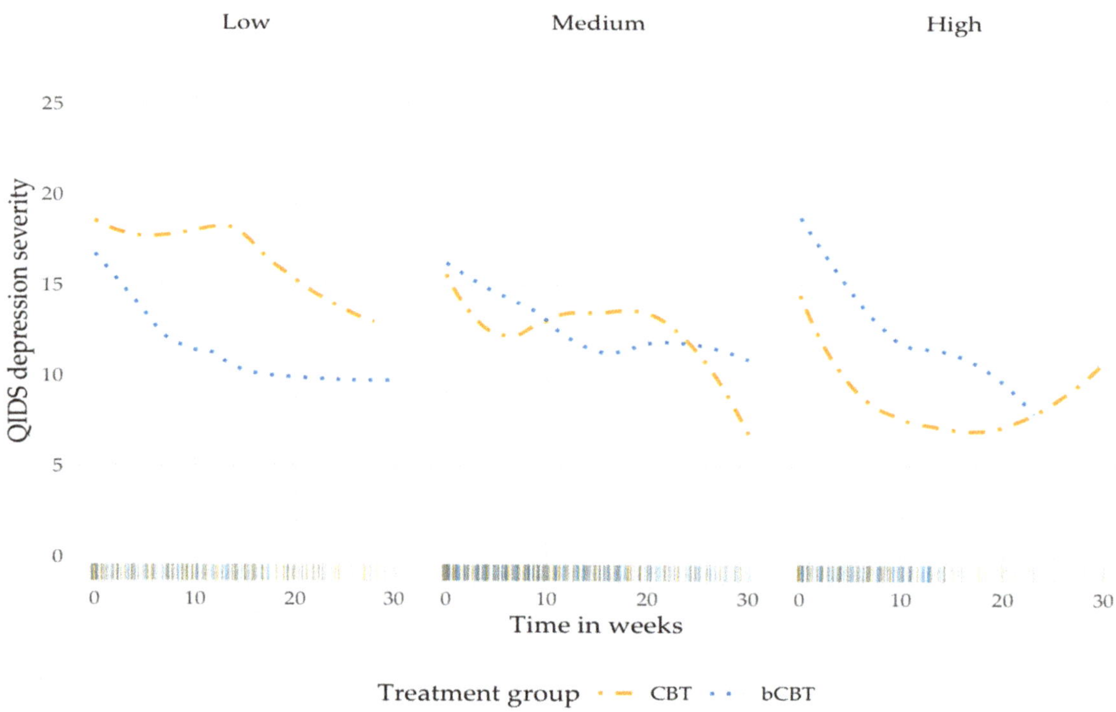

Figure 1. Observed change in depression over time for both treatment groups, clustered in low, medium, and high patient-rated working alliance (measured at week 10). bCBT: blended Cognitive Behavioral Therapy; CBT: Cognitive Behavioral Therapy (face-to-face only); QIDS: Quick Inventory of Depressive Symptomatology.

The graphs in Figure 1 suggest that depression severity in the face-to-face CBT group was associated with patient evaluations of working alliance. In the bCBT group, a similar pattern of decreasing depression severity appeared to occur in all three alliance categories. Post hoc subgroup analyses supported this theory. In bCBT, no alliance–outcome association was found. In the face-to-face CBT group, patients who provided higher ratings had significantly lower QIDS scores—$b = -7.78$ (95% CI −13.10; −1.95), t (27.21) = −2.68, uncorrected $p = 0.012$—than patients giving lower ratings. Control for therapist time invested in treatment did not alter the findings. Table 4 shows the results of the linear mixed model assessing patient-rated working alliance.

Table 4. Results of the linear mixed model with patient-rated working alliance.

Predictors	Dependent Variable				
	Estimates	SE	95% CI	Statistic	*p*-value
(Intercept)	14.96	0.88	13.25; 16.68	17.08	<0.001
Time × group × working alliance	0.61	0.14	0.33; 0.89	4.25	<0.001
Quadratic time × group × working alliance	−0.03	0.00	−0.04; −0.02	−5.34	<0.001

Notes: SE: Standard error. Random effects: residual (σ^2) = 6.63; intercept (τ_{00}) = 20.70; slope (τ_{11}) = 0.08; intercept–slope covariance (ϱ_{01}) = −0.17; intraclass correlation coefficient (ICC) = 0.76; $N = 70$; Observations 1118; Marginal R^2/Conditional R^2 = 0.191/0.804; log likelihood = −2861.15.

Therapist-rated alliance was not significantly associated with outcome ($p > 0.05$). LMM revealed similar significant interactions between treatment group and the linear and quadratic trends, suggesting a steeper decrease in depression severity during the first ten weeks of treatment in the bCBT group versus a more linear pattern of decrease of severity in the face-to-face CBT group. Rounding centered alliance scores for descriptive purposes showed that therapists provided lower overall alliance ratings in 2 cases (range 2.9 to 3.0), medium ratings in 58 cases (range 3.1 to 3.9), and high ratings in 30 cases (range 4.0 to 5.0). Explorative analysis revealed no association between the level of agreement (convergence) between patients' and therapists' working alliance ratings and outcome ($p > 0.05$).

4. Discussion

This study examined working alliance between patients and their therapists in blended cognitive behavioral therapy (bCBT) for depression, as provided in specialized mental healthcare settings, and compared it with the working alliance in face-to-face CBT.

4.1. Working Alliance between Patients and Therapists

No differences were found between treatment groups in the way patients and therapists evaluated the working alliance, nor in the associations between patient and therapist ratings of working alliance within either group. This suggests that providing part of treatment online, rather than face-to-face, did not have a negative impact on working alliance between patients and therapists. This is an important finding, because prior research found that therapists voiced this as one of their concerns when considering blended treatment [18]. In general, patients and therapists in both treatment groups were satisfied with the working alliance. Because the current study was one of the first to examine working alliance in bCBT compared with face-to-face CBT, these results cannot be related to outcomes from other studies yet. The high alliance ratings are similar to those reported in other studies that examined patient- and therapist-rated alliance, for example, the trial by Preschl and colleagues ($N = 53$) which compared online CBT with face-to-face CBT for depression [33], and the uncontrolled study by Vernmark and colleagues ($N = 73$) in blended CBT for depression [34].

While both patients and therapists provided positive ratings on average in the current study, no significant association was found between patient and therapist evaluations on general alliance (composite score), and on the Goal and Bond components. On the Task component a moderate positive association was found in the full study sample ($\varrho = 0.41$, 95% CI: 0.20; 0.59), suggesting that higher patient ratings on the Task domain concurred with higher therapist ratings. Further exploration of general working alliance showed that over half of the patients (43 out of 71, 61%) provided less positive evaluations than their therapist, with an average of minus 1 point on a five-point scale. While this is a notable finding, the level of agreement between patients and therapists was not associated with change in depression severity or vice versa. This suggests the degree of convergence after ten weeks of treatment did not impact the treatment effect in the current study.

4.2. Association between Working Alliance and Depressive Symptoms

For patient-rated alliance, an alliance–outcome association was found in the face-to-face group, but not in the bCBT group. In face-to-face CBT, higher depression severity was accompanied by lower alliance ratings, and vice versa. The results for bCBT concurred with the findings of the above-cited study by Vernmark and colleagues [34], which likewise found no alliance–outcome association for patient-rated working alliance in bCBT. That study, however, did not include a comparison group in the analyses. The cause of the disparity in the alliance–outcome association between our study groups cannot be determined here, and more research is needed. Because patients in both groups received CBT, the difference in the alliance–outcome association is more likely to be related to treatment *form* rather than to *content* or therapeutic techniques. One possible explanation is that in bCBT, more emphasis was placed on self-efficacy and autonomy by letting patients work through part of the treatment protocol on their own via the online platform. Hence, patients in bCBT were possibly less dependent on their therapist to achieve a change in depression severity than patients in the face-to-face CBT group.

In this study, no association between therapist-rated alliance and outcome was found in both groups. A possible explanation is that therapists were predominantly positive about the working alliance with their patients, thus restricting variance in this variable and limiting the feasibility of detecting associations between change in depression severity and working alliance. Comparison to other work is complicated, as therapist ratings are often not included in studies. The meta-analytic synthesis by Flückiger and colleagues [28], for example, identified 295 study samples that examined alliance in adult psychotherapy for various mental health problems, but only 40 (14%) of these included therapist ratings. Overall, the synthesis found similar alliance–outcome associations for the alliance ratings of both patients and therapists, suggesting that our current findings are not consistent with general findings on this issue. The same holds for the findings in the Vernmark study, where a significant association was found for therapist ratings and outcome in bCBT, but not for patient ratings, with each point increase in therapist ratings being associated with a 0.5 point reduction per week on the PHQ-9 (Patient Health Questionnaire-9) (95% CI −0.74; −0.26).

4.3. Change in Depressive Symptoms

Over the full study period (30 weeks), both of our treatment groups showed a similar overall improvement in depressive symptoms. Compared with patients in standard face-to-face CBT, those in bCBT reported a steeper decrease in depression severity in the first fifteen weeks of treatment, after which depression scores stabilized. In the face-to-face group, a more linear pattern was observed. This difference is an indication that the higher treatment intensity in bCBT might lead to additional health benefits. Our planning of bCBT treatment intensity was based on the 2013 meta-regression analysis by Cuijpers and colleagues [53], which focused on the amount of psychotherapy required to treat depression. The study suggested that, rather than treatment duration and dosage, the intensity in which sessions are offered per week positively impacts the effect of treatment. While the original goal of providing 18 bCBT sessions in ten weeks [35] was not met in the current study, patients did receive an average of 78% of treatment during that time frame, while those in the less intensive face-to-face CBT group received 37% of the treatment protocol during this period. However, such results should be interpreted with caution, as the current study was not designed to specifically examine the relationship between treatment intensity and treatment effects. Future studies should explore this further, along with the possible role a blended approach could play in achieving higher effectiveness through higher intensity.

4.4. Strengths and Limitations

The current study was one of the first to examine working alliance in a blended cognitive behavioral treatment format in routine practice, and to compare it with alliance in standard face-to-face CBT. By assessing depression severity at a weekly basis, the study also sheds light on the changing severity of depression over the course of treatment, revealing patterns of change rather than absolute differences measured before and after therapy. Moreover, the study included both patient and therapist evaluations of working alliance, providing insights into the degree of convergence between the actors and its possible effects on treatment outcome.

There are also some limitations to be considered while interpreting the results. First, working alliance was treated as a stable factor and was therefore measured only once. That time point was chosen in relation to the expected ten-week duration of the bCBT protocol. Future studies could consider performing an additional measurement at an early stage of treatment, or integrating a weekly assessment of working alliance into the treatment. That would help clarify changes and dynamics in therapeutic alliance over time. Repeated measures would enable more detailed comparison of patterns of depression severity and alliance ratings.

Second, the study had a relatively small sample size, which limited the power to detect small to moderate effects. These have therefore not been revealed by our study. Larger studies could also examine factors that potentially moderate or mediate associations, such as patient demographics, number of prior episodes, and prior experiences with treatment.

Third, the current study specifically focused on patients in outpatient special mental health care for depression. In order to further establish the potential value of bCBT, it is important to evaluate bCBT in other settings, such as primary care, and in different countries. Results from a large European study are forthcoming, examining the comparative effectiveness of bCBT versus treatment as usual in eight different European countries [16].

Additionally, it would be interesting to differentiate between online and face-to-face working alliance within bCBT. Patients might have different expectations of agreement on goals and tasks in the face-to-face sessions than in the online sessions. In the current study, for example, patients and therapists could modify general tasks and goals during their face-to-face sessions, while the content of the online sessions was fixed. Further, it would be interesting to examine whether patients evaluate the online affective bond differently from the bond with their therapist.

Fourth, 16 out of 33 therapists in our study treated patients in both treatment arms, allowing them to compare their experiences with both types of treatment. This could potentially cause bias. Because of the limited sample size, no subgroup analyses were done to examine a possible effect on the evaluation of working alliance when therapists treat patients in both treatment groups.

Finally, because this was one of the first studies to examine bCBT, therapists were relatively inexperienced with the format. It would be interesting to examine whether working alliance ratings in blended treatment increase with the therapists' level of experience.

5. Conclusions

This study shows that bCBT and face-to-face CBT are associated with similarly high working alliance ratings by both patients and therapists when provided to patients with depression in specialized mental health care. Replacing a proportion of the face-to-face sessions with online sessions and online therapist feedback evidently has no negative effect on working alliance and treatment effect. We did find that a more positive evaluation of working alliance was associated with lower depression severity in face-to-face CBT, whereas no such alliance–outcome association was seen in bCBT. The reason for that difference between treatment groups is still unclear. Replication of these results in larger samples to also enable assessment of possible moderators and mediators is warranted.

Author Contributions: All authors were involved in conceptualization, study design, methodology, and writing the original draft. Data curation, L.K. and J.R.; formal analysis, L.K. and J.R.; funding acquisition, P.v.O. and H.R.; project administration, L.K. and J.W.; supervision, J.R., J.W., P.v.O. and H.R.; visualization, L.K. and J.R.; writing—review & editing, L.K., J.W., P.v.O. and H.R. J.R. died in July 2019, before submission of the manuscript. All authors have read and agreed to the published version of the manuscript.

Acknowledgments: In loving memory of Jeroen Ruwaard. The authors gratefully acknowledge the contribution of all therapy participants, research assistants, therapists and all others who contributed to the study.

References

1. Kessler, R.C.; Chiu, W.T.; Demler, O.; Merikangas, K.R.; Walters, E.E. Prevalence, severity, and comorbidity of 12-month DSM-IV disorders in the National Comorbidity Survey Replication. *Arch. Gen. Psychiatry* **2005**, *62*, 617–627. [CrossRef]
2. Kohn, R.; Saxena, S.; Levav, I.; Saraceno, B. The treatment gap in mental health care. *Bull. World Health Organ.* **2004**, *82*, 858–866. [PubMed]
3. Demyttenaere, K.; Bruffaerts, R.; Posada-Villa, J.; Gasquet, I.; Kovess, V.; Lepine, J.P.; Angermeyer, M.C.; Bernert, S.; de Girolamo, G.; Morosini, P.; et al. Prevalence, severity, and unmet need for treatment of mental disorders in the World Health Organization World Mental Health Surveys. *JAMA* **2004**, *291*, 2581–2590. [PubMed]
4. Bremmer, F.; van Es, M. *Een Analyse van de Verwachte Kosten en Baten Van Ehealth: Blended Behandelen en Begeleiden*; GGZ Nederland: Amersfoort, The Netherlands, 2013.
5. Van't Hof, E.; Cuijpers, P.; Stein, D.J. Self-help and Internet-guided interventions in depression and anxiety disorders: A systematic review of meta-analyses. *CNS Spectr.* **2009**, *14*, 34–40. [PubMed]

6. Cuijpers, P.; Donker, T.; van Straten, A.; Li, J.; Andersson, G. Is guided self-help as effective as face-to-face psychotherapy for depression and anxiety disorders? A systematic review and meta-analysis of comparative outcome studies. *Psychol. Med.* **2010**, *40*, 1943–1957. [CrossRef]
7. Mohr, D.C.; Lyon, A.R.; Lattie, E.G.; Reddy, M.; Schueller, S.M. Accelerating digital mental health research from early design and creation to successful implementation and sustainment. *J. Med. Internet Res.* **2017**, *19*, e153. [CrossRef]
8. Schröder, J.; Berger, T.; Westermann, S.; Klein, J.P.; Moritz, S. Internet interventions for depression: New developments. *Dialogues Clin. Neurosci.* **2016**, *18*, 203–212.
9. Andersson, G.; Cuijpers, P.; Carlbring, P.; Riper, H.; Hedman, E. Guided Internet-based vs. face-to-face cognitive behavior therapy for psychiatric and somatic disorders: A systematic review and meta-analysis. *World Psychiatry* **2014**, *13*, 288–295. [CrossRef]
10. Cuijpers, P.; Riper, H. Internet Interventions for depressive disorders: An overview. *Revista de Psicopatología y Psicol. Clínica* **2014**, *19*, 209–216. [CrossRef]
11. Richards, D.; Richardson, T. Computer-based psychological treatments for depression: A systematic review and meta-analysis. *Clin. Psychol. Rev.* **2012**, *32*, 329–342. [CrossRef]
12. Andrews, G.; Basu, A.; Cuijpers, P.; Craske, M.G.; McEvoy, P.; English, C.L.; Newby, J.M. Computer therapy for the anxiety and depression disorders is effective, acceptable and practical health care: An updated meta-analysis. *J. Anxiety Disord.* **2018**, *55*, 70–78. [CrossRef] [PubMed]
13. Carlbring, P.; Andersson, G.; Cuijpers, P.; Riper, H.; Hedman-Lagerlöf, E. Internet-based vs. face-to-face cognitive behavior therapy for psychiatric and somatic disorders: An updated systematic review and meta-analysis. *Cogn. Behav. Ther.* **2018**, *47*, 1–18. [CrossRef] [PubMed]
14. Cuijpers, P.; Donker, T.; Johansson, R.; Mohr, D.C.; van Straten, A.; Andersson, G. Self-guided psychological treatment for depressive symptoms: A meta-analysis. *PLoS ONE* **2011**, *6*, e21274. [CrossRef] [PubMed]
15. Andersson, G.; Rozental, A.; Shafran, R.; Carlbring, P. Long-term effects of internet-supported cognitive behaviour therapy. *Expert Rev. Neurother.* **2017**, *18*, 21–28. [CrossRef] [PubMed]
16. Kleiboer, A.; Smit, J.; Bosmans, J.; Ruwaard, J.; Andersson, G.; Topooco, N.; Berger, T.; Krieger, T.; Botella, C.; Baños, R.; et al. European COMPARative Effectiveness research on blended Depression treatment versus treatment-as-usual (E-COMPARED): Study protocol for a randomized controlled, non-inferiority trial in eight European countries. *Trials* **2016**, *17*, 387. [CrossRef]
17. Høifødt, R.S.; Lillevoll, K.R.; Griffiths, K.M.; Wilsgaard, T.; Eisemann, M.; Waterloo, K.; Kolstrup, N. The clinical effectiveness of web-based cognitive behavioral therapy with face-to-face therapist support for depressed primary care patients: Randomized controlled trial. *J. Med. Internet Res.* **2013**, *15*, e153. [CrossRef]
18. Van der Vaart, R.; Witting, M.; Riper, H.; Kooistra, L.; Bohlmeijer, E.T.; van Gemert-Pijnen, L.J.E.W.C. Blending online therapy into regular face-to-face therapy for depression: Content, ratio and preconditions according to patients and therapists using a Delphi study. *BMC Psychiatry* **2014**, *14*, 355. [CrossRef]
19. Kenter, R.M.F.; van de Ven, P.M.; Cuijpers, P.; Koole, G.; Niamat, S.; Gerrits, R.S.; Willems, M.; van Straten, A. Costs and effects of Internet cognitive behavioral treatment blended with face-to-face treatment: Results from a naturalistic study. *Internet Interv.* **2015**, *2*, 77–83. [CrossRef]
20. Kooistra, L.C.; Ruwaard, J.; Wiersma, J.E.; van Oppen, P.; van der Vaart, R.; van Gemert-Pijnen, J.E.W.C.; Riper, H. Development and initial evaluation of blended cognitive behavioural treatment for major depression in routine specialized mental health care. *Internet Interv.* **2016**, *4*, 61–71. [CrossRef]
21. Erbe, D.; Eichert, H.-C.; Riper, H.; Ebert, D.D. Blending face-to-face and Internet-based interventions for the treatment of mental disorders in adults: Systematic review. *J. Med. Internet Res.* **2017**, *19*, e306. [CrossRef]
22. Thase, M.E.; Wright, J.H.; Eells, T.D.; Barrett, M.S.; Wisniewski, S.R.; Balasubramani, G.K.; McCrone, P.; Brown, G.K. Improving the efficiency of psychotherapy for depression: Computer-assisted versus standard CBT. *Am. J. Psychiatry* **2018**, *175*, 242–250. [CrossRef] [PubMed]
23. Berger, T.; Krieger, T.; Sude, K.; Meyer, B.; Maercker, A. Evaluating an e-mental health program ("deprexis") as adjunctive treatment tool in psychotherapy for depression: Results of a pragmatic randomized controlled trial. *J. Affect. Disord.* **2018**, *227*, 455–462. [CrossRef] [PubMed]
24. Kooistra, L.C.; Wiersma, J.E.; Ruwaard, J.; Neijenhuijs, K.; Lokkerbol, J.; van Oppen, P.; Smit, F.; Riper, H. Costs and effectiveness of blended versus standard cognitive behavioral therapy for depressed outpatients in routine specialized mental health care: Pilot randomized controlled trial. *J. Med. Internet Res.* **2019**, *21*, e14261. [CrossRef] [PubMed]

25. Wampold, B.E. How important are the common factors in psychotherapy? An update. *World Psychiatry* **2015**, *14*, 270–277. [CrossRef] [PubMed]
26. Horvath, A.O.; Del Re, A.C.; Flückiger, C.; Symonds, D. Alliance in individual psychotherapy. *Psychotherapy* **2011**, *48*, 9–16. [CrossRef]
27. Zilcha-Mano, S. Is the alliance really therapeutic? Revisiting this question in light of recent methodological advances. *Am. Psychol.* **2017**, *72*, 311–325. [CrossRef]
28. Flückiger, C.; Del, A.C.; Wampold, B.E.; Horvath, A.O. The alliance in adult psychotherapy: A meta-analytic synthesis. *Psychotherapy* **2018**, *55*, 316–340. [CrossRef]
29. Cameron, S.K.; Rodgers, J.; Dagnan, D. The relationship between the therapeutic alliance and clinical outcomes in cognitive behaviour therapy for adults with depression: A meta-analytic review. *Clin. Psychol. Psychother.* **2018**, *25*, 446–456. [CrossRef]
30. Laws, H.B.; Constantino, M.J.; Sayer, A.G.; Klein, D.N.; Kocsis, J.H.; Manber, R.; Markowitz, J.C.; Rothbaum, B.O.; Steidtmann, D.; Thase, M.E.; et al. Convergence in patient-therapist therapeutic alliance ratings and its relation to outcome in chronic depression treatment. *Psychother. Res.* **2017**, *27*, 410–424. [CrossRef]
31. Lorenzo-Luaces, L.; Driessen, E.; DeRubeis, R.J.; Van, H.L.; Keefe, J.R.; Hendriksen, M.; Dekker, J. Moderation of the alliance-outcome association by prior depressive episodes: Differential ffects in cognitive-behavioral therapy and short-term psychodynamic supportive psychotherapy. *Behav. Ther.* **2017**, *48*, 581–595. [CrossRef]
32. Berger, T. The therapeutic alliance in internet interventions: A narrative review and suggestions for future research. *Psychother. Res.* **2017**, *27*, 511–524. [CrossRef] [PubMed]
33. Preschl, B.; Maercker, A.; Wagner, B. The working alliance in a randomized controlled trial comparing online with face-to-face cognitive-behavioral therapy for depression. *BMC Psychiatry* **2011**, *11*, 189. [CrossRef] [PubMed]
34. Vernmark, K.; Hesser, H.; Topooco, N.; Berger, T.; Riper, H.; Luuk, L.; Backlund, L.; Carlbring, P.; Andersson, G. Working alliance as a predictor of change in depression during blended cognitive behaviour therapy. *Cogn. Behav. Ther.* **2019**, *48*, 285–299. [CrossRef] [PubMed]
35. Kooistra, L.C.; Wiersma, J.E.; Ruwaard, J.; van Oppen, P.; Smit, F.; Lokkerbol, J.; Cuijpers, P.; Riper, H. Blended vs. face-to-face cognitive behavioural treatment for major depression in specialized mental health care: Study protocol of a randomized controlled cost-effectiveness trial. *BMC Psychiatry* **2014**, *14*, 290. [CrossRef] [PubMed]
36. Sheehan, D.V.; Lecrubier, Y.; Sheehan, K.H.; Amorim, P.; Janavs, J.; Weiller, E.; Hergueta, T.; Baker, R.; Dunbar, G.C. The Mini-International Neuropsychiatric Interview (M.I.N.I.): The development and validation of a structured diagnostic psychiatric interview for DSM-IV and ICD-10. *J. Clin. Psychiatry* **1998**, *59* (Suppl. 2), 22–33, quiz 34–57. [PubMed]
37. Van Vliet, I.M.; De Beurs, E. Het Mini Internationaal Neuropsychiatrisch Interview (MINI). Een kort gestructureerd diagnostisch psychiatrisch interview voor DSM-IV en ICD-10-stoornissen. *Tijdschr. Psychiatr.* **2007**, *49*, 393–397.
38. Bockting, C.L.H.; Huibers, M.J.H. Protocollaire Behandeling Van Patienten Met Een Depressieve Stoornis. In *Protocollaire Behandelingen Voor Volwassenen Met Psychische Klachten 1*; Keijsers, G.P.J., van Minnen, A., Hoogduin, C.A.L., Eds.; Uitgeverij Boom: Amsterdam, The Netherlands, 2011; pp. 251–288. ISBN 9789461057723.
39. Beck, A.T.; Rush, A.J.; Shaw, B.F.; Emery, G. *Cognitive Therapy of Depression*; Guilford: New York, NY, USA, 1979; ISBN 0898620007.
40. Rush, A.J.; Trivedi, M.H.; Ibrahim, H.M.; Carmody, T.J.; Arnow, B.; Klein, D.N.; Markowitz, J.C.; Ninan, P.T.; Kornstein, S.; Manber, R.; et al. The 16-Item Quick Inventory of Depressive Symptomatology (QIDS), clinician rating (QIDS-C), and self-report (QIDS-SR): A psychometric evaluation in patients with chronic major depression. *Biol. Psychiatry* **2003**, *54*, 573–583. [CrossRef]
41. Bordin, E.S. The generalizability of the psychoanalytic concept of the working alliance. *Psychother. Theory, Res. Pract.* **1979**, *16*, 252–260. [CrossRef]
42. Horvath, A.O.; Greenberg, L.S. Development and validation of the Working Alliance Inventory. *J. Couns. Psychol.* **1989**, *36*, 223–233. [CrossRef]
43. Hatcher, R.L.; Gillaspy, J.A. Development and validation of a revised short version of the working alliance inventory. *Psychother. Res.* **2006**, *16*, 12–25. [CrossRef]

44. Stinckens, N.; Ulburghs, A.; Claes, L. De werkalliantie als sleutelelement in het therapiegebeuren: Meting met behulp van de WAV-12, de Nederlandstalige versie. *Tijdschr. Klin. Psychol.* **2009**, *39*, 44–60.
45. Munder, T.; Wilmers, F.; Leonhart, R.; Linster, H.W.; Barth, J. Working alliance inventory-short revised (WAI-SR): Psychometric properties in outpatients and inpatients. *Clin. Psychol. Psychother.* **2010**, *17*, 231–239. [CrossRef] [PubMed]
46. Shapiro, S.S.; Wilk, M.B. An analysis of variance test for normality (complete samples). *Biometrika* **1965**, *52*, 591–611. [CrossRef]
47. Revelle, W. *Psych: Procedures for Psychological, Psychometric and Personality Research*; Northwestern University: Evanston, IL, USA, 2018.
48. R Core Team. *R: A Language and Environment for Statistical Computing*; R Core Team: Vienna, Austria, 2017.
49. Hesser, H. Modeling individual differences in randomized experiments using growth models: Recommendations for design, statistical analysis and reporting of results of internet interventions. *Internet Interv.* **2015**, *2*, 110–120. [CrossRef]
50. White, I.R.; Carpenter, J.; Horton, N.J. Including all individuals is not enough: Lessons for intention-to-treat analysis. *Clin. Trials* **2012**, *9*, 396–407. [CrossRef]
51. Holm, S. A simple sequentially rejective multiple test procedure. *Scand. J. Stat.* **1979**, *6*, 65–70.
52. Bates, D.; Maechler, M.; Bolker, B.; Walker, S.; Christensen, R.H.B.; Singmann, H.; Dai, B.; Eigen, C. *Linear Mixed-Effects Models using "Eigen" and S4; R package, version 1-1.21*; 2017.
53. Cuijpers, P.; Huibers, M.; Ebert, D.D.; Koole, S.L.; Andersson, G. How much psychotherapy is needed to treat depression? A metaregression analysis. *J. Affect. Disord.* **2013**, *149*, 1–13. [CrossRef]

11

Experienced Burden of and Adherence to Smartphone-Based Ecological Momentary Assessment in Persons with Affective Disorders

Claire R. van Genugten [1,2,*], Josien Schuurmans [1,2], Femke Lamers [2], Harriëtte Riese [3], Brenda W. J. H. Penninx [1,2], Robert A. Schoevers [3], Heleen M. Riper [1,2,4,5] and Johannes H. Smit [1,2]

1 Department of Research and Innovation, GGZ inGeest, Specialized Mental Health Care, 1081 Amsterdam, The Netherlands; j.schuurmans@ggzingeest.nl (J.S.); b.penninx@amsterdamumc.nl (B.W.J.H.P.); h.riper@vu.nl (H.M.R.); jh.smit@ggzingeest.nl (J.H.S.)

2 Department of Psychiatry, Amsterdam Public Health Research Institute, Amsterdam UMC, Vrije Universiteit, 1081 Amsterdam, The Netherlands; f.lamers@ggzingeest.nl

3 Interdisciplinary Centre for Psychopathology and Emotion Regulation, Department of Psychiatry, University Medical Centre Groningen, University of Groningen, 9713 Groningen, The Netherlands; h.riese@umcg.nl (H.R.); r.a.schoevers@umcg.nl (R.A.S.)

4 Department of Clinical, Neuro and Developmental Psychology, Clinical Psychology Section, Vrije Universiteit Amsterdam and the Amsterdam Public Health Research Institute, 1081 Amsterdam, The Netherlands

5 Institute of Telepsychiatry, University of Southern Denmark, 5000 Odense, Denmark

* Correspondence: c.genugten@ggzingeest.nl

Abstract: (1) Background: The use of smartphone-based ecological momentary assessment (EMA) questionnaires in affective disorder research has rapidly increased. Though, a thorough understanding of experienced burden of and adherence to EMA is crucial in determining the usefulness of EMA. (2) Methods: Persons with current affective disorders (n = 100), remitted persons (n = 190), and healthy controls (n = 94) participated in a smartphone-based EMA two-week monitoring period. Our primary outcomes were (momentary) perceived burden of and adherence to EMA. (3) Results: In the whole sample, lower positive and higher negative affect were associated with slightly higher levels of perceived momentary burden (B = −0.23 [95%CI = −0.27–0.19], B = 0.30 [95%CI = 0.24–0.37], respectively). The persons with current affective disorders reported slightly higher levels of experienced momentary burden (Mdn = 1.98 [IQR = 1.28–2.57]), than the remitted persons (Mdn = 1.64 [IQR = 1.11–2.24]) and healthy controls (Mdn = 1.28 [IQR = 1.04–1.92]). Nevertheless, the persons with current affective disorders still showed very high adherence rates (Mdn = 94.3% [IQR = 87.9–97.1]), at rates on a par with the remitted persons (Mdn = 94.3% [IQR = 90.0–97.1]) and healthy controls (Mdn = 94.3% [IQR = 90.0–98.6]). (4) Discussion: Frequent momentary questionnaires of mental well-being are slightly more burdensome to the persons with current affective disorders, but this does not seem to have a negative impact on adherence. Their high rate of adherence to EMA—which was similar to that in remitted persons and healthy controls —suggests that it is feasible to apply (short-duration) EMA.

Keywords: affective disorders; depression; anxiety disorders; ecological momentary assessment; burden; adherence

1. Background

In recent decades, we have witnessed a surge in research acknowledging the importance of real-life context and diurnal variation of affective states in persons with affective disorders [1–4]. Ecological momentary assessment (EMA) is a valuable addition to the traditional methods of studying these dynamics [5–8]. EMA questionnaires were initially administered via paper-and-pencil diaries. Nowadays, online tools or apps on devices such as mobile telephones are designed to capture momentary ratings. With EMA, participants are asked to self-report information on their momentary affect throughout the day in natural settings [7–9], rather than recalling and summarizing their affect within a certain time interval (e.g., last week/month), as is done in retrospective questionnaires [9].

Advocates of EMA argue that assessing affective states more frequently is a more appropriate way to measure affect dynamics, as retrospective distortions are minimized [6,10–13]. EMA questionnaires provide us with the essential information that needs to be measured in order to generate insights in the temporal variability of anxiety and mood symptoms, the importance of real-life context, phenomenology, and the interrelatedness of symptoms [14–16]. These nuances are hard to capture when using traditional retrospective questionnaires, for the reasons mentioned above.

Measuring affect more frequently means that persons are repeatedly asked to provide information on their own mental well-being. However, since symptoms such as a lack of motivation to act and problems concentrating are core features of the clinical presentation of depression [17,18], adhering to these repeated questionnaires is not self-evident for persons with affective disorders. Also, repeatedly assessing affective states in persons who suffer from a persistently negative mood might lead to high levels of perceived burden. Nevertheless, systematic reviews showed encouraging results regarding the burden experienced and adherence rates by persons with affective disorders [8,14,15]. However, studies only investigated burden in terms of a reflection on the whole monitoring period; momentary burden, e.g., perceived burden at the moment of measuring, was not taken into account in any of these studies. Moreover, the majority of studies reporting on adherence rates used EMA methods such as paper-and-pencil diaries and personal digital assistants (PDAs) instead of smartphone-based EMA questionnaires. Adherence to smartphone-based EMA might differ from other EMA methods; nowadays the use of telephones is incorporated in the daily lives of many persons, as opposed to paper-and-pencil diaries and PDAs that were distributed for study-purposes only. A better understanding of experiences of users is crucial when considering the usefulness of smartphone-based EMA questionnaires for persons with affective disorders.

The aim of this study was to explore perceived burden and adherence to smartphone-based EMA questionnaires in persons with affective disorders sampled from the Ecological Momentary Assessment (EMA) and Actigraphy sub-study (NESDA-EMAA) [19,20]. As well as persons with affective disorders, the cohort also included remitted persons and healthy controls. All (n = 384) participated in an interview, including a clinical assessment and an intensive two-week smartphone-based EMA monitoring period with five EMA questionnaires a day. Due to this design, we were able to make a direct comparison in adherence and perceived burden between the persons with current affective disorders and the other two groups in a single cohort.

2. Methods

2.1. Study Design and Participants

The participants of the Ecological Momentary Assessment (EMA) and Actigraphy sub-study (NESDA-EMAA) were selected from the Netherlands Study of Depression and Anxiety (NESDA). In brief, NESDA is an ongoing longitudinal multi-site naturalistic cohort study which aims to examine the biological, social, and psychological factors contributing to the long-term course of depressive and anxiety disorders [21]. NESDA participants were initially recruited for the baseline measurement between 2004 and 2007 (n = 2981) and were invited for a fifth interview on the occasion of the nine-year follow-up measurement (Wave 6; 2014-2017; $n = 1776$). At Wave 6, siblings ($n = 367$) of a subsample of NESDA participants were also recruited and included in the NESDA cohort.

Wave 6 comprised a large number of measurements, administered by trained research staff. These included a structured clinical diagnostic interview. After measurement, the participants were invited to join the NESDA-EMAA. For the NESDA-EMAA we invited NESDA participants who participated in at least two of the previous waves, consented to be approached for the NESDA-EMAA, participated in the interview no more than 31 days prior starting with the EMA questionnaires, were familiar with smartphone use and willing to wear a wrist-worn actigraphy device. Siblings were invited if they did not meet the criteria of a current or past diagnosis of depressive and/or anxiety disorder or other severe psychiatric disorder [19,20]. A flowchart showing the enrolment processes is given in Figure 1.

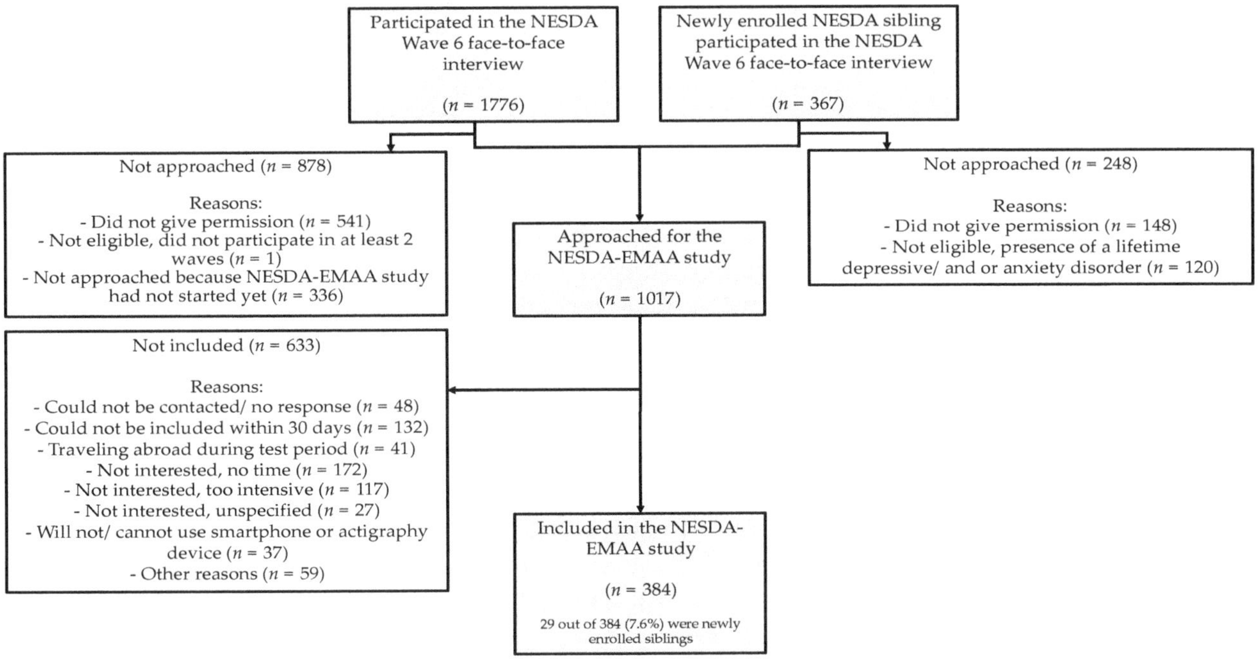

Figure 1. Flowchart of the Ecological Momentary Assessment (EMA) and Actigraphy sub-study (NESDA-EMAA).

This resulted in a sample of 384 included participants (of whom 29 were newly enrolled siblings). The sample was divided into three groups: 1) a group with at least one current affective disorder ($n = 100$) (i.e., persons who met the criteria for a depressive or anxiety disorder in the past six months, per to the Diagnostic and Statistical Manual of Mental Disorders, Fourth Edition, Text Revision (DSM-IV-TR) criteria); 2) a group with an affective disorder in remission ($n = 190$) (persons with a life-time diagnosis of depressive and/or anxiety disorder, but who did not meet DSM-IV-TR criteria in the past six months); and 3) a healthy control group ($n = 94$) (persons with no lifetime history of psychiatric disorders). The in- and exclusion criteria are described in more detail elsewhere [19,20].

The study was carried out in accordance with the latest version of the Declaration of Helsinki. The Ethical Review Board of VU University Medical Centre Amsterdam and the local review boards of the participating centres provided ethical approval and all participants provided written consent. The NESDA and the NESDA-EMAA are described in more detail elsewhere [19–21].

2.2. *Smartphone-Based Ecological Momentary Assessment Protocol*

All the NESDA-EMAA participants were invited to conduct five EMA questionnaires a day for 14 days. These were conducted during the day, using a time-based sampling protocol with fixed time intervals of three hours. The questionnaires were in the form of self-reported answers with a maximum of 31 questions, focusing on momentary affective states, as well as a number of additional items such as hours of sleep since the last questionnaire. Data were collected via smartphones; at an appointed time, the participants received an invitation by text message to conduct and submit the questionnaire. Participants were instructed to complete the questionnaire as soon as possible after receiving the text message, preferably within 15 minutes, but at least within 60 minutes. After completing the questionnaires, the participant's answers were saved automatically to the secured web-based server (RoQua) [22].

In addition to the automatic reminder, several measures were taken to motivate the participants and to provide support when needed. Research assistants called them on at least two separate occasions: one day and one week after the moment they started with the questionnaires. Additionally, participants received a gift voucher worth €20 and a personalized report of their EMA questionnaires afterwards.

2.3. *Measurements*

2.3.1. Baseline Characteristics

Basic demographics and clinical characteristics were requested during the Wave 6 measurement. We obtained information about age, gender, and educational level through standard questions. Number of current weekly working hours was assessed by the use of the Treatment Inventory of Costs in Patients with psychiatric disorders (TiC-P) [23]. Presence of lifetime and/or current depressive (dysthymia and major depressive disorder) and anxiety disorders (social anxiety disorder, panic disorder with or without agoraphobia, agoraphobia, and generalized anxiety disorder) was defined according to DSM-IV criteria [24]. Diagnoses were established using the Composite International Diagnostic Interview (CIDI Version 2.1) [25]. This has high validity for the assessment of mental disorders [26].

2.3.2. Momentary Affective States

Momentary affective states were measured repeatedly through the daily EMA questionnaires. The participants provided information about their mental well-being by completing a thirteen-item questionnaire. Twelve of these items were derived from the affect-questionnaire in the Uncovering Positive Potential of Emotional Reactivity (UPPER) study [27]. For this study we added a thirteenth item on feelings of anxiety. The list included seven items covering the negative affective state, whilst the other six covered the positive state. The negative affect items (At this moment I feel upset, irritated, listless/apathic, down, nervous, bored, anxious) were averaged to form a negative affect (NA) subscale and the positive affect ones (At this moment I feel satisfied, relaxed, cheerful, energetic, enthusiastic, calm) were averaged to form a positive affect (PA) subscale. The items were rated on seven-point Likert scales (1 = not at all, 4 = moderate, 7 = very); higher scores meant respectively higher levels of negative and positive affect.

2.4. *Outcomes*

2.4.1. Momentary Burden

Experienced burden as a result of the daily EMA questionnaires was one of the main outcomes of this study. We assessed momentary burden; participants were asked about their experienced burden as a result of the EMA questionnaire itself. They did so by answering the following standard question "How disturbing is filling out a questionnaire right now?". The question was rated on a seven-point Likert scale (1 = not at all, 4 = moderate, 7 = very).

2.4.2. Experienced Burden Over the Whole Monitoring Period

We also assessed the participants' overall experience. Immediately after the last daily EMA questionnaire, participants received a text message with a link to an addendum questionnaire, which included four items to evaluate experienced burden over the whole EMA monitoring period. Questions about the study duration; the number of questions; assessment frequency; and overall experience were rated on a seven-point Likert scale (1 = not at all, 4 = moderate, 7 = very). The average of these four items represented the evaluation score (sum possibilities ranging from 1 to 7). The four items showed excellent internal consistency in this sample (Cronbach's $\alpha = 0.924$).

2.4.3. Adherence to the Daily EMA Questionnaires

The other main outcome of this study was adherence to the daily EMA questionnaires. This was calculated by counting the percentage of completed EMA questionnaires out of the total of 70 each participant was invited to undertake. Moreover, at the last EMA questionnaire participants were asked to report their main reasons for missing a questionnaire, if they had done so. Possible reasons listed in the questionnaire were: being busy with an activity; no network connection; being asleep; technical problems; not hearing the smartphone; not bringing the smartphone; could not making themselves do it; and "other" reasons. The participants were allowed to select more than one reason. In addition, we counted the absolute number of omissions due to technical issues.

2.5. Statistical Analyses

We calculated descriptive statistics for the majority of our variables. Because data appeared to be non-normally distributed based on Kolmogorov–Smirnov tests, we report the median (Mdn) and the interquartile range (IQR) for the continuous variables. Differences between the three diagnosis groups in terms of demographic characteristics, absolute number of uploaded assessments, the retrospective evaluation sum-score, and reported reasons for missing assessments were analyzed; for this we used Kruskall–Wallis tests, Bonferroni-adjusted Mann–Whitney tests, Pearson chi-square tests, and likelihood ratio tests as appropriate.

To analyze the EMA data, we conducted several tests. We looked at whether the groups differed in respect of mean momentary burden as reported through the daily EMA questionnaires. In order to do this, we first calculated the person-mean of this variable by averaging the scores across the participants' EMA questionnaires. We then compared the averages of the person-mean scores for the three diagnosis groups using a Kruskall–Wallis test and conducted pairwise comparisons using Bonferroni-adjusted Mann–Whitney tests. In addition, we produced a number of generalized estimated equation (GEE) models for the overall sample. We chose GEE models because EMA data have a hierarchical structure; this type of model adjusts for dependency of repeated measures within one participant and can handle non-normally distributed data. GEE models are also suitable for dealing with missing data; it is not required to exclude participants with missing questionnaires, nor should missing questionnaires be imputed beforehand. A more detailed description about GEE models is described in detail elsewhere [28,29]. We used the GEE models to analyze the association between positive and negative affect on the one hand, and momentary burden as a result of the measurement itself on the other. The variables diagnosis group, gender, age, weekly working hours, and educational level were separately added to the GEE models as independent variables to check for possible confounding. Next, the variables were added as interaction terms to the model to check for possible effect modification. A GEE model was also used to analyze the stability of the reported levels of momentary burden across the EMA questionnaires. To see whether levels of burden changed as the study period progressed, we added the variable time to the unadjusted model. All analyses were carried out using SPSS (version 25.0) and two-sides p values < 0.05 were considered significant ($p < 0.017$ after Bonferroni correction).

3. Results

3.1. Sample Characteristics

Table 1 shows the demographic and clinical characteristics that were assessed across the three diagnosis groups. In the overall sample, 67.0% (238 out of 384) of the participants were female, the median age was 51.0 years (IQR = 38.00–61.00), the average of weekly working hours was 20

(IQR = 0.00–35.5), and most individuals had intermediate (50.3% [193 out of 384]) or high (46.4% [178 out of 384]) education. In general, a considerable number of persons with current affective disorder and remitted persons suffered multiple affective disorder at the time of the EMA questionnaires or in their history, respectively. In total, 39.0% (39 out of 100) of the persons with current affective disorders suffered from more than one affective disorder (range 2–7) at the time of the EMA questionnaires. In the group of persons with remitted persons, 66.3% (126 out of 190) suffered from more than one affective disorder (range 2–7), in parallel or in sequence, in their life span.

Table 1. Demographics of the study sample.

	Persons with Current Affective Disorder(S) Persons (n = 100)	Remitted Persons (n = 190)	Healthy Controls (n = 94)	Total (n = 384)	Test Value	p Value
Demographic characteristics						
Age	50.5 (41.5–59.0)	48.5 (36.0–61.0)	54.0 (4.0–62.0)	51.0 (38.0–61.0)	H(2) = 4.25	0.12
Gender						
Female	64 (64.0)	132 (69.5)	51 (54.3)	238 (67.0)	$\chi^2(2) = 6.35$	0.04
Male	36 (36.0)	58 (30.5)	43 (45.7)	117 (33.0)		
Educational level						
Basic	8 (8.0)	4 (2.1)	1 (1.1)	13 (3.4)	$\chi^2(4) = 14.51$	0.01
Intermediate	49 (49.0)	106 (55.8)	38 (40.4)	193 (50.3)		
High	43 (43.0)	80 (42.1)	55 (58.5)	178 (46.4)		
Working hours (a week)	10.0 (0.0–32.0)	20.0 (0.0–32.0)	30.0 (0.0–37.0)	20.0 (0.0–35.5)	H(2) = 10.22	0.01
DSM-IV-R Diagnosis	**Current**	**Lifetime**				
One more or anxiety disorder	71(71.0)	142 (74.7)				
One or more depressive disorder	61 (61.0)	163 (85.8)				
Generalized anxiety disorder	12 (12.0)	69 (36.3)				
Social phobia	35 (35.0)	86 (45.3)				
Panic disorder with agoraphobia	6 (6.0)	41 (21.6)				
Panic disorder without agoraphobia	13 (13.0)	31 (16.3)				
Agoraphobia	22 (22.0)	32 (16.8)				
Major depressive disorder	57 (57.0)	160 (84.2)				
Dysthymia	15 (15.0)	52 (27.4)				
Number of affective disorders*	**Current**	**Lifetime**				
1	61 (61.0)	64 (33.7)				
2	23 (23.0)	45 (23.7)				
3	12 (12.0)	39 (20.5)				
4	3 (3.0)	22 (11.6)				
5	1 (1.0)	10 (5.3)				
6	0 (0.0)	8 (4.2)				
7	0 (0.0)	2 (1.1)				

Note: Data are n (%), mean (SD) or median (IQR). Kruskall–Wallis, Pearson's chi-square and likelihood ratio tests were used as appropriate. * Affective disorders include depressive disorders (major depressive disorder, dysthymia) and anxiety disorders (social anxiety disorder, panic disorder with or without agoraphobia, agoraphobia, and generalized anxiety disorder).

3.2. Burden

3.2.1. Person-Mean Momentary Burden

To examine perceived burden as a result of the daily EMA questionnaires, we looked at momentary burden and at an evaluation of experienced burden over the whole two-week EMA monitoring period. Figure 2 shows the distribution of the person-means of the momentary burden in the three diagnosis groups. Tests showed a significant difference between the three groups (H[2] = 17.31, $p < 0.0001$). Subsequent, Bonferroni-corrected pairwise comparisons showed that, on average, the person-means of momentary burden reported by the persons with current affective disorders (Mdn = 1.98, IQR = 1.28–2.57) were significantly higher than in both the remitted persons (Mdn = 1.64, IQR = 1.11–2.24; U = 7229.50, p = 0.01) and the healthy controls (Mdn = 1.28, IQR = 1.04–1.92; U = 3098.50, $p < 0.0001$).

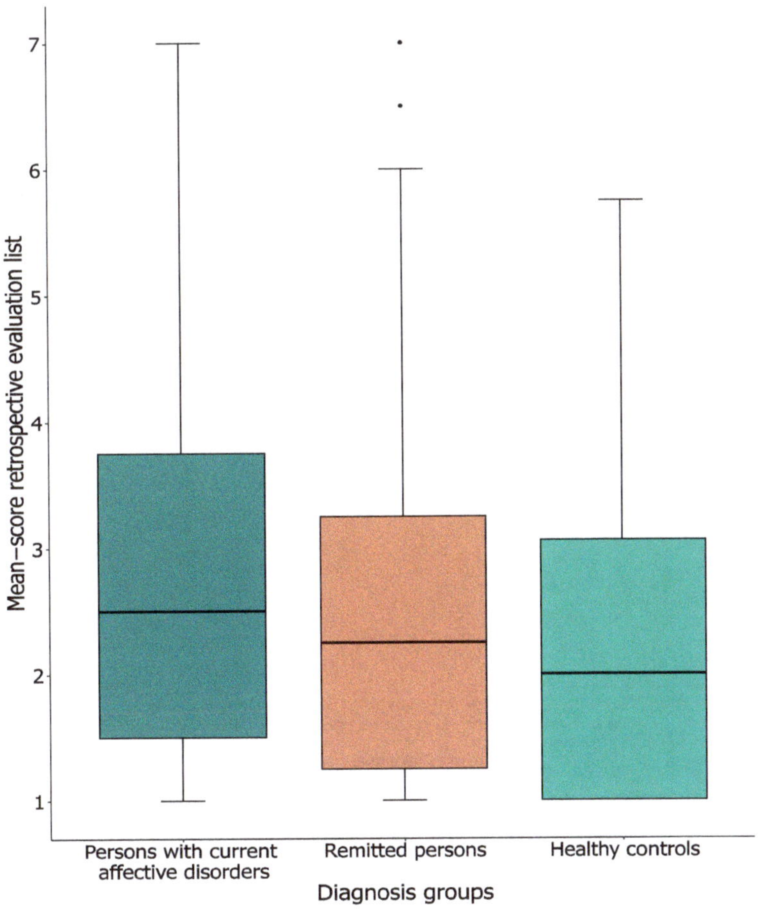

Figure 3. Mean scores of the retrospective evaluation of experienced burden. Note: Mean scores of the retrospective evaluation; a reflection of experienced burden over the whole EMA monitoring period. Score range between 1 and 7, higher score indicates more burden. Thick black line shows the median, error bars show the interquartile range (IQR), whiskers show +/−1.5 IQR, and ● = outlier, deviates by ≥ 1.5× IQR.

3.2.4. Adherence Rates

Adherence to the daily EMA questionnaires was our other main outcome. We looked at adherence rates, self-reported main reasons for missing questionnaires, and the number of omissions due to technical issues. Figure 4 shows the median (Mdn) and inter-quartile range (IQR) of the adherence rates to the EMA questionnaires. All groups showed the same median adherence rate (66 out of 70 [94.3%]) to the EMA measures, meaning that there is no significant difference between the persons with current affective disorders (IQR = 63.5–69.0), the remitted persons (IQR = 63.0–68.0), and the healthy controls (IQR = 62.0–69.0; (H[2] = 0.08, p = 0.98). These results show that adherence rates in our sample were high.

3.2.5. Reasons for Missing Daily EMA Questionnaires

After the last daily EMA questionnaire, participants were asked to list their main reasons for missing questionnaires. In total, 369 participants (out of 384) completed this addendum questionnaire-321 of which missed at least one EMA questionnaire. For 57.2% of them (184 out of 321), it appears that 'being busy with an activity' was one of their main reasons for missing a questionnaire. Other reasons frequently reported were 'no network connection' (reported by 22.4% [72 out of 321]), and 'being asleep' (reported by 21.2% [68 out of 321]). There are no statistically significant group differences for these and the other reasons as listed in Table 3.

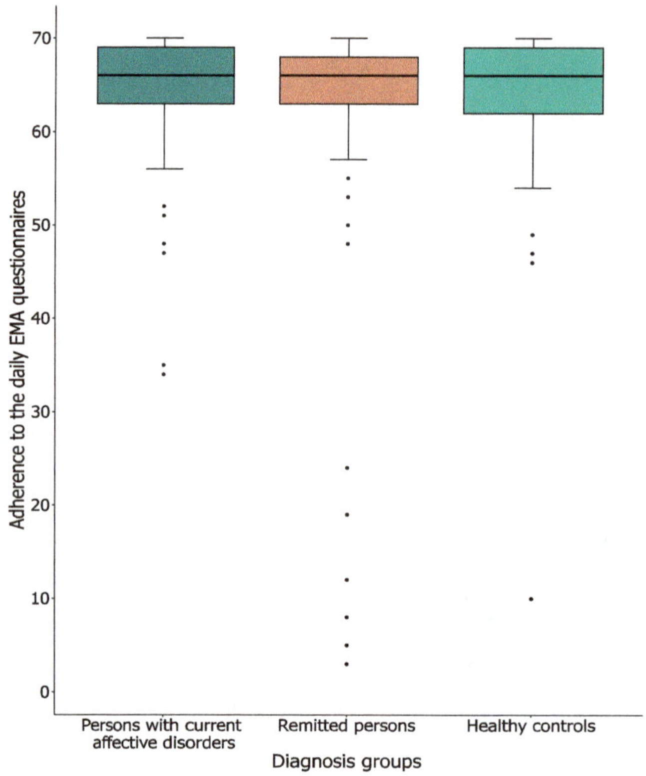

Figure 4. Adherence to the EMA questionnaires. Note: Participants were invited to conduct a total of 70 EMA questionnaires. Thick black line shows the median, error bars show the interquartile range (IQR), whiskers show +/−1.5 IQR, and ● = outlier, deviates by ≥ 1.5× IQR.

Table 3. Self-reported main reasons for missing EMA questionnaires.

	Persons with Current Affective Disorders (n = 77)	**Remitted Persons (n = 156)**	**Healthy Controls (n = 75)**	**Total (n = 321)**	**Test Value**	**p Value**
Amount of reasons	2 (1–2)	2 (1–2)	1 (1–2)	2 (1-3)	H(2) = 3.10	0.21
Main reasons for missing questionnaires						
Being busy with an activity	52 (67.5)	86 (55.1)	46 (61.3)	184 (57.3)	$\chi^2(2) = 3.40$	0.18
No network connection	18 (23.4)	38 (24.4)	16 (21.3)	72 (22.4)	$\chi^2(2) = 0.26$	0.88
Being asleep	22 (28.6)	36 (23.1)	10 (13.3)	68 (21.2)	$\chi^2(2) = 5.31$	0.07
Technical problems	14 (18.2)	29 (18.6)	15 (20.0)	58 (18.1)	$\chi^2(2) = 0.94$	0.95
Did not hear the smartphone	17 (22.1)	24 (15.4)	14 (18.7)	55 (17.1)	$\chi^2(2) = 1.62$	0.45
Did not bring the smartphone	12 (15.6)	26 (16.7)	7 (9.3)	45 (14.0)	$\chi^2(2) = 2.26$	0.32
Could not make themselves do it	1 (1.3)	0 (0.0)	0 (0.0)	1 (0.3)	$\chi^2(2) = 3.01$	0.22
Other reason	15 (19.5)	40 (25.6)	18 (24.0)	73 (22.7)	$\chi^2(2) = 1.09$	0.58

Note: Data are n (%) or median (IQR). Only individuals who missed at least one EMA questionnaire and completed the addendum questionnaire were taken into account in this table. Participants were allowed to select more than one option. Likelihood ratio or Pearson's chi-square tests were used as appropriate.

Next, we checked whether EMA questionnaires were missed due to technical issues with the server. In the group of persons with current affective disorders, this was the case for 0.14% (10 out of 7000) of the questionnaires. The equivalent figure for the group of remitted persons was 0.19% (25 out of 13,300) and for the healthy controls it was 0.30% (20 out of 6,580 measures). It thus appears that, across the sample, technical issues accounted for only a small number of the missed questionnaires.

4. Discussion

The results of this study show that, when asked at the moment of assessing, perceived burden as a result of the ecological momentary assessment (EMA) questionnaires was slightly higher when affect was worse. Adhering to the measure was thus more burdensome for persons diagnosed with an affective disorder, than it was for remitted persons and healthy controls. Nevertheless, when asked to evaluate the overall experienced burden of the whole two-week monitoring period, no significant inter-group differences were found. Moreover, the persons with current affective disorders showed very high adherence rates regardless.

Our findings show that when asked "in the moment", higher negative affect and lower positive affect were associated with slightly higher levels of perceived burden as a result of the EMA questionnaires. This was the case for all diagnosis groups and regardless the number of weekly working hours, age, gender, and educational background of the participant. The persons with current affective disorders thus reported higher levels of burden by comparison to the other two groups. These findings could possibly be explained by the fact that the clinical picture of the current affective disorders involves a persistent depressed mood and/or diminished interest or pleasure in general [17,18]. Adhering to EMA questionnaires might therefore be more intrusive to persons with current affective disorders, than for persons without such a disorder. Nevertheless, across the two-week EMA monitoring period the experienced burden remained stable, and for the overall experienced burden of the whole two-week EMA inter-group differences were no longer found.

Importantly, the higher levels of "in the moment burden" amongst the persons with current affective disorders did not result in nonadherence; on average, they completed over 94% of the EMA questionnaires—a rate on a par with the other two groups in this cohort. Moreover, the adherence rates found in this study are even higher than in previous ones with a similar population, although these studies used different EMA methods (e.g., paper-and-pencil diaries, PDAs) [8,14,15]. Previous studies using a smartphone-based method in other psychiatric populations also had lower adherence. A meta-analysis showed a pooled average adherence rate of 71% in substance abusers [30]. Note, however, the adherence rates in our study might have been influenced by the fact that participants were allowed to answer the questionnaires within 60 minutes after being prompted. Other studies often only allow for a short period of time to complete the questionnaires (e.g., up till 30 minutes) [31].

Our study does have some limitations, though, which should be considered when interpreting our findings. Most notably, it can be reasonably assumed that the participants in the NESDA-EMAA sample are highly motivated as they have been taking part in the NESDA study for over nine years. In addition, the results of our a relatively short EMA monitoring period might not be readily generalized to other settings that rely on longer EMA monitoring periods. Another point is that momentary burden was collected with one single item. As a result, the psychometric properties of this main outcome measure could not be assessed. In future work, it is advised to include (multiple item) questionnaires in order to report psychometric properties of the momentary burden assessment. Still, the results of the present study have important clinical implications for clinical practice. In most clinical settings, some form of real-time data is already gathered via paper-and-pencil methods (e.g., thought diaries, assessment of mood fluctuation in bipolar patients, or assessments of the frequency and intensity of panic attacks). The number of studies investigating the clinical usefulness of EMA methods via a smartphone in routine practice is also rising [32–34]. User experiences should also be explored in clinical settings when considering whether EMA can indeed be translated into a tool, beneficial for patients with affective disorders.

5. Conclusions

In conclusion, even though the persons with current affective disorders did report experiencing more burden as a result of the EMA questionnaires when asked about this at the moment of assessment, this was not the case when asked to evaluate the whole monitoring period, and they were still able and willing to provide real-time information on their mental well-being. This study is, to the best of our knowledge, the first to systematically examine user experiences of EMA questionnaires in persons with current affective disorders while making a direct comparison with remitted persons and healthy controls in a single cohort. Although our conclusions highlight the need to examine this topic further, they do already provide important insights into the acceptability of (short-duration) EMA methods for persons with affective disorders.

Author Contributions: All authors have contributed substantially to the work reported. All authors critically revised the paper. Conceptualization, C.R.v.G., J.S., H.M.R. and J.H.S.; methodology, C.R.v.G., J.S., H.M.R. and J.H.S.; writing—original draft preparation, C.R.v.G.; writing—review and editing, J.S., F.L., H.R., B.W.J.H.P., R.A.S., H.M.R. and J.H.S.; supervision: J.S., H.M.R. and J.H.S. All authors have read and agreed to the published version of the manuscript.

Acknowledgments: This work was financially supported by Innovative Medicines Initiative 2 Joint undertaking under grant agreement no. 115902. Femke Lamers has received funding from the European Union Seventh Framework Programme (FP7/2007–2013) under grant agreement no. PCIG12-GA-2012–334065. The infrastructure for the NESDA study (www.nesda.nl) is funded through the Geestkracht program of the Netherlands Organization for Health Research and Development (ZonMw, grant number no. 10-000-1002) and financial contributions by participating universities and mental health care organizations (Amsterdam UMC location VUmc, GGZ inGeest, Leiden University Medical Centre, Leiden University, GGZ Rivierduinen, University Medical Centre Groningen, University of Groningen, Lentis, GGZ Friesland, GGZ Drenthe, Rob Giel Onderzoekscentrum).

References

1. Houben, M.; van den Noortgate, W.; Kuppens, P. The Relation between Short-Term Emotion Dynamics and Psychological Well-Being: A Meta-Analysis. *Psychol. Bull.* **2015**, *141*, 901–930. [CrossRef] [PubMed]
2. Lamers, L.; Swendsen, J.; Cui, L.; Husky, M.; Johns, J.; Zipunnikov, V.; Merikangas, K.R. Mood Reactivity and Affective Dynamics in Mood and Anxiety Disorders. *J. Abnorm. Psychol.* **2018**, *127*, 659–669. [CrossRef] [PubMed]
3. Nelson, J.; Klumparendt, A.; Doebler, P.; Ehring, T. Everyday Emotional Dynamics in Major Depression. *Emotion* **2018**. [CrossRef] [PubMed]
4. Thompson, R.J.; Mata, J.; Jaeggi, S.M.; Buschkuehl, M.; Jonides, J.; Gotlib, I.H. The everyday emotional experience of adults with major depressive disorder: Examining emotional instability, inertia, and reactivity. *J. Abnorm. Psychol.* **2012**, *121*, 819–829. [CrossRef] [PubMed]
5. Marzano, L.; Bardill, A.; Fields, B.; Herd, K.; Veale, D.; Grey, N.; Moran, P. The Application of MHealth to Mental Health: Opportunities and Challenges. *Lancet Psychiatry* **2015**, *2*, 942–948. [CrossRef]
6. Myin-Germeys, I.; Kasanova, Z.; Vaessen, T.; Vachon, H.; Kirtley, O.; Viechtbauer, W.; Reininghaus, U. Experience Sampling Methodology in Mental Health Research: New Insights and Technical Developments. *World Psychiatry* **2018**, *17*, 123–132. [CrossRef]
7. Trull, T.J.; Ebner-Priemer, U.W. Using Experience Sampling Methods/Ecological Momentary Assessment (ESM/EMA) in Clinical Assessment and Clinical Research: Introduction to the Special Section. *Psychol. Assess.* **2009**, *21*, 457–462. [CrossRef]
8. Wenze, S.J.; Miller, I.W. Use of Ecological Momentary Assessment in Mood Disorders Research. *Clin. Psychol. Rev.* **2010**, *30*, 794–804. [CrossRef]
9. Shiffman, S.; Stone, A.A.; Hufford, M.R. Ecological Momentary Assessment. *Ann. Rev. Clin. Psychol.* **2008**, *4*, 1–32. [CrossRef]
10. Ben-Zeev, D.; Young, M.A.; Madsen, J.W. Retrospective Recall of Affect in Clinically Depressed Individuals and Controls. *Cogn. Emot.* **2009**, *23*, 1021–1040. [CrossRef]
11. Gloster, A.T.; Miché, M.; Wersebe, H.; Mikoteit, T.; Hoyer, J.; Imboden, C.; Bader, K.; Meyer, A.H.; Hatzinger, M.; Lieb, R. Daily Fluctuation of Emotions and Memories Thereof: Design and Methods of an Experience Sampling Study of Major Depression, Social Phobia, and Controls. *Int. J. Methods Psychiatr. Res.* **2017**, *26*, 1–12. [CrossRef] [PubMed]
12. Myin-Germeys, I.; Oorschot, M.; Collip, D.; Lataster, J.; Delespaul, P.; van Os, J. Experience Sampling Research in Psychopathology: Opening the Black Box of Daily Life. *Psychol. Med.* **2009**, *39*, 1533–1547. [CrossRef] [PubMed]

13. Armey, M.F.; Schatten, H.T.; Haradhvala, N.; Miller, I.W. Ecological momentary assessment (EMA) of depression-related phenomena. *Curr. Opin. Psychol.* **2015**, *4*, 21–25. [CrossRef] [PubMed]
14. Aan het Rot, M.; Hogenelst, K.; Schoevers, R.A. Mood Disorders in Everyday Life: A Systematic Review of Experience Sampling and Ecological Momentary Assessment Studies. *Clin. Psychol. Rev.* **2012**, *32*, 510–523. [CrossRef]
15. Colombo, D.; Fernández-Álvarez, J.; Patané, A.; Semonella, M.; Kwiatkowska, M.; García-Palacios, A.; Cipresso, P.; Riva, G.; Botella, C. Current State and Future Directions of Technology-Based Ecological Momentary Assessment and Intervention for Major Depressive Disorder: A Systematic Review. *J. Clin. Med.* **2019**, *8*, 465. [CrossRef]
16. Walz, L.C.; Nauta, M.H.; Aan Het Rot, M. Experience Sampling and Ecological Momentary Assessment for Studying the Daily Lives of Patients with Anxiety Disorders: A Systematic Review. *J. Anxiety Disord.* **2014**, *28*, 925–937. [CrossRef]
17. American Psychiatric Association. *Diagnostic and Statistical Manual of Mental Disorders*, 5th ed.; American Psychiatric Association: Washington, DC, USA, 2013.
18. Beck, A.T.; Alford, B.A. *Depression: Causes and Treatment*, 2nd ed.; University of Pennsylvania Press: Philadelphia, PL, USA, 2009.
19. Difrancesco, S.; Lamers, F.; Riese, H.; Merikangas, K.R.; Beekman, A.T.F.; Hemert, A.M.; Schoevers, R.A.; Penninx, B.W.J.H. Sleep, Circadian Rhythm, and Physical Activity Patterns in Depressive and Anxiety Disorders: A 2-week Ambulatory Assessment Study. *Depress. Anxiety* **2019**. [CrossRef]
20. Schoevers, R.A.; Van Borkulo, C.D.; Lamers, F.; Servaas, M.N.; Bastiaansen, J.A.C.J.; Beekman, A.T.; Van Hemert, A.M.; Smit, J.H.; Penninx, B.W.J.H.; Riese, H. Momentary affect fluctuations differ between patients with current depression and anxiety disorders, remitters and healthy controls. *Psychol. Med.* (under review).
21. Penninx, B.W.J.H.; Beekman, A.T.; Smit, J.H.; Zitman, F.G.; Nolen, W.A.; Spinhoven, P.; Cuijpers, P.; De Jong, P.J.; Van Marwijk, H.W.; Assendelft, W.J.; et al. The Netherlands Study of Depression and Anxiety (NESDA): Rationale, Objectives and Methods. *Int. J. Methods Psychiatr. Res.* **2008**, *17*, 121–140. [CrossRef]
22. Sytema, S.; van der Krieke, L. Routine Outcome Monitoring: A Tool to Improve the Quality of Mental Health Care. In *Improving Mental Health Care: The Global Challenge*, 1st ed.; Thornicroft, G., Ruggeri, M., Goldberg, D., Eds.; John Wiley & Sons: Chichester, UK, 2013.
23. Bouwmans, C.; De Jong, K.; Timman, R.; Zijlstra-Vlasveld, M.; Van Der Feltz-Cornelis, C.; Tan, S.S.; Hakkaart-Van Roijen, L. Feasibility, reliability and validity of a questionnaire on healthcare consumption and productivity loss in patients with a psychiatric disorder (TiC-P). *BMC Health Serv. Res.* **2013**, *13*, 217. [CrossRef]
24. American Psychiatric Association. *Diagnostic and Statistical Manual of Mental Disorders*, 4th ed.; American Psychiatric Association: Washington, DC, USA, 1994.
25. WHO. *Composite International Diagnostic Interview*, version 2.1; World Health Organization: Geneva, Switzerland, 1991.
26. Wittchen, H.U.; Robins, L.N.; Cottler, L.B.; Sartorius, N.; Burke, J.D.; Regier, D. Cross-Cultural Feasibility, Reliability and Sources of Variance of the Composite International Diagnostic Interview (CIDI). *Br. J. Psychiatr.* **1991**, *159*, 645–653. [CrossRef]
27. Bennik, E. Every Dark Cloud Has a Colored Lining: The Relation between Positive and Negative Affect and Reactivity to Positive and Negative Events. Ph.D. Thesis, University of Groningen, Groningen, The Netherlands, 2015.
28. Lu, B.; Preisser, J.S.; Qaqish, B.F.; Suchindran, C.; Bangdiwala, S.I.; Wolfson, M. A comparison of two bias-corrected covariance estimators for generalized estimating equations. *Biometrics* **2007**, *63*, 935–941. [CrossRef] [PubMed]
29. Twisk, J.; de Vente, W. Attrition in Longitudinal Studies: How to Deal with Missing Data. *J. Clin. Epidemiol.* **2002**, *55*, 329–337. [CrossRef]
30. Jones, A.; Remmerswaal, D.; Verveer, I.; Robinson, E.; Franken, I.H.A.; Wen, C.K.F.; Field, M. Compliance with Ecological Momentary Assessment Protocols in Substance Users: A Meta-Analysis. *Addiction* **2018**, *114*, 609–619. [CrossRef] [PubMed]
31. Janssens, K.A.M.; Bos, E.H.; Rosmalen, J.G.M.; Wichers, M.C.; Riese, H. A Qualitative Approach to Guide Choices for Designing a Diary Study. *BMC Med. Res. Methodol.* **2018**, *18*. [CrossRef] [PubMed]

32. Bos, F.M.; Snippe, E.; Bruggeman, R.; Wichers, M.; van der Krieke, L. Insights of patients and clinicians on the promise of the experience sampling method for psychiatric care. *Psychiatr. Serv.* **2019**, *70*, 983–991. [CrossRef]
33. Loo Gee, B.; Griffiths, K.M.; Gulliver, A. Effectiveness of Mobile Technologies Delivering Ecological Momentary Interventions for Stress and Anxiety: A Systematic Review. *J. Am. Med. Inform. Assoc.* **2016**, *23*, 221–229. [CrossRef]
34. Schueller, S.M.; Aguilera, A.; Mohr, D.C. Ecological Momentary Interventions for Depression and Anxiety. *Depress. Anxiety* **2017**. [CrossRef]

12

Minding the Gatekeepers: Referral and Recruitment of Postpartum Mothers with Depression into a Randomized Controlled Trial of a Mobile Internet Parenting Intervention to Improve Mood and Optimize Infant Social Communication Outcomes

Kathleen M. Baggett [1,*], Betsy Davis [2], Lisa B. Sheeber [2], Robert T. Ammerman [3], Elizabeth A. Mosley [1], Katy Miller [1] and Edward G. Feil [2]

1 Mark Chaffin Center for Healthy Development, Georgia State University, Atlanta, GA 30303, USA; emosley@gsu.edu (E.A.M.); kspinks@gsu.edu (K.M.)
2 Oregon Research Institute, Eugene, OR 97403, USA; betsy@ori.org (B.D.); lsheeber@ori.org (L.B.S.); edf@ori.org (E.G.F.)
3 Cincinnati Children's Hospital Medical Center, University of Cincinnati College of Medicine, Cincinnati, OH 45229, USA; robert.ammerman@cchmc.org
* Correspondence: Kbaggett@gsu.edu

Abstract: Mothers in the United States (U.S.) who are of non-dominant culture and socioeconomically disadvantaged experience depression during postpartum at a rate 3 to 4 times higher than mothers in the general population, but these mothers are least likely to receive services for improving mood. Little research has focused on recruiting these mothers into clinical intervention trials. The purpose of this article is to report on a study that provided a unique context within which to view the differential success of three referral approaches (i.e., community agency staff referral, research staff referral, and maternal self-referral). It also enabled a preliminary examination of whether the different strategies yielded samples that differed with regard to risk factors for adverse maternal and child outcomes. The examination took place within a clinical trial of a mobile intervention for improving maternal mood and increasing parent practices that promote infant social communication development. The sample was recruited within the urban core of a large southern city in the U.S. and was comprised primarily of mothers of non-dominant culture, who were experiencing severe socioeconomic disadvantage. Results showed that mothers self-referred at more than 3.5 times the rate that they were referred by either community agency staff or research staff. Moreover, compared to women referred by research staff, women who self-referred and those who were referred by community gatekeepers were as likely to eventually consent to study participation and initiate the intervention. Results are discussed with regard to implications for optimizing referral into clinical intervention trials.

Keywords: maternal depression; referral; recruitment; mobile intervention; clinical trials

---

1. Introduction

Ramifications of depressive conditions are quite severe, with depression being a leading cause of disability for women and contributing significantly to the overall burden of disease globally [?]. During the first year after childbirth, women are more likely to develop depression and anxiety than at any other time in their life [?]. Perhaps some of the greatest costs of maternal depression are borne by the children. Perinatal mood and anxiety disorders compromise parenting and adversely affect children's physical and emotional development [? ? ?]. In particular, maternal depression can undermine sensitive and responsive caregiving, parenting behaviors that are key to supporting healthy child development [?]. Hence, it is crucial to provide interventions that both address maternal depression and strengthen skills involved in sensitive and responsive parenting as early as possible in a child's life to promote subsequent maternal and child health and development [?].

Unfortunately, delivering intervention to mothers and children most in need has proven difficult, and few depressed mothers receive treatment [?]. Mothers living in socioeconomic disadvantage and those who are of non-dominant culture are more likely to experience depression compared to higher resourced mothers of the dominant culture [?], but they are far less likely to receive treatment [?]. In the U.S., women of European origin use mental health services at more than twice the rate of Black or Latinx women [?]. This finding is consistent with the more general finding that racial and ethnic minorities are less likely to receive mental health services when compared to non-Latinx White persons after controlling for multiple demographic characteristics and disorder severity [?]. The American Academy of Pediatrics (AAP) and the American College of Obstetricians and Gynecologists (ACOG) [?] have called for women to receive depression screening and referral to intervention during the first year postpartum [?]. Evidence suggests, however, that the majority of women with depressive symptoms do not receive screening and appropriate treatment [?], even within systems reportedly conducting universal screening [?].

According to the Maternal, Infant, and Early Childhood Home Visiting Technical Assistance Coordinating Center [?], mothers who are least likely to enroll and engage in services are those experiencing depression and, because of structural and systemic biases [?], are of non-dominant culture and living within socioeconomic disadvantage. Moreover, in the U.S., redistribution of social safety net resources away from the very poor affect their ability to receive needed mental health and other family services [?]. Issues of diversity and access also come into play in research examining efficacy and effectiveness of interventions [?]. Systemic and structural barriers to recruitment into clinical trials of potential participants from non-dominant cultures exist, including distrust in research as well as costs and logistics that impede participation [?]. Moreover, even when members of non-dominant ethnic and racial groups are included in samples, frequent failure to report ethnic and racial characteristics restricts understanding about service delivery to these populations [?]. In a review of clinical trials for depression spanning a 36-year period [?], researchers reported that over time, participation by persons of low socioeconomic status (SES) and those of minority ethnic and racial backgrounds has increased. Nonetheless, persons of European backgrounds remained the most highly represented group. Moreover, within National Institutes of Health (NIH)-funded clinical trials where racial/ethnic representation in samples is expected and reported [?], researchers often do not examine racial/ethnic status as moderators of treatment effects, such that limited data are available that speak to effectiveness of intervention within these populations [?]. These limitations in the literature leave in question whether access to effective interventions is equitable across populations.

Recruitment of depressed participants, in general, into clinical trials is difficult, spurring conceptual work seeking to understand important gatekeeper-patient factors in recruitment [?] as well as intervention work seeking to modify recruitment behaviors within gatekeeper systems [?]. However, lower resourced individuals are not well-represented within these efforts. One study that directly assessed family general practitioner gatekeeper referrals found substantial disparities in referral and access to mental health services both within and outside of family general practitioner gatekeeper systems [?]. Individuals with greater resource levels were more likely to bypass the gatekeeper system to access directly mental health services, and if these individuals first went to the gatekeeper for referral, they were more likely and more quickly referred to mental health services compared to individuals with lower resource levels [?]. However, this study occurred outside of the U.S. in a country with a profoundly different health service context. In the U.S., large numbers of individuals from non-dominant cultures are under- or uninsured, contributing barriers to health-related service receipt [?] as well as inclusion in clinical trials [?].

Given the ubiquity of digital technologies, mobile health interventions can serve as a way to increase intervention access for those who are traditionally missed [?]. However, there are issues related to what we know about connecting individuals to these interventions. While online recruitment is frequently used in mobile health interventions, very little systematic research exists on this recruitment method [?]. One study comparing recruitment approaches found online paid advertising was more cost effective and timely than provider referral for recruitment to a mobile health early parenting obesity prevention intervention [?]. Another study compared non-paid and paid recruitment approaches to a mobile health smoking cessation intervention and found that online paid advertising and survey panel approaches were best for increasing racial/ethnic diversity in their sample to reach at minimum 25% [?]. Their resultant sample, however, was still primarily White. A recent study describing the recruitment of depressed individuals into a multi-site trial noted that Black participants self-referred into their study at 1.5 times the rate of the local population [?]. However, while self-referral appears an important mechanism for increasing access, the study pertained to a community-based group intervention rather than a mobile health intervention.

At present, existing recruitment studies are extremely limited with regard to implications for referral and recruitment into mobile health intervention trials among non-dominant culture mothers who are depressed and experiencing significant socioeconomic disadvantage. Efforts are needed to identify referral methods that best connect these mothers with intervention and to examine the extent to which various methods are successful at engaging mothers in intervention. We are currently conducting a clinical trial evaluating the efficacy of an integrated internet-based parenting and depression intervention. The intervention is designed to reduce maternal symptomatology and increase sensitive and responsive parenting in mothers of infants. This study, which takes place within the urban core of a large southern city within the U.S., provides a valuable in situ context within which to examine referral and recruitment efforts. Results have the potential to provide information with relevance to improving access to interventions for both depressed women and for women who are socioeconomically disadvantaged, of culturally non-dominant groups, and who continue to have severely unequal access to needed services.

This current study compared three referral approaches to examine their relative success at engaging potential participants in the study. Because researchers may succeed at or fail at engaging women who could benefit from an intervention at multiple points in the recruitment process, we compared the relative success of the referral approaches at several points between initial referral and engagement in the intervention, as described more specifically below. The current study used data from the ongoing clinical trial to examine a year-long period of referral to and recruitment into the intervention trial. The trial provides a unique context within which to compare the success of three referral approaches and examine, in a preliminary way, whether samples referred to the study by different approaches differ on variables associated with adverse maternal and infant outcomes as well as ability to access treatment. The questions we address are:

(1) Are the three referral approaches (i.e., community agency referral, research-team referral, and maternal self-referral) differentially successful as defined by: (a) number of mothers referred; (b) number who complete eligibility screening; (c) number of screenings resulting in eligible participants; (d) number of mothers who consent to participation; and ultimately, (e) number of mothers who initiate intervention?

(2) Do samples referred to the study by different approaches differ on variables associated with maternal or infant outcomes and ability to access treatment, including educational level, relationship status, maternal knowledge of infant development, and severity of maternal symptomatology. Notably, we could not examine income or racial/ethnic differences between groups because of homogeneity in the sample.

2. Materials and Methods

The design of the intervention trial, from which the data presented here were derived, called for recruitment of depressed mothers of infants under one year of age. We focused our recruitment efforts to generate a sample inclusive of mothers from non-dominant cultures who were experiencing socioeconomic disadvantage and elevated maternal depressive symptoms. Inclusion criteria were intended to produce a sample of mother–infant dyads, in which infants were at elevated risk for poor social communication development as a function of maternal depression and adverse mother–infant interactions that exacerbate the detrimental effects of poverty. Prior to initiating human subject activity, all study procedures were approved by the Georgia State University IRB. Potentially eligible women were contacted by research staff who described the project, conducted eligibility screening, and obtained informed consent.

Consented participants were randomized into one of two parallel intervention arms: (1) Mom and Baby Net (MBN) or (2) Depression and Developmental Awareness (DDAS). MBN is a 14-session, coach-facilitated, online intervention that teaches mothers both cognitive-behavioral strategies to reduce depressive symptoms and specific skills for engaging with their infants to promote infant social-communication competencies. DDAS is an informational program designed to improve maternal awareness of depression and understanding of infant developmental milestones. The MBN is a skill-based program designed to promote parental competencies to address affective symptoms and interact positively with their infants. DDAS, on the other hand, is an informational program that provides relevant content but does not shape new skills directly. The two mobile interventions were identical with regard to number of sessions, session length, and delivery mechanisms. For more information about the interventions, see Baggett el al. [**?**].

In this report, we compared three recruitment strategies for enrolling women into the intervention study. The enrollment period examined herein began one year after initiating outreach to build recruitment capacity and continued for an additional 12 months. Recruitment strategies included the following: (1) community agency referrals; (2) research staff outreach visits to community agencies and community events (i.e., research staff referrals); and (3) maternal self-referral. Outcomes compared across the referral conditions included the following: number referred, number screened, number of eligible screens, number of consented, and number that completed initial session to connect with intervention. We also examined a number of individual characteristics that present risk for maternal depression, adverse mother–infant interactions, and poor infant social communication development. These factors included education level, absence of social support, depression symptom severity, and knowledge about infant social communication development.

2.1. Sample

Participants referred were mothers of infants aged 0–12 months ($N = 203$). Mothers were included in the study sample if they had a score of 3 or more on the Patient Health Questionnaire-2 (PHQ-2) [**?**] at screening, were a minimum of 18 years old, spoke English, and lived in the local metropolitan area of a large southern city in the U.S. Exclusion criteria included history of psychotic symptoms, residence in homeless or domestic violence shelter, infant receiving intensive medical treatment, and not having permanent legal guardianship of infant. Demographic characteristics for the sample of 86 enrolled mothers are presented in Table **??**.

Table 1. Demographic characteristics of the sample recruited into the study.

Variable	Value
Maternal age in years, mean (SD); range	28.12 (5.85); 19.00 to 44.00
Child age in months, mean (SD); range	5.16 (2.82); 2.00 to 12.00
Number of children in the home, mean (SD); range	2.67 (1.45); 1.00 to 6.00
Maternal race (Black) % (*n*)	95.35% (82)
Maternal ethnicity (Latinx), % (*n*)	3.49% (3)
Maternal Education (<college degree), % (*n*)	84.88% (73)
Maternal income, %(*n*) </=138% Federal Poverty Guideline	85.00% (68)

2.2. *Referral*

At the onset of study referral, we anticipated enrolling approximately 50 women per year based on referral agreements secured from agencies serving socioeconomically disadvantaged mothers and their infants. However, after one year of community outreach and recruitment capacity building, we had obtained only 5 referrals from community agencies. Moreover, we had received 10 maternal self-referrals, and 19 referrals of women our research team recruited at community events and occasional visits to community agencies to provide support to agency staff making referrals. At this point, we broadened our recruitment strategy to include online maternal self-referral. Referral strategies are described below.

Agency referral: Consistent with the original research plan, the research team encouraged ongoing referral from community agencies serving mothers and infants, such as WIC (Special Supplemental Nutrition Program for Women, Infants, and Children), the regional children's hospital, and medical clinics serving low income women. Partnerships with these agencies were established prior to study initiation for the purpose of participant recruitment. This approach had the potential benefit of reaching women at convenient access points, where they intersected with community agencies designed to promote the health and safety of their children as well as their own well-being. Agencies were provided with information about the project and agreed to screen women with the PHQ-2 and refer potential participants to the project via any of the following mechanisms, as per agency staff preference: (1) use of the project's online screening and referral system; (2) phone; or (3) secure email. However, many agency staff referred mothers without conducting depression screening; in these cases, the research team completed depression screening as part of the overall eligibility assessment and recruitment process.

Research staff outreach and referral: Research staff visited community agencies and attended community events, such as resource fairs, at which service agencies advertise their programs. Staff provided interested women with information about the intervention project, screened for inclusion criteria, and referred mothers to the project coordinator for enrollment.

Online maternal self-referral: The project maintained a self-referral mechanism through its website, which provided the following: (1) access to a brief video describing the intervention programs; (2) information about the project team; (3) depression screening; and (4) a form for providing contact information to research staff. To promote awareness of the online self-referral mechanism, the research team posted information on local community agency websites, social media platforms, and in print material available at local community agencies. We did not use any paid advertising mechanism.

2.3. *Measures*

To assess maternal progression from referral through successful recruitment into the study intervention, the following variables were documented by date of occurrence or disposition within the project database: referred, screened for eligibility, and eligible after screening. The PHQ-2 was administered online to screen for depression with the established criteria of a score of 3 or higher defined as a positive depression screen. The PHQ-2 is an efficient and well-established measure with strong psychometric characteristics for identifying individuals with depression [?]. At pre-intervention assessment, participants completed a demographic questionnaire to facilitate characterization of the sample with regard to mother's age, ethnicity, race, educational level, income, significant relationship status, and number of children in the home. We also obtained child age in months and child sex.

Additional participant intrapersonal risk characteristics were also assessed at pre-intervention. The Patient Health Question-9 (PHQ-9) was administered to assess depression severity. Endorsement of the PHQ-9 item, "Thoughts that you would be better off dead or of hurting yourself", was viewed as an indicator of self-harm thoughts [?]. The PHQ-9 possesses strong psychometric properties for assessing depression severity; a score at or above 20 is suggestive of severe depression [?]. Participants were also administered the Knowledge of Infant Social communication Development and Competency Promotion, which has demonstrated high internal consistency and sensitivity to intervention change [?].

2.4. *Analysis*

Using data collected between 21 September 2018 and 20 September 2019 on 203 referred mothers, we viewed the following five progression points into intervention: number of mothers referred from each of the three approaches, the number of mothers screened for eligibility, the number of mothers found to be eligible in screening, the number of mothers who consented to participate in the clinical trial, and the number of mothers who initiated the intervention. For number referred, we do not know the number of mothers within each approach, who could possibly have been referred in order to calculate a relative rate of referral within each approach. We will, therefore, report each approach's contribution of referred mothers to the overall recruited sample and calculate a multiplicative index to reflect any referral number differences between approaches (e.g., one approach contributed 2.7 times the number of referred mothers from other approaches across the same time period). The examination of other successive efficiency progression points is dependent upon the sample sizes resulting from each referral approach. Utilizing G*Power [?] with an overall n of 203, assuming equal numbers of mothers within each referral condition, with $p < 0.05$ two-tailed, we calculated that we would have less than 80% power (i.e., 71%) to detect moderately small effect sizes (d = 0.40), between the three conditions. If sample sizes diverge between the referral approach groups, parametric power would be reduced even further. Hence, to reduce the power burden, we took a conservative approach and limited analysis a priori to a two-group comparison, comparing maternal self-referral and agency referral groups. The a-priori group comparison was based on the fact that the two referral conditions selected are the most salient for referral into intervention research. The Chi Square test was used for the first research question and the Mann–Whitney tests were used for the second research question, given categorical versus ordinal variables, respectively. Working with an equal n two-group design (n = approximately 136), using wmwpow [?] at 80% power, small effect size (d = 0.40), $p < 0.05$ two-tail, and assuming a normal distribution for the two groups, we estimated power = 0.80, an acceptable criterion. If groups sizes differed, however, power was reduced and we focused on reporting effect size estimates, viewing d = 0.30 or higher as potentially meaningful for subsequent examination.

3. Results

With regard to the first research question on referral success, the number of self-referred mothers far surpassed that of mothers referred from traditional agency and research referral gatekeepers, with more than 3.5 times more referrals generated from the self-referral group as compared to referrals from community agency staff or research staff referral groups (see Figure **??**).

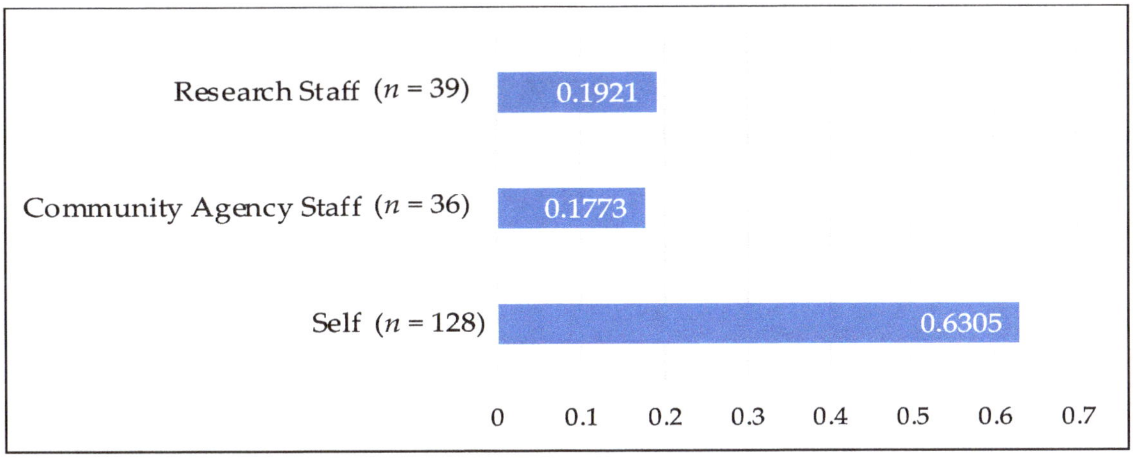

Figure 1. Percentage of each referral group contribution to the total referred sample.

The large difference in the number of cases generated through self-referral, as compared to agency and research staff, had significant impact on the number of cases to be examined at each successive point. Hence, we moved to our most conservative test to reduce burden on power, as described earlier. We conducted four Chi Square tests of between-group examinations and restricted comparisons to the self-referral and agency-referral groups. Table **??** presents the number of mothers within each referral group at each successive point.

Table 2. Number of mothers by referral group meeting each progression point.

Variable	Agency Referral	Research Staff Referral	Mother Self-Referral	Total Referrals
Number referred	36	39	128	203
Number/% screened for eligibility	30 83.33%	28 71.79%	106 82.81%	164 80.79%
Number/% eligible based on screening	20 (66.67%)	24 (85.71%)	92 (86.79%)	136 (82.93%)
Number/% who consented	12 (60%)	10 (41.67%)	64 (69.56%)	86 (63.23%)
Number/% who completed initial intervention session	12 (100%)	9 (90%)	62 (96.88%)	83 (96.51%)

Overall, agency-referred and self-referred mothers moved at similar percentage rates through four of the five successive points. The number of women who were eligible to participate based on the screening, however, was significantly higher for the self-referred group as compared to the agency-referred group. This difference reflected a small effect (Chi Square = 6.52, $p = 0.01$, d = 0.45). Figure **??** presents an overall view of the proportion of mothers moving through each point of the recruitment process by referral strategy.

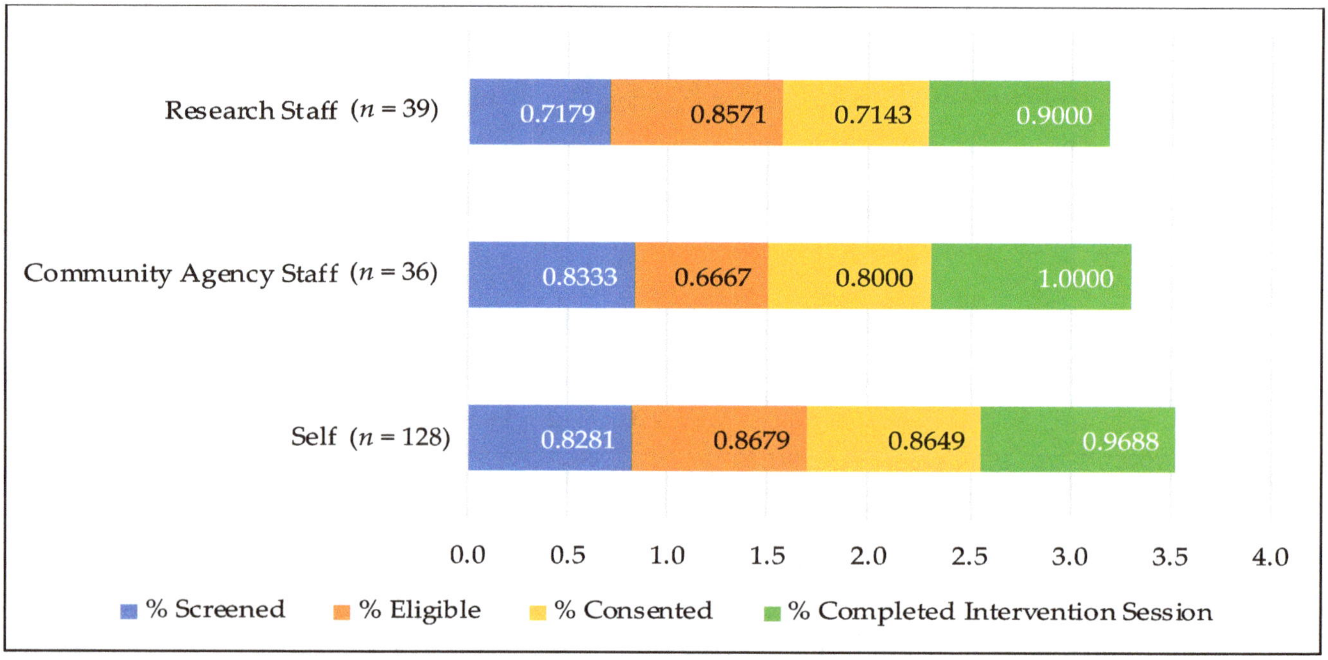

Figure 2. Success of referral to intervention engagement by referral strategy.

Our second question focused on intrapersonal risks experienced by referred mothers. As displayed in the demographics shown in Table **??** above, we achieved our intended sample of mothers, who were primarily of non-dominant culture (Black race) and socioeconomically disadvantaged who, as established in the literature review, experience extreme inequity in accessing depression-focused intervention. We, therefore, created a cumulative intrapersonal risk index to view the level of other risk variables over race and poverty among mothers in our recruited sample (See Table **??**). Each of the five risk variables was dichotomized based on the criterion specified in the table, with 1 representing presence of the characteristic. These variables were summed to produce a risk index range of 0–5.

Table 3. Intrapersonal risk characteristics by referral approach group.

Variable	Agency Referral	Research Staff Referral	Mother Self-Referral
* *N*/% Less than college degree	12 100%	10 100%	51 79.69%
N/% Severe symptom range	5 41.67%	2 20%	21 32.81%
* *N*/%Thoughts of self-harm	6 50%	0 0%	11 17.19%
No significant other	9 75%	7 70%	46 71.88%
N/% < 60% Parent knowledge of infant SE development and promotion	11 91.67%	10 100%	53 82.81%

* Significance level <0.05.

Figure ?? presents a plot of the risk index for mothers recruited using each referral strategy. Descriptively, mothers referred by research staff had the lowest and most restricted range of risk. The self-referred mothers had the largest range of risk. Agency-referred mothers demonstrated a slightly higher 75th percentile value (approximately 4.5/5 risks) than those of self-referred mothers (approximately 4/5 risks). For staff-referred, the 75th percentile risk level was approximately the same as the median risk value for agency-referred mothers. We followed the conservative approach to examination and conducted a Mann–Whitney between-group comparison of agency-referred and self-referred mothers. This examination resulted in a small effect size difference (U = 268; $p = 0.08$, d = 0.39), with agency-referred mothers reporting slightly higher levels of risk.

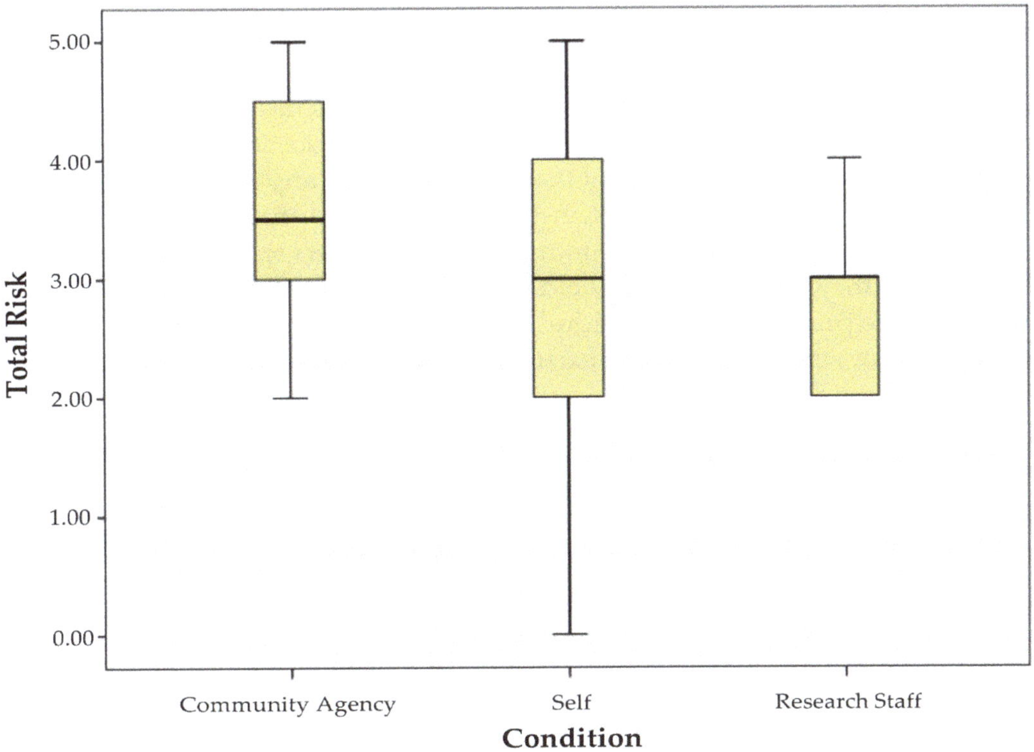

Figure 3. Boxplot of risk for agency, self-referral, and research staff approaches.

4. Discussion

4.1. Summary

The gatekeeper referral systems that relied on agency- and research-staff referrals were less successful compared to mother self-referral. They resulted in substantially fewer initial referrals and experienced losses of potential participants at rates equivalent to or sometimes greater than that of the self-referral system at each stage of the process up through initiation of the intervention. A substantial proportion of mothers across referral groups consented to participation and initiated the intervention. As planned, the final sample across referral groups reflected the population from which they were recruited: non-dominant culture, experiencing severe socioeconomic disadvantage, not having a significant other, and having limited knowledge of infant social-emotional development.

In our preliminary examination of risk factors experienced by mothers, mothers in the self-referred group had the greatest range of risk levels. Though this almost certainly reflects the relatively larger size of the group relative to those referred through other mechanisms, it nonetheless suggests that this approach has potential to result in a somewhat diverse group of participants with regard to these factors. It is important to note that mothers referred by agency staff evidenced a somewhat higher level of risk factors. Though the effect size was small, and the small sample size renders the finding preliminary, it is consistent with prior evidence that individuals with greater resources are more likely to bypass gatekeeper systems to access mental health services directly [?]. We think these findings suggest the potential importance of continuing to try to engage community agency gatekeepers in the referral process. It seems plausible that busy agency staff may be reserving their efforts for women whom they see as most vulnerable. It is also possible that though self-referral is excellent with regard to creating a smooth path to entry for most women (including those who are depressed, of non-dominant culture, and socioeconomically disadvantaged), it is not yet clear the threshold of vulnerability at which entry may require too much initiative for mothers.

4.2. Contributions

Although online recruitment is common in mobile health interventions, there is limited research on recruitment [?]. To our knowledge, this is a first systematic examination of referral processes as they relate to recruitment into intervention for depressed mothers. The existing research on online recruitment into parenting interventions for mothers of newborns has focused nearly exclusively on paid advertising such as through ads on parenting sites and via Facebook [?]. In contrast, our study provides an examination of online recruitment that did not require any paid advertising—a potentially important consideration for cost containment. Although published studies have been reported on the use of non-paid advertising for recruiting into mobile health interventions focused in areas such as smoking cessation [?], they have tended to yield less diverse samples, reflecting primarily dominant culture groups [?]. The present study is unique in that it focuses on a target sample of postpartum women with depression, who are lacking in existing study samples, namely women who identify as non-dominant culture and who are socioeconomically disadvantaged.

4.3. Limitations and Implications for Future Research

The current study has important limitations to note, which reflect that this was a secondary analysis of existing data to address an important research question that was distinct from those of the original parent study. First, relative to race, ethnicity, and income demographics of the sample, our clinical trial is being conducted within an area of concentrated poverty in the urban center of a large southern city, where the population is predominantly Black. Moreover, because we sought to refer and recruit within agencies serving low income individuals within one of the most income disparate cities in the U.S. with a long history of structural and systemic racism [?], the majority of our sample is severely socioeconomically disadvantaged. As such, we cannot adequately examine race and income sample differences by referral group. The current results may not be generalizable to other referral and recruitment efforts taking place within target populations that contain greater diversity in race and income. Of course, it seems unlikely that an approach that worked this successfully in a highly stressed and low resourced population would not be feasible in other samples.

A second limitation is the lack of clinical diagnostic measures. As the aims of the larger study did not necessitate diagnostic interviews, depression is defined here by a well-established questionnaire measure, which, though it has strong concordance with clinically derived diagnoses, is not equivalent and does not provide indices of cooccurring disorders. As such, we do not know how many of the participants met diagnostic criteria for current mood disorders or whether the presence of depressive or comorbid diagnoses influence the success of one or more of the referral processes. Nonetheless, the current results suggest that women experiencing depressive symptoms at levels likely to indicate disorder were enrolled successfully.

Another limitation is the relatively small sample. Clearly, future research on larger samples within more regionally, socioeconomically, and racially diverse target populations is needed to determine generalizability of the current findings and, in particular, to provide stronger data regarding the extent to which diverse recruitment strategies yield equivalent samples. However, based on the current results, we note evidence in support of the possibility that mothers who are Black and socioeconomically disadvantaged can and do self-seek services beyond typical gatekeeper systems to address depression. Studies are needed within community settings, outside of the clinical intervention trial structure, to determine if self-referral into intervention will result in greater racial and ethnic equity in accessing needed community services to reduce depression and strengthen parenting. It is also important to note that our examination of referral progression toward intervention access took place within the framework of a clinical intervention trial. As such, the outcomes may not generalize to processes of community agency and self-referral into community-based clinical intervention services, where there may be less support for moving mothers toward intervention access.

Expanding beyond the current study, other important future research directions to consider include the following: (1) examination of other factors that might influence referral such as insurance status, number of children in the home, or feelings about online interventions; (2) examination of cost effectiveness of various referral approaches; (3) documentation of how self-referring mothers access recruitment websites to self-refer (for example, whether by content searches, service searches, in response to friend suggestions in social communications, or responding to print or electronic links from trusted service providers), and (4) studies that extend beyond the relationship between referral approach and intervention access to include exploration of the relationship between referral approach and study retention, especially with regard to intervention dosage.

5. Conclusions

Results showed that mothers self-referred at more than 3.5 times the rate of referral by community agency staff and research staff. The resultant sample across referral groups reflected mothers of Black race experiencing severe socioeconomic disadvantage. Compared to traditional referral gatekeeper groups, self-referred mothers were equally successful with regard to recruitment into the study intervention.

Author Contributions: Conceptualization, K.M.B., B.D. and L.B.S.; methodology, K.M.B., B.D. and L.B.S.; software, K.M.; formal analysis, K.M.B., B.D., E.A.M. and K.M.; investigation, K.M.B., B.D. and E.G.F.; resources, K.M.B., B.D. and E.G.F.; writing—original draft preparation, K.M.B., B.D., L.B.S., R.T.A. and E.A.M.; writing—review and editing, K.M.B., B.D., L.B.S., R.T.A. and E.A.M.; supervision, K.M.B.; project administration, K.M.B. and B.D.; funding acquisition, K.M.B. All authors have read and agreed to the published version of the manuscript.

References

1. World Health Organization. Depression. World Health Organization: Geneva, Switzerland, January 2020. Available online: https://www.who.int/en/news-room/fact-sheets/detail/depression (accessed on 16 September 2020).
2. Miller, L.J.; LaRusso, E.M. Preventing Postpartum Depression. *Psychiatr. Clin. N. Am.* **2011**, *34*, 53–65. [CrossRef]
3. Mental Health America. Position Statement 49: Perinatal Mental Health. 2018. Available online: https://www.mhanational.org/issues/position-statement-49-perinatal-mental-health (accessed on 30 November 2020).
4. Goodman, S.H.; Simon, H.F.M.; Shamblaw, A.L.; Kim, C.Y. Parenting as a Mediator of Associations between Depression in Mothers and Children's Functioning: A Systematic Review and Meta-Analysis. *Clin. Child Fam. Psychol. Rev.* **2020**, *23*, 427–460. [CrossRef] [PubMed]
5. Rogers, A.; Obst, S.; Teague, S.J.; Rossen, L.; Spry, E.A.; Macdonald, J.A.; Sunderland, M.; Olsson, C.A.; Youssef, G.; Hutchinson, D. Association Between Maternal Perinatal Depression and Anxiety and Child and Adolescent Development: A Meta-analysis. *JAMA Psychiatry* **2020**, *174*, 1082–1092. [CrossRef]
6. Center on the Developing Child at Harvard University, Maternal Depression Can Undermine the Development of Young Children: Working Paper No. 8. 2009. Available online: https://developingchild.harvard.edu/resources/maternal-depression-can-undermine-the-development-of-young-children/ (accessed on 30 November 2020).

7. Goodman, S.H.; Garber, J. Evidence-Based Interventions for Depressed Mothers and Their Young Children. *Child Dev.* **2017**, *88*, 368–377. [CrossRef] [PubMed]
8. Baker, C.E.; Brooks-Gunn, J.; Gouskova, N. Reciprocal Relations between Maternal Depression and Child Behavior Problems in Families Served by Head Start. *Child Dev.* **2020**, *91*, 1563–1576. [CrossRef] [PubMed]
9. National Center for Health Statistics. *Health, United States, 2015: With Special Feature on Racial and Ethnic Health Disparities*; Centers for Disease Control and Prevention: Hyattsville, MD, USA, 2016. Available online: https://www.cdc.gov/nchs/data/hus/hus15.pdf (accessed on 30 November 2020).
10. Grote, N.K.; Zuckoff, A.; Swartz, H.; Bledsoe, S.E.; Geibel, S. Engaging Women Who Are Depressed and Economically Disadvantaged in Mental Health Treatment. *Soc. Work* **2007**, *52*, 295–308. [CrossRef] [PubMed]
11. *Substance Abuse and Mental Health Services Administration, Racial/Ethnic Differences in Mental Health Service Use among Adults*; Substance Abuse and Mental Health Services Administration: Rockville, MD, USA, 2015. Available online: http://www.samhsa.gov/data/ (accessed on 30 November 2020).
12. Ramos, G.; Chavira, D.A. Use of Technology to Provide Mental Health Care for Racial and Ethnic Minorities: Evidence, Promise, and Challenges. *Cogn. Behav. Pract.* **2019**. [CrossRef]
13. Rafferty, J.; Mattson, G.; Earls, M.F.; Yogman, M.W. Incorporating Recognition and Management of Perinatal Depression into Pediatric Practice. *Pediatrics* **2019**, *143*, 31. [CrossRef]
14. American Academy of Pediatrics; American College of Obstetricians and Gynecologists (Eds.) *Guidelines for Perinatal Care*, 8th ed.; American Academy of Pediatrics; The American College of Obstetricians and Gynecologists: Washington, DC, USA, 2017.
15. Allbaugh, L.J.; Marcus, S.M.; Ford, E.C.; Flynn, H.A. Development of a screening and recruitment registry to facilitate perinatal depression research in obstetrics settings in the USA. *Int. J. Gynecol. Obstet.* **2015**, *128*, 260–263. [CrossRef]
16. Byatt, N.; Simas, T.A.M.; Lundquist, R.S.; Johnson, J.V.; Ziedonis, D.M. Strategies for improving perinatal depression treatment in North American outpatient obstetric settings. *J. Psychosom. Obstet. Gynecol.* **2012**, *33*, 143–161. [CrossRef]
17. Maternal, Infant, and Early Childhood Home Visiting Technical Assistance Coordinating Center (MIECHV TACC). *MIECHV Issue Brief on Family Enrollment and Engagement*; Health Resources and Services Administration: Rockville, MD, USA, 2015. Available online: https://mchb.hrsa.gov/sites/default/files/mchb/MaternalChildHealthInitiatives/HomeVisiting/tafiles/enrollmentandengagement.pdf (accessed on 30 November 2020).
18. Bailey, Z.D.; Krieger, N.; Agénor, M.; Graves, J.; Linos, N.; Bassett, M.T. Structural racism and health inequities in the USA: Evidence and interventions. *Lancet* **2017**, *389*, 1453–1463. [CrossRef]
19. Moffitt, R.A. The Deserving Poor, the Family, and the U.S. Welfare System. *Demography* **2015**, *52*, 729–749. [CrossRef]
20. Oh, S.S.; Galanter, J.; Thakur, N.; Pino-Yanes, M.; Barcelo, N.E.; White, M.J.; de Bruin, D.M.; Greenblatt, R.M.; Bibbins-Domingo, K.; Wu, A.H.; et al. Diversity in Clinical and Biomedical Research: A Promise Yet to Be Fulfilled. *PLoS Med.* **2015**, *12*, e1001918. [CrossRef]
21. Durant, R.W.; Wenzel, J.A.; Scarinci, I.C.; Paterniti, D.A.; Fouad, M.N.; Hurd, T.C.; Martin, M.Y. Perspectives on barriers and facilitators to minority recruitment for clinical trials among cancer center leaders, investigators, research staff, and referring clinicians: Enhancing minority participation in clinical trials (EMPaCT): Perspectives on Minority Recruitment. *Cancer* **2014**, *120*, 1097–1105. [CrossRef]
22. Williams, M.; Tellawi, G.; Wetterneck, C.T.; Chapman, L.K. Recruitment of Ethnoracial Minorities for Mental Health Research. *Drugs* **2013**, *67*, 236–244.
23. Polo, A.J.; Makol, B.A.; Castro, A.S.; Colón-Quintana, N.; Wagstaff, A.E.; Guo, S. Diversity in randomized clinical trials of depression: A 36-year review. *Clin. Psychol. Rev.* **2019**, *67*, 22–35. [CrossRef]
24. Kanakamedala, P.; Haga, S.B. Characterization of Clinical Study Populations by Race and Ethnicity in the Biomedical Literature. *Ethn. Dis.* **2013**, *22*, 96.
25. Geller, S.E.; Koch, A.; Pellettieri, B.; Carnes, M. Inclusion, Analysis, and Reporting of Sex and Race/Ethnicity in Clinical Trials: Have We Made Progress? *J. Womens Health* **2011**, *20*, 315–320. [CrossRef]
26. Hughes-Morley, A.; Young, B.; Waheed, W.; Small, N.; Bower, P. Factors affecting recruitment into depression trials: Systematic review, meta-synthesis and conceptual framework. *J. Affect. Disord.* **2015**, *172*, 274–290. [CrossRef]

27. Amorrortu, R.P.; Arevalo, M.; Vernon, S.W.; Mainous, A.G.; Diaz, V.; McKee, M.D.; Ford, M.E.; Tilley, B.C. Recruitment of racial and ethnic minorities to clinical trials conducted within specialty clinics: An intervention mapping approach. *Trials* **2018**, *19*, 115. [CrossRef]
28. Steele, L.; Glazier, R.; Agha, M.; Moineddin, R. The Gatekeeper System and Disparities in Use of Psychiatric Care by Neighbourhood Education Level: Results of a Nine-Year Cohort Study in Toronto. *Healthc. Policy Polit. Santé* **2009**, *4*, e133–e150. [CrossRef]
29. Lillie-Blanton, M.; Hoffman, C. The Role of Health Insurance Coverage in Reducing Racial/Ethnic Disparities in Health Care. *Health Aff. (Millwood)* **2005**, *24*, 398–408. [CrossRef]
30. Cho, H.L.; Danis, M.; Grady, C. The ethics of uninsured participants accessing healthcare in biomedical research: A literature review. *Clin. Trials* **2018**, *15*, 509–521. [CrossRef]
31. Anderson-Lewis, C.; Darville, G.; Mercado, R.E.; Howell, S.; Di Maggio, S. Mobile health Technology Use and Implications in Historically Underserved and Minority Populations in the United States: Systematic Literature Review. *JMIR Mob. Health UHealth* **2018**, *6*, e128. [CrossRef]
32. Lane, T.S.; Armin, J.; Gordon, J.S. Online Recruitment Methods for Web-Based and Mobile Health Studies: A Review of the Literature. *J. Med. Internet Res.* **2015**, *17*, e183. [CrossRef]
33. Laws, R.A.; Litterbach, E.K.V.; Denney-Wilson, E.A.; Russell, C.G.; Taki, S.; Ong, K.L.; Campbell, K.J. A Comparison of Recruitment Methods for an mobile health Intervention Targeting Mothers: Lessons from the Growing Healthy Program. *J. Med. Internet Res.* **2016**, *18*, e248. [CrossRef]
34. Watson, N.L.; Mull, K.E.; Heffner, J.L.; McClure, J.B.; Bricker, J.B. Participant Recruitment and Retention in Remote eHealth Intervention Trials: Methods and Lessons Learned From a Large Randomized Controlled Trial of Two Web-Based Smoking Interventions. *J. Med. Internet Res.* **2018**, *20*, e10351. [CrossRef]
35. Brown, J.S.L.; Murphy, C.; Kelly, J.; Goldsmith, K. How can we successfully recruit depressed people? Lessons learned in recruiting depressed participants to a multi-site trial of a brief depression intervention (the 'CLASSIC' trial). *Trials* **2019**, *20*, 131. [CrossRef]
36. Baggett, K.M.; DiPetrillo, B.; Beacham, C.; Patterson, A.; Miller, K.; Davis, B.; Feil, E.; Sheeber, L. Built Pathways to Resilience: Engaging Mothers with Depression in a Mobile Intervention to Improve Infant Social-Emotional Outcomes. In Proceedings of the Conference on Research Innovations in Early Intervention, San Diego, CA, USA, 27–29 February 2020.
37. Kroenke, K.; Spitzer, R.L.; Williams, J.B.W. The Patient Health Questionnaire-2: Validity of a Two-Item Depression Screener. *Med. Care* **2003**, *41*, 1284–1292. [CrossRef]
38. Wisner, K.L.; Sit, D.K.; McShea, M.C.; Rizzo, D.M.; Zoretich, R.A.; Hughes, C.L.; Eng, H.F.; Luther, J.F.; Wisniewski, S.R.; Costantino, M.L.; et al. Onset Timing, Thoughts of Self-harm, and Diagnoses in Postpartum Women With Screen Positive Depression Findings. *JAMA Psychiatry* **2013**, *70*, 490. [CrossRef]
39. Kroenke, K.; Spitzer, R.L.; Williams, J.B.W. The PHQ-9: Validity of a brief depression severity measure. *J. Gen. Intern. Med.* **2001**, *16*, 606–613. [CrossRef]
40. Feil, E.G.; Baggett, K.; Davis, B.; Landry, S.; Sheeber, L.; Leve, C.; Johnson, U. Randomized control trial of an internet-based parenting intervention for mothers of infants. *Early Child. Res. Q.* **2020**, *50*, 36–44. [CrossRef]
41. Franz, F.; Erdfelder, E.; Lang, A.-G.L.; Buchner, A. G*Power 3: A flexible statistical power analysis program for the social, behavioral and biomedical sciences. *Behav. Res. Methods.* **2007**, *39*, 175–191.
42. Mollan, K.R.; Trumble, I.M.; Reifeis, S.A.; Ferrer, O.; Bay, C.P.; Baldoni, P.L.; Hudgens, M.G. Exact Power of the Rank-Sum Test for a Continuous Variable. *arXiv* **2019**, arXiv:1901.04597.
43. Sommeiller, E.; Price, M.; Wazeter, E. *Income Inequality in the U.S. by State, Metropolitan Area, and County*; Economic Policy Institute: Washington, DC, USA, 2016; Available online: https://files.epi.org/pdf/107100.pdf (accessed on 30 November 2020).

13

The Effect of a Virtual-Reality Full-Body Illusion on Body Representation in Obesity

Federica Scarpina [1,2,*,†], Silvia Serino [3,*,†], Anouk Keizer [4], Alice Chirico [5], Massimo Scacchi [6,7], Gianluca Castelnuovo [2,5], Alessandro Mauro [1,8] and Giuseppe Riva [3,5]

1 Istituto Auxologico Italiano, IRCCS, U.O. di Neurologia e Neuroriabilitazione, Ospedale S. Giuseppe, 28824 Piancavallo, Italy
2 Istituto Auxologico Italiano, IRCCS, Laboratorio di Psicologia, Ospedale S. Giuseppe, 28824 Piancavallo, Italy
3 Istituto Auxologico Italiano, IRCCS, Laboratorio Sperimentale di Ricerche Tecnologiche Applicate alla Psicologia, 20149 Milano, Italy
4 Experimental Psychology/Helmholtz Institute, Faculty of Social and Behavioural Sciences, Utrecht University, 3584 Utrecht, The Netherlands
5 Psychology Department, Università Cattolica del Sacro Cuore, 20123 Milan, Italy
6 Istituto Auxologico Italiano, IRCCS, U.O. di Medicina Generale, Ospedale S. Giuseppe, 28824 Piancavallo, Italy
7 Department of Clinical Sciences and Community Health, University of Milan, 20122 Milan, Italy
8 "Rita Levi Montalcini" Department of Neuroscience, University of Turin, 10124 Turin, Italy
* Correspondence: federica.scarpina@gmail.com (S.F.); s.serino@auxologico.it (S.S.)
† These authors equally contributed to this work.

Abstract: Background. The effective illusory ownership over an artificial body in modulating body representations in healthy and eating disorders population has been repeatedly reported in recent literature. In this study, we extended this research in the field of obesity: specifically, we investigated whether ownership over a virtual body with a skinny abdomen might be successfully experienced by participants affected by obesity. **Methods**. Fifteen participants with obesity and fifteen healthy-weight participants took part at this study in which the VR-Full-Body Illusion was adopted. The strength of illusion was investigated through the traditional Embodiment Questionnaire, while changes in bodily experience were measured through a body size estimation task. **Results**. Participants with obesity as well as healthy-weight participants reported to experience the illusion. About the body size estimation task, both groups reported changes only in the estimation of the abdomen's circumference after the experimental condition, in absence of any another difference. **Discussion**. Participants with obesity reported to experience the illusion over a skinny avatar, but the modulation of the bodily experience seems controversial. Future lines of research exploiting this technique for modulating body representations in obesity, specifically in terms of potential therapeutic use, were discussed.

Keywords: body representation; obesity; health; virtual reality; full body illusion

---

1. Introduction

The efficacy of the illusory ownership over an artificial body (i.e., body-ownership illusion) as a method for modulating body representations in both healthy such as [1–6] and clinical population (such as individuals suffering of eating disorders [7,8], Complex Regional Pain Syndrome [9] and Disturbed Body Integrity [10,11] has been repeatedly reported in recent literature. Indeed, since from the traditional Rubber Hand Illusion [12], it was speculated if bodily illusions might be adopted in therapeutic settings [13–17] for enhancing positive rehabilitative outcomes. More recently, the research about body ownership illusions moves from the embodiment of a single body part (such as the hand [12] or the foot [10], towards the entire body. For example, in the Virtual Reality-Full Body Illusion (VR-FBI) [2–5] participants experience the illusion of ownership towards a full-body avatar. Traditionally, the avatar is showed with different physical dimensions (i.e., thinner or larger) respect to the participants. Interestingly, when participants experience successfully the illusion, they generally perceive themselves as fatter or thinner than they really are, according to the characteristics of embodied virtual body [2–5]. An example was offered by Normand and colleagues (2011) [18], who induced embodiment over a virtual body with a larger abdomen in a sample of males; immediately after this experience, participants perceived their own body as larger than the real physical dimensions, congruently with the embodied avatars' characteristics. The illusion seemed to work also in the opposite direction: female participants who embodied avatars with skinny bodies tended to perceive their own bodies as slimmer [2–5].

As concerns eating disorders, there are in literature some interesting but preliminary studies investigating the use of body-ownership illusions as a method for exploring the boundaries of bodily self in affected individuals. For example, Eshkevari and colleagues [19] found an increased malleability of the bodily experience for individuals with eating disorders, who rated to experience the Rubber Hand Illusion higher than the healthy controls. Keizer and colleagues [7] applied the VR-FBI in a sample of individuals affected by Anorexia Nervosa, revealing that participants who experience ownership over a different virtual body reported a significant decrease in their body-size distortions too. In the 2016, our group presented a single-case study about a female individual affected by severe obesity, who experienced high level of body dissatisfaction and showed consistent distortions in the estimation of her own body-size parts [20]. We reported that both components (body dissatisfaction and body-size distortions) improved after experiencing the VR-FBI. In our knowledge, this single case study is still the only unique attempt to exploit this illusion in the context of obesity; thus, if body-ownership illusion could successfully modulate body representation in individuals affected by obesity is still an open question.

In the current study, we used a VR-FBI [1,2,20] as a technique for inducing illusory ownership over a virtual body with a skinny abdomen in a sample of individuals affected by obesity, compared to a group of healthy-weight individuals. Thus, in this study, participants saw the slim abdomen of the avatar through VR googles. When the experimenter stroked participants on their abdomen, delivering a tactile stimulation, they saw this stroking on the avatar's abdomen (i.e., the visual input). In line with previous studies [1,2,20], two conditions were administered for all participants: the experimental condition, in which the touch and the vision of the touch were *synchronized*; the temporal coherence between the sensory input onset generally elicits the illusory ownership over the artificial body; and the control condition, in which the two perceived stimuli are *asynchronized*, since there was a temporal delay between the visual and tactile input onset. To measure the potential changes in the perceptual component of body parts representations, we adopted the Body Part Size Estimation Task [1,20]. Participants were asked to estimate their height, and the width and the circumference of three different body parts (shoulders, abdomen, and hips), at three time points: before the VR-FBI, representing the baseline, and after both the two (synchronous and asynchronous) conditions of visuo-tactile stimulation. Moreover, in line with the traditional literature [1–12,20,21], we adopted the Embodiment Questionnaire [1]: this questionnaire, administered after both stimulation conditions, allows to measure the strength of illusion in terms of: (1) *Ownership* over the virtual body; (2) *Self-location*, i.e., being in the same location of the virtual body; and (3) *Sense of agency* over the virtual body.

Considering the previous results about healthy individuals [1–5,18], we might expect that all participants experienced successfully the VR-FBI after the synchronous visuo-tactile stimulation (i.e., the experimental condition), but not after the asynchronous (i.e., control) condition. Moreover, about the Body Part Size Estimation Task [1,20], there would be a decrease in body size estimations compared to the baseline (i.e., before the VR-FBI took place); indeed, when the illusion emerged, healthy-weight individuals should perceive themselves slimmer than real physical dimensions, accordingly with the avatar's dimension. Similarly, if the illusion might be efficiently induced also for individuals affected by obesity, we might expect to find a difference in the estimation of their body parts after the synchronous, but not the asynchronous condition.

2. Methods

The study was conducted in compliance with the Helsinki's Declaration (of 1975, as revised in 2008), was approved by the Ethics Review Board of the Università Cattolica del Sacro Cuore (Catholic University of the Sacred Heart, Milan, Italy). Subjects volunteered to participate; they received verbal explanation of the procedures and gave informed written consent, were free to withdraw at will and were naïve to the rationale of the experiment.

Participants. All participants were female and right-handed. None of them had previously experience with bodily illusions and were naïve to the rationale of this experiment. Fifteen individuals affected by obesity and fifteen female healthy-weight individuals took part in the study (Table 1). Participants affected by obesity were individuals at the first week of a diagnostic hospitalization, before a rehabilitative treatment for losing weight. We adopted the same inclusion criteria of our previous studies [22–24]. All subjects were nonsmokers and free from gastrointestinal, cardiovascular, psychiatric, or metabolic disorders or any concurrent medical condition not related to obesity, according to routinely clinical assessment. In addition, weight and height were measured to the nearest 0.1 kg and 0.1 cm, respectively, using standard methods. BMI was expressed as body mass (kg)/ height (m^2). Obesity was defined for any BMI over 30 kg/m^2. Healthy-weight participants were recruited through convenience and snowball sampling—In particular, students from the Catholic University of Milan were invited during lessons and asked to refer friends. No economical compensation was given. The same above-mentioned inclusion criteria were adopted, except for the BMI that was between 18.5 and 25 kg/m^2.

VR-FBI. In this experiment we used the same protocol of our previous studies [1–20]. During the entire procedure, participants were kindly asked to avoid any movements; this set-up did not track participants' movement and the avatar was not responsive. All participants were invited to stand upright and wear the head-mounted display (Oculus Rift DK2) to experience the VR-FBI. The Oculus Rift DK2D (compatible with the developed application) was connected to a portable computer (HP TRUE VISION with CPU Intel® Core™i7). The virtual room was developed with the software Unity3D (www.unity3d.com), while the avatar was modelled using the software MakeHuman (http://www.makehuman.org/). To experience the illusion, all participants were exposed to two different conditions. During the *synchronous* condition (i.e., the experimental condition), the experimenter provided a visuo-tactile stimulation on participants' abdomen with a brush attached to the motion-tracking device (i.e., Razer Hydra) for 90 s, while a synchronous stimulation was delivered on virtual abdomen (i.e., the virtual touch provided on the abdomen of the virtual body). In the *asynchronous* condition (i.e., the control condition) the experimenter provided the same visuo-tactile stimulation on participants' abdomen for 90 s, but there was a delay in the corresponding virtual touch (i.e., absence of synchronization between tactile and visual stimulation). In particular, in the asynchronous condition the touch on participants' abdomen was actually recorded by pressing a button on the Razer Hydra at the beginning of the movement. This procedure stopped the image seen by the participants as soon as the touch ended, and then it was replayed in VR when the experimenter finished each touch. Also, this stimulation lasted for 90 s.

All participants were exposed to these two conditions in a counterbalanced order in a within subject-design. They were requested to wear the head-mounted display (i.e., Oculus) to visualize in a first-person perspective the virtual body of a female avatar by looking down at the abdomen of virtual body (i.e., the stimulated body part). They saw the body of a young woman (approximately 25 years old) with a thin abdomen (i.e., with a different shape/size in comparison to the actual body of participants) standing upright in a stimulus-free room was used to induce the full body illusion (Figure 1).

The waist circumference of the avatar was 73.95 cm: the waist circumference of the avatar was significantly smaller respect to the mean waist circumference of both the healthy-weight participants [t(14) = 23.021; $p < 0.001$; mean = 100.18; SD = 4.41)] and participants affected by obesity [t(14) = 18.094; $p < 0.001$; mean = 140.18; SD = 14.24)]. Thus, the avatar was perceptively skinner respect to both groups of participants.

Table 1. Means and standard deviation (in brackets) were reported about demographical and clinical information, percentage of misestimation at the baseline for both groups. In bold, when p value was <0.05. Age and Education are reported in years; body parts physical dimensions were reported in cm.

	Participants with Obesity	Healthy Weight Participant	*t*	*p* Value	*d*
Age	32 (6)	29 (8)	0.97	0.33	0.4
Education	14 (3)	16 (1)	1.97	0.058	0.35
BMI	45 (6.69)	22 (1.66).	12.63	**<0.001**	4.71
		Body parts physical dimensions			
Height	161.91 (8.15)	164.52 (9.31)	0.81	0.42	0.29
		Width			
Shoulders	48.15 (7.8)	39.7 (1.82)	4.079	**<0.001**	1.49
Abdomen	42.57 (7.12)	29.7 (3.81)	6.16	**<0.001**	2.25
Hips	48.44 (6.12)	35.64 (2.6)	7.44	**<0.001**	2.72
		Circumference			
Shoulders	121.15 (12.87)	88.7 (6.86)	8.61	**<0.001**	3.14
Abdomen	130.24 (14.73)	83.27 (9.8)	10.27	**<0.001**	3.75
Hips	140.46 (14.23)	100.17 (4.41)	10.46	**<0.001**	3.82
		Body Parts Size Estimation Task: percentage of misestimation—Baseline			
Height	3.2 (3.73)	0.74 (4.31)	1.86	0.76	0.61
		Width			
Shoulders	−10.8 (21.86)	−2.19 (14.54)	1.71	0.1	0.46
Abdomen	−1.6 (20.92)	0.13 (23.12)	0.22	0.82	0.07
Hips	6.8 (23.66)	10.37 (22.24)	0.62	0.5	0.15
		Circumference			
Shoulders	16.2 (27.6)	39.45 (18.94)	2.69	**0.012**	0.98
Abdomen	6.5 (30.61)	24.43 (15.03)	3.96	**<0.001**	0.74
Hips	7.5 (22.07)	26.08 (15.84)	2.64	**0.013**	0.96

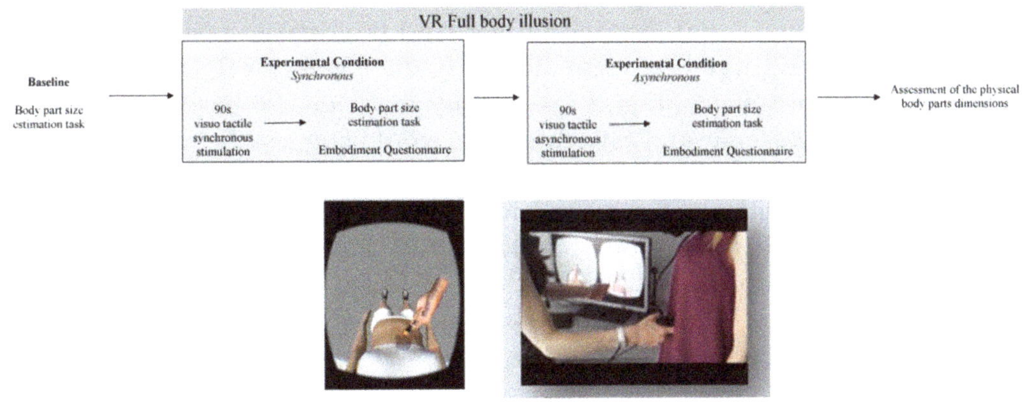

Figure 1. Graphical representation of the VR experimental time-line (upper part) and set-up (below up).

Embodiment Questionnaire. After both the synchronous visuo-tactile stimulation (experimental condition) and the asynchronous visuo-tactile stimulation (control condition), participants were required to fill the Embodiment Questionnaire [1], that it is routinely adopted to assess how participants subjectively experienced the illusion. It consisted of 20 items. Participants rated each statement on a 7-point Likert scale (range from 1 to 7), with higher scores indicating a stronger illusion. The questionnaire allows us to investigate the strength of illusion in terms of: (1) *ownership*, i.e., over the virtual body; (2) *self-location*, i.e., being in the same location of the virtual body; and (3) *sense of agency* over the virtual body. The three components were obtained by calculating the mean scores from the corresponding items.

Body Part Size Estimation Task. Before the illusion (i.e., the baseline) and after both the synchronous visuo-tactile stimulation (experimental condition) and the asynchronous visuo-tactile stimulation (control condition), participants were asked to estimate their own body parts, according to the procedure explained in our previous work [1]. Participants were asked to stand in front of a wall and to estimate the horizontal width of their own shoulders, abdomen, and hips by placing adhesive stickers: the stickers should represent the estimated distance between the left and the right side of the target body part. They were explicitly asked to not look at their body to avoid that they used it as a "reference" for making the estimates. Furthermore, they were asked to estimate the circumference of the above-mentioned three parts of their body by placing a piece of rope in a circle/oval on the floor. Moreover, participants estimated their height using an adhesive marker they placed on the wall. Also, in this case, they were explicitly asked to not use their own body as a reference to estimate their height. At the end of the entire experiment, the experimenter measured the actual width and circumference of the targeted body parts. The order of body parts (height, shoulders, abdomen, hips) and type of estimation (width, circumference) was counterbalanced over participants. For each body part and type of estimation, we calculated the percentage of misestimation according to the formula proposed by Keizer and colleagues [7]:

$$\textit{percentage of misestimation} = [(\text{estimated size} - \text{actual size})/\text{actual size}] \times 100$$

According to the formula, a negative result suggested an underestimation, while a positive result an overestimation.

Data Analyses. Differences in demographical and clinical aspects were examined through an Independent samples t-test. For the embodiment questionnaire a Repeated Measure ANOVA with the within factors of *Condition* (i.e., synchronous vs. asynchronous) and of *Subscale* (i.e., ownership, location and agency) and the between factor of *Group* (participants with obesity vs. healthy weight participants) was conducted.

For the Body Part Size Estimation Task, we first explored any possible difference between the two groups in the estimation of the body parts at the baseline through an independent sample *t*-test. Successively, for each body part, a Repeated Measure ANOVA was run with the within factor of *Condition* (i.e., baseline, synchronous asynchronous) and the between factor of *Group* (participants with obesity vs. healthy weight participants), to verify the effect of VR_FBI on the body estimation. A significant main effect of *Condition*, and specifically between the baseline and the synchronous condition, but not between baseline and asynchronous, would suggest the effect of VR-FBI on the body size estimation; in case of significant interaction *Group*Condition*, the effect of *Condition* would emerge differently between individuals affected by obesity and healthy-weight individuals. In this case, for the two groups independently we performed post-hoc two independent sample t-tests: in the first one, the error in the synchronous condition was compared to the baseline; in the second, the error in the asynchronous condition. A difference was considered significant if the p value was below the Bonferroni's corrected threshold of 0.025 (0.05/2).

3. Results

Demographical and clinical aspects. Obese and healthy weight participants did not differ in *Age* and *Education level*, as showed in Table 1. As expected, participants affected by obesity had a significantly higher *BMI* than healthy weight participants. Moreover, for all considered body parts, except for height, individuals affected by obesity had higher physical dimensions than controls.

Embodiment Questionnaire. No main effect of *Group* (participants with obesity M = 3.58; SD = 1.87; healthy-weigh participants M = 3.82; SD = 1.39) emerged [F(1,28) = 0.25; p = 0.62; $\eta\rho^2$ = 0.009). The main effect of *Subscale* (ownership M = 3.56; SD = 1.48; location M = 4.04; SD = 1.49; agency M = 3.49; SD = 1.85) [F(2, 56) = 3.13; p = 0.051; $\eta\rho^2$ = 0.1) was marginally significant, but not the main effect of *Condition* (synchronous M = 3.86; SD = 1.53; asynchronous M = 3.54; SD = 1.71) [F(1, 28) = 1.71; p = 0.2; $\eta\rho^2$ = 0.05). Interestingly, an interaction *Condition**Subscale* [F(2, 56) = 3.8; p = 0.028; $\eta\rho^2$ = 0.12) emerged. Thus, we performed three paired sample t-tests in which for each subscale (ownership, location and agency) we compared the scores at the two *Conditions* (synchronous vs. asynchronous). A significant difference (Bonferroni corrected p-value 0.05/3 = 0.016) emerged for the *location* subscale [t(29) = 2.69; p = 0.012], but not for the *ownership* subscale [t(29) = 1.32; p = 0.19] or for the *agency* subscale [t(29) = 0.41; p = 0.68] (Figure 2).

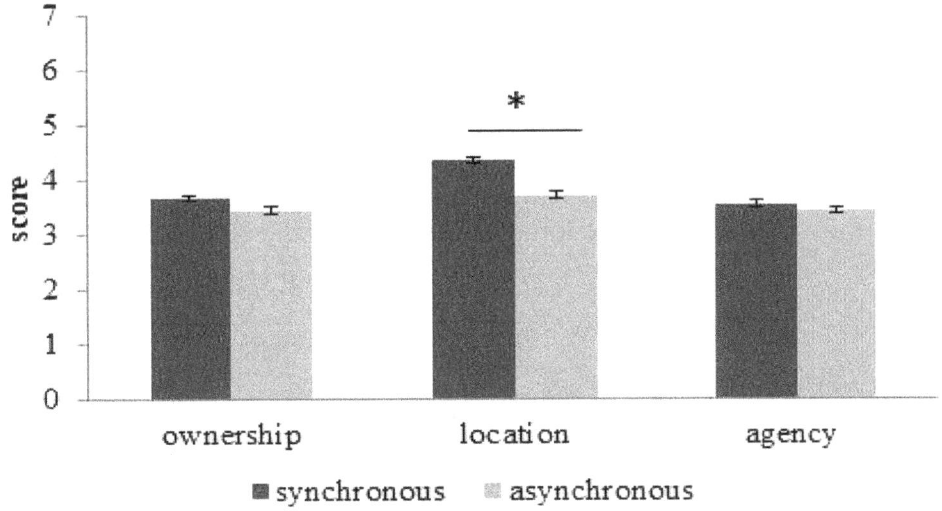

Figure 2. About the Embodiment questionnaire, means of the score and standard error (bars) were showed for each subscale (ownership, location and agency) in the synchronous (dark grey) and asynchronous (light grey) conditions. * indicates a significant difference according to the Bonferroni-corrected p value of 0.016.

The interactions *Condition**Group* [F(1,28) = 0.26; p = 0.61; $\eta\rho^2$ = 0.009) and *Subscale**Group* [F(2, 56) = 0.14; p = 0.86; $\eta\rho^2$ = 0.005) were not significant. Finally the second level-interaction *Group**Condition*Subscale* was not significant [F(2,56) = 0.52; p = 0.59; $\eta\rho^2$ = 0.018]. The absence of any difference between groups suggested that both participants with obesity and healthy-weight participants reported similar scores in the Embodiment Questionnaire after the induction of the VR-FBI, but it should be noticed that it is true independently from the condition (experimental/synchronous vs. control/asynchronous). However, all participants reported a stronger illusion in the experimental/synchronous condition with respect to the control/asynchronous condition in terms of self-location: in other words, when in the experimental condition, participants reported a stronger feeling to be in the same spatial location of the avatar with respect to the control condition.

Body Parts Size Estimation Task. As reported in the Table 1, at the baseline, analyses revealed a significant difference between the two groups in the estimation of the circumference of the shoulders, abdomen and hips, but not in the estimation of their width; moreover, no difference emerged in the estimation of the height. Specifically, as suggested by means reported in the Table 1, the healthy-weight participants showed a significant larger percentage of misestimation of the circumference of the three body parts than the participants with obesity.

Focusing on height, a significant main effect of *Group* emerged (F(1, 26) = 4.67; p = 0.04; $\eta\rho^2$ = 0.15), showing that individuals affected by obesity (M = 3.16; SD = 1.07) had a significant overestimation compared to the controls (M = –0.004; SD = 0.99), in absence of main effect of *Condition* (baseline

M = 1.9; SD = 3.72; synchronous M = 1; SD = 4.91; asynchronous M = 1.6; SD = 4.47) (F(2, 52) = 1.82; $p = 0.17$; $\eta\rho^2 = 0.06$) or a significant interaction *Group*Condition* (F(2,52) = 2.88; $p = 0.88$; $\eta\rho^2 = 0.41$). Thus, the VR-FBI did not change the height estimation for both groups.

For shoulder width estimation no main effect of *Group* (participants with obesity M = −10.24; SD = 4.32; healthy-weigh participants M = −4.58; SD = 4.67) (F(1, 24) = 0.78; $p = 0.38$; $\eta\rho^2 = 0.032$) or *Condition* (baseline M = −5.35; SD = 3.65; synchronous M = −8.52; SD = 3.42; asynchronous M = −8.36; SD = 3.15) (F(2,48) = 1.38; $p = 0.26$; $\eta\rho^2 = 0.055$) was found. Instead, a significant interaction *Group*Condition* (F(2,48) = 3.5; $p = 0.038$; $\eta\rho^2 = 0.12$) emerged. Post-hoc comparison for participants affected by obesity did not show a difference in the horizontal estimation of the shoulders between the baseline and the synchronous condition (t(13) = 0.049; $p = 0.62$), nor between the baseline and the asynchronous condition (t(13) = 1.13; $p = 0.27$). Instead, in the controls a significant difference emerged between the baseline and the synchronous condition (t(12) = 2.58; $p = 0.024$), but not between the baseline and the asynchronous condition (t(12) = 2.36; $p = 0.035$), when we adopted the Bonferroni corrected p value threshold (0.05/2 = 0.025) (Figure 3). Thus, these results show that the illusion affected shoulder width estimation of healthy-weight controls but not of individuals affected by obesity. However, as shown in Figure 3, it should be noticed that controls show a larger error after the synchronous and the asynchronous (even though the difference did not reach the significance) stimulation with respect to the baseline: this result was in contrast with the previous literature [1,2,5,18], in which it was generally reported a reduction of the error after the VR-FBI manipulation.

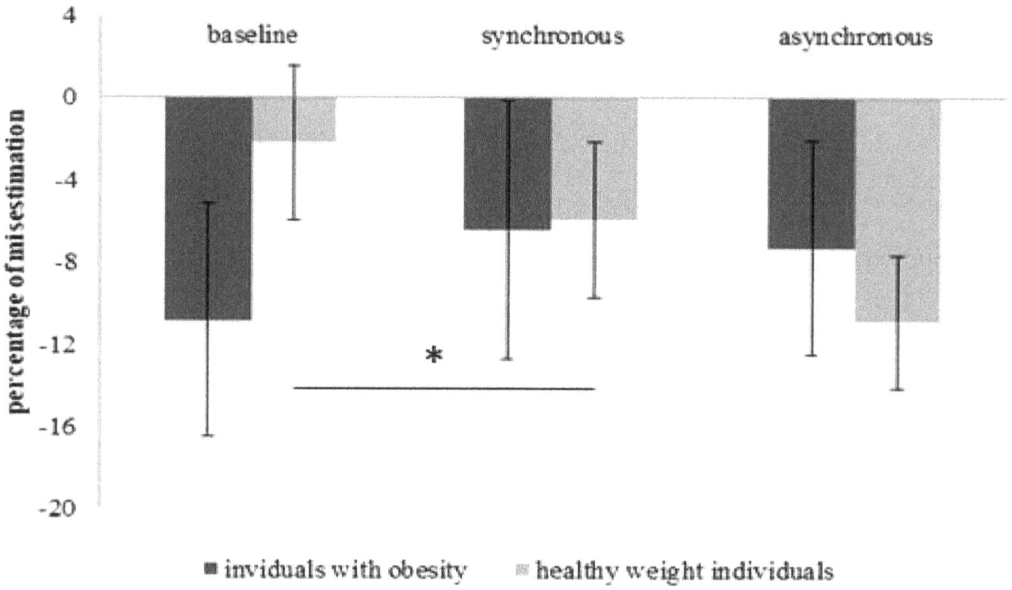

Figure 3. About the horizontal estimation of the shoulders, means of the percentage of misestimation and standard error (bars) were showed for participants affected by obesity (dark grey bars) and healthy-weight participants (light grey) for the three experimental conditions. * indicates a significant difference according to the Bonferroni-corrected p value of 0.025.

For width estimation of the abdomen, no main effect of *Group* (participants with obesity M = −4.49 SD = 5.39; healthy-weigh participants M = −1.29; SD = 5.79) (F(1, 26) = 0.16; $p = 0.68$; $\eta\rho^2 = 0.006$) or *Condition* (baseline M = −0.006; SD = 3.77; synchronous M = −4.93; SD = 4.29; asynchronous M = −3.73; SD = 4.53) (F(2, 52) = 2.12; $p = 0.13$; $\eta\rho^2 = 0.07$) emerged; moreover no significant interaction *Group*Condition* (F(2, 52) = 1.21; $p = 0.3$; $\eta\rho^2 = 0.04$) was found. Thus, the FBI did not change the width estimation of the abdomen for both groups.

For width estimation of the hips, we found a main effect of *Group* (F(1, 24) = 8.33; $p = 0.008$; $\eta\rho^2 = 0.25$): participants affected by obesity (M = 15.03; SD = 3.55) overestimated this body part with respect to the controls (M = 0.49; SD = 3.55). However, no main effect of *Condition* (baseline M = −9.47;

SD = 2.91; synchronous M = 4.94; SD = 2.54; asynchronous M = 8.87; SD = 3.02) ($F(2, 48) = 2.37$; $p = 0.1$; $\eta\rho^2 = 0.09$) or interaction *Group*Condition* ($F(2, 48) = 2.54$; $p = 0.08$; $\eta\rho^2 = 0.09$) emerged. This result suggested that VR-FBI did not change the width estimation of the hips for both groups.

For circumference estimation of shoulders, a significant main effect of *Group* was found ($F(1, 28) = 4.86$; $p = 0.036$; $\eta\rho^2 = 0.14$) confirming the previous results; in general, healthy-weight participants (M = 31.98; SD = 5.48) overestimated this body part compared to the participants affected by obesity (M = 14.88; SD = 5.48). Interestingly, a significant main effect of *Condition* emerged ($F(2, 56) = 3.17$; $p = 0.049$; $\eta\rho^2 = 0.10$): however, when the post-hoc t-test comparisons adopting the Bonferroni corrected p value threshold (0.05/2 = 0.025) were performed, no significant difference between the baseline (M = 27.81; SD = 4.32) and the synchronous condition (M = 19.91; SD = 4.53) ($t(29) = 2.2$; $p = 0.036$) or the baseline and the asynchronous condition (M = 22.58; SD = 4) ($t(29) = 1.41$; $p = 0.16$) emerged. Moreover, no significant interaction *Group*Condition* emerged ($F(1, 26) = 1.64$; $p = 0.2$; $\eta\rho^2 = 0.05$).

For estimation of the circumference of the abdomen, a significant main effect of *Group* emerged ($F(1, 23) = 19.95$; $p < 0.001$; $\eta\rho^2 = 0.46$): in line with the previous results, healthy-weight participants (M = 21.84; SD = 3) reported a significant overestimation of their body size compared to participants with obesity (M = 2.44; SD = 3.13), in absence of any main effect of *Condition* (baseline M = 13.14; SD = 2.91; synchronous M = 11.07; SD = 2.81; asynchronous M = 12.2; SD = 2.14) ($F(2, 46) = 0.31$; $p = 0.73$; $\eta\rho^2 = 0.013$) or a significant interaction *Group*Condition* ($F(2, 46) = 0.97$; $p = 0.38$; $\eta\rho^2 = 0.04$).

For estimation of the circumference of the hips, no main effect of *Group* (participants with obesity corrected M = 16.73; SD = 4.13; healthy-weight participants corrected M = 6.61; SD = 3.84) ($F(1, 26) = 3.21$; $p = 0.08$; $\eta\rho^2 = 0.11$) was found. However, we observed a main effect of *Condition* ($F(2, 52) = 3.51$; $p = 0.037$; $\eta\rho^2 = 0.11$): a significant difference between the baseline (M = 15.51; SD = 3.6) and the synchronous condition (M = 8.89; SD = 3.07) ($t(28) = 2.6$; $p = 0.014$) was found. Instead, no difference emerged between the baseline and the asynchronous condition (M = 10.6; SD = 2.86) ($t(28) = 1.94$; $p = 0.06$) (Figure 4). No significant interaction *Group*Condition* ($F(2, 52) = 2.17$; $p = 0.12$; $\eta\rho^2 = 0.07$) was found. Thus, according to these results, for both groups, changes in the estimation of the hips circumference emerged after the synchronous (but not the asynchronous) condition, with respect to the baseline. Specifically, as shown in Figure 4, after the illusion was induced in the synchronous condition, all participants reported a reduction of the error in the estimation of the hips' circumference, in line with our hypothesis.

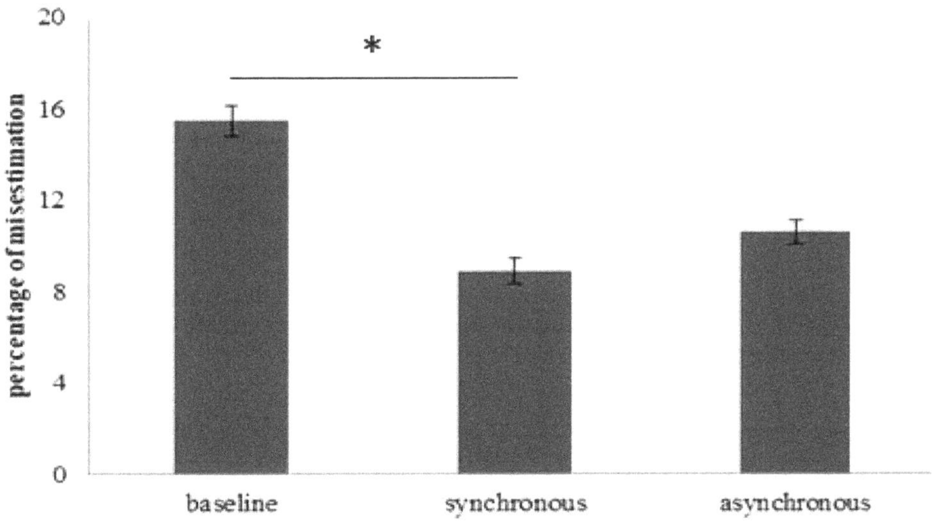

Figure 4. About the circumference estimation of the hips, means of the percentage of misestimation and standard error (bars) were showed for the three experimental condition (baseline, synchronous and asynchronous). * indicates a significant difference according to the Bonferroni-corrected p value of 0.025.

4. Discussion

The aim of the present work was to investigate for the first time in literature the potential changes in body representations induced by the illusionary ownership over a virtual skinny body (i.e., the VR-FBI) in a sample of individuals affected by obesity in comparison with a group of healthy weight individuals. We adopted two measures: the Embodiment Questionnaire [1] to study the strength of the bodily illusion; and the Body Part Size Estimation Task [1] to verify if the illusion might induce a modulation of body representations in our participants.

First, we found that VR-FBI was efficiently induced in individuals with obesity with the same strength of the healthy weight individuals. Indeed, there was no significant difference between the two groups as concerns the scores obtained from the Embodiment Questionnaire [1]. However, for all participants, it should be noted that we found a significant difference in the *self-location* subscale, but not in the *ownership* and *agency* subscales, between the two experimental conditions, suggesting that also in the asynchronous condition (and thus not only the synchronous one) all individuals experience the illusion of ownership. To this regard, it was already reported that a first-person perspective of a realistic virtual body substituting participants' own body might be sufficient to generate an illusory feeling of ownership, with changes in body representations, in absence of any multisensory stimulation [25], as reported also for the Rubber Hand Illusion [26]. Thus, the asynchronous stimulation is not a *"neutral condition"*, since it can affect body representations [27]. As concerns the self-location subscale, we did not expect specific differences between the two conditions, since our paradigm did not experimentally manipulate the spatial location. However, higher scores in self-location subscale could drive higher embodiment over the virtual body, as Maselli and Slater [25] emphasized a strict relationship between the sense of ownership and the feeling of self-location towards the virtual body. Moreover, there is an ongoing debate about what subjective components, such as body dissatisfaction [5] or bodily sensory experience [2,28–30]—That were not directly measured by the questionnaire—might enhance or impede to experience the bodily illusion [2,28–31]. Moreover, as recently stated by Tamè and colleagues [28] about the Rubber Hand Illusion, even though individuals report the *feeling* like the fake hand is part of their own body, *"they do not believe that it really is"*: this aspect should be taken in account also when individuals are asked to rate their experience of ownership towards an avatar.

The second other main result regarded the possible modulation of body representations, when measured through the Body Part Size Estimation Task [1], due to the bodily illusion. According to the results, an interesting pattern emerged considering the estimation of the circumference of the hips: both healthy weight individuals and individuals affected by obesity shown a reduction of the error after the synchronous, but not the asynchronous, condition, with respect to the baseline. This result seems to suggest that the illusion can efficiently modulate body representations in individuals affected by obesity, specifically in terms of the circumference of the hips, as well as in controls. In other words, affected individuals perceived themselves to have skinner hips after they have embodied a skinny avatar. However, such an effect did not emerge for the other body parts investigated in this study. How might this pattern of results be interpreted? We might observe that the hips represent a very significant and critical body part, not only in obesity but also in healthy weight participants, and specifically in women, in which there is a propensity to accumulate fat on the hips and buttocks (the "feminine gynecoid" type) instead of a more central distribution on the abdomen, that is typically observed in males [32–34]. Thus, it makes sense to believe that from a clinical point of view this body part is quite important and perhaps more sensitive than other body parts, such as the shoulders. Second, it should be noted that during the experimental procedure, participants looked toward the avatar's lower part, that was clearly skinner than the own physical body dimension. Considering that, it should be carefully clarified the psychological meaning of this difference. Indeed, it cannot be excluded that the presence of a skinny avatar would might enhance (and not mitigate) the negative feelings towards the body. In this sense, the therapeutic applicability of bodily illusions in obesity should require future investigation in which also psychological and clinical factors, as well as the outcome of the weight loss program, should be taken in account. For example, it should be investigated

if the alteration of body parts size estimation might be related to other psychological factors, such as fear and worries about the success of the treatment as well as the subjective level of perceived social stigma [35,36] since they could be negative consequences on efficacy of rehabilitative intervention, as well as the most recent study about the effect of bodily illusions on social cognition [31]. Indeed, Guardia and colleagues [37] described the single case of an individual affected by obesity who did not update her body image to the "new" physical body dimensions after a massive weight loss; in other words, the patient continued to describe her body as larger as before the treatment [37–39].

Overall, this study provided preliminary evidence that individuals with obesity can experience the VR-FBI, and that the illusion can induce a modulation of body representations only for specific body parts.

However, some caveats should be considered not only in the interpretation of our data but also for future investigation. First, a higher number of participants is mandatory to verify the reproducibility of our results.

When we investigate the application of the bodily illusion in the obesity, we should take in account not only the psychological and emotional components associated to this procedure, but also the cognitive process on which bodily illusions ground, that is the *multisensory integration* [40]. Specifically, the illusion can be efficiently induced only when the two stimuli (in this case, tactile and visual input) are perceived temporally synchronous; in other words, they are perceived as unique temporal event. For humans, multisensory integration is very critical, since it seems to be implicated in several cognitive processes, such as taste perception [41], flavor perception [42–44], but also bodily awareness [45,46] and sense of agency [47]. Focusing on bodily illusions, and specifically the asynchronous stimulation, the recognition of the delay between stimuli might depend on the subjective efficacy of the multisensory integration process, with effect on the induction and the strength of the illusion e.g., [25,27,48,49]. In obesity, the research about alteration of primary [50–52] and multiple sensory inputs [24–56] is still in its infancy. However, it was reported that individuals affected by obesity show an alteration of multisensory process, with possible effects of the ability in recognizing two stimuli (and overall, two events) as concurrent and concomitant [24–56]. Thus, future research needs to fully explore the relationship between the alteration in the experience of bodily illusions and altered multisensory integration.

Focusing on the VR-FBI, two aspects should be taken in account. The first regards the dimension of the avatar. In this work, we adopted an avatar with a skinny body, in line with our previous studies [1,20]. However, it should be verified if different dimensions of avatar (thus, a larger avatar as well as an avatar with bodily dimensions equivalent to the physical one) would affect differently body parts size estimation. In fact, in healthy individuals, while it was reported that a correct feeling of ownership was observed for images of hands with veridical and enlarged dimension respect to the physical one in healthy individuals, but absent in case of reduced dimensions, in the Rubber Hand Illusion [57,58]. Instead, the illusion emerged with both large and small full bodies in VR-FBI [55,59]. We reported that the two groups differed in the estimation of body size at the baseline. Interestingly, the healthy weight participants reported a significant larger error for the circumference of the three body parts of shoulders, abdomen and hips in respect to the participants with obesity. As expected, for all considered body parts, except for the height, individuals affected by obesity had higher physical dimensions than controls; thus, bodily dimensions were dramatically different between groups. However, the distortion of the body parts circumference observed in the healthy weight participants was quite different respect to that of the participants with obesity. As previously mentioned, the physical reduction of body size dimensions is a goal of the rehabilitative program for losing weight, and it is reasonable to think that individuals with obesity might be more aware about their own physical body than healthy weight individuals, who otherwise are generally described to have a negative feeling and high level of concerns about their own body [60]. Moreover, it should be noted the body size distortions are highly present also in healthy population [60]. However, as reviewed by Costantini and Haggard [40], pre-existing body representations play a crucial in body ownership. Indeed, the ownership towards an external object is due not only to the simultaneity of the sensory (visual-tactile) stimulation, but also to the match between the visual image of the body part/whole body adopted in the illusion and its existing subjective cognitive representation, i.e., the perceptual body representation [61] or offline stored knowledge about own body [62]. Nevertheless, when we ask individuals to judge the dimension of body parts, perhaps we are measuring the perceptual dimension together *plus* the feelings, concerns and preoccupation about those body parts [22–63], affecting the judgement itself. The second aspect regards the fact that during this experiment, in line with previous research [2–5], participants did not move as well as avatar was static. However, brain seems to be more responsive to human action than to static images [64], with possible implications on changes in body representations [65,66]. Thus, in the future perspectives, body representations changes might be investigated when embodiment towards an avatar is induced through a visuo-motor integration (the virtual body is seen to move synchronously with the own body), instead of a visuo-tactile integration (as done in the present study), taking advantage of motion sensors technology. Nevertheless, in case of motion, the presence of cybersickness during the VR experiment should be carefully measured, specifically when clinical condition like obesity, in which dizziness and falls are generally experience [67], are tested.

Finally, even though it is out of the scope of this work, we would like to underline some criticisms relative to the two measures (i.e., Body size estimation task and Embodiment Questionnaire) adopted in this study. About the Body parts size estimation task, it should be noticed that height (i.e., a vertical measurement taken from the top of the body to its base), horizontal (from the left of the body to the right) and circumferential (a measurement taken around the body) estimations ground on different neural mechanisms about spatial processing [68]. For example, a task in which we are required to identify the midline of a horizontal line would be solved adopting counting strategies, that instead might not be so useful when we have to estimate where is the center of a circle [69]. This aspect should be taken in account when a task about the estimation of body parts or whole body is chosen as measure of the illusion. Moreover, it should be noted that in the Body Size Estimation Task [1–20], participants are explicitly required to estimate the horizontal distance between the left and right side of each body part placing adhesive stickers on the wall. To avoid that they used their body as a reference for giving a correct body size estimation, we explicitly required participants to do not look at their own body during the task. This task has clear advantages: it's economical and traditionally adopted in clinical settings [70,71]. However, participants are fully aware that they have to focus on their own body to solve the task, and possible overcome side effect of negative attitudes on the judgment might reduce the illusion effect. Adopting more implicit measures in which a lower level of subjective awareness about the judgment [72] is required, should strengthen our results. A similar criticism can be arisen about the Embodiment Questionnaire [1], since it allows us to assess exclusively the subjective (and thus explicit and aware) experience of the illusion.

5. Conclusions

In this manuscript we presented the first investigation on the effect of a VR-FBI [2–5,17,18,20] on body representations in obesity. Indeed, only one single case study about VR-FBI on body representations in obesity [20] was reported in literature. Our results revealed that individuals affected by obesity might efficiently experience the illusory ownership over an entire virtual body, with possible changes on the estimation of the circumference of the hips. Thus, VR-FBI might be a promising tool to be adopted in rehabilitative settings [8,17], also in obesity. However, this work represents the first step in the field: future research should verify if and in which clinical and psychological circumstances as well as experimental conditions the illusion can efficiently modulate body representation in obesity.

Author Contributions: Conceptualization, S.F., S.S. and R.G.; Data curation, C.A., S.M., C.G. and M.A.; Formal analysis, S.F.; Funding acquisition, R.G.; Investigation, S.F., S.S. and C.A.; Methodology, S.F., S.S. and K.A.; Software, C.A.; Supervision, M.A.; Writing—Original draft, S.F. and S.S.; Writing—Review & editing, K.A., S.M., C.G., M.A. and R.G.

Acknowledgments: This paper was partially supported by the Italian MIUR (Ministero dell'Università e della Ricerca Italiana) research project "Unlocking the memory of the body: Virtual Reality in Anorexia Nervosa" (Grant no. 201597WTTM).

References

1. Serino, S.; Scarpina, F.; Dakanalis, A.; Keizer, A.; Pedroli, E.; Castelnuovo, G.; Chirico, A.; Catallo, V.; Di Lernia, D.; Riva, G. The Role of Age on Multisensory Bodily Experience: An Experimental Study with a Virtual Reality Full-Body Illusion. *Cyberpsychol. Behav. Soc. Netw.* **2018**, *21*, 304–310. [CrossRef] [PubMed]
2. Petkova, V.I.; Ehrsson, H.H. If I were you: Perceptual illusion of body swapping. *PLoS ONE* **2008**, *3*, e3832. [CrossRef]
3. Slater, M.; Spanlang, B.; Sanchez-Vives, M.V.; Blanke, O. First person experience of body transfer in virtual reality. *PLoS ONE* **2010**, *5*, e10564. [CrossRef] [PubMed]
4. Serino, S.; Pedroli, E.; Keizer, A.; Triberti, S.; Dakanalis, A.; Pallavicini, F.; Chirico, A.; Riva, G. Virtual Reality Body Swapping: A Tool for Modifying the Allocentric Memory of the Body. *Cyberpsychol. Behav. Soc. Netw.* **2016**, *19*, 127–133. [CrossRef] [PubMed]
5. Preston, C.; Ehrsson, H.H. Implicit and explicit changes in body satisfaction evoked by body size illusions: Implications for eating disorder vulnerability in women. *PLoS ONE* **2018**, *13*, e0199426. [CrossRef] [PubMed]
6. Valzogher, C.; Mazzurega, M.; Zampini, M.; Pavani, F. Incongruent multisensory stimuli alter bodily self-consciousness: Evidence from a first-person perspective experience. *Acta Psychol.* **2018**, *191*, 261–270. [CrossRef] [PubMed]
7. Keizer, A.; van Elburg, A.; Helms, R.; Dijkerman, H.C. A Virtual Reality Full Body Illusion Improves Body Image Disturbance in Anorexia Nervosa. *PLoS ONE* **2016**, *11*, e0163921. [CrossRef] [PubMed]
8. Serino, S.; Polli, N.; Riva, G. From avatars to body swapping: The use of virtual reality for assessing and treating body-size distortion in individuals with anorexia. *J. Clin. Psychol.* **2019**, *75*, 313–322. [CrossRef] [PubMed]
9. Jeon, B.; Cho, S.; Lee, J.H. Application of virtual body swapping to patients with complex regional pain syndrome: A pilot study. *Cyberpsychol. Behav. Soc. Netw.* **2014**, *17*, 366–370. [CrossRef]
10. Lengeenhager, B.; Hilti, L.M.; Brugger, P. Disturbed body integrity and the "rubber foot illusion". *Neuropsychology* **2015**, *29*, 205–211. [CrossRef]
11. Kaplan, R.A.; Enticott, P.G.; Hohwy, J.; Castle, D.J.; Rossell, S.L. Is body dysmorphic disorder associated with abnormal bodily self-awareness? A study using the rubber hand illusion. *PLoS ONE* **2014**, *9*, e99981. [CrossRef]
12. Botvinick, M.; Cohen, J. Rubber hands 'feel' touch that eyes see. *Nature* **1998**, *391*, 756. [CrossRef] [PubMed]
13. Moseley, G.L.; Gallace, A.; Spence, C. Bodily illusions in health and disease: Physiological and clinical perspectives and the concept of a cortical 'body matrix'. *Neurosci. Biobehav. Rev.* **2012**, *36*, 34–46. [CrossRef] [PubMed]
14. Gutiérrez-Maldonado, J.; Wiederhold, B.K.; Riva, G. Future Directions: How Virtual Reality Can Further Improve the Assessment and Treatment of Eating Disorders and Obesity. *Cyberpsychol. Behav. Soc. Netw.* **2016**, *19*, 148–153. [CrossRef] [PubMed]
15. Riva, G. Virtual reality in the treatment of eating and weight disorders. *Psychol. Med.* **2017**, *47*, 2567–2568. [CrossRef] [PubMed]
16. Freeman, D.; Reeve, S.; Robinson, A.; Ehlers, A.; Clark, D.; Spanlang, B.; Slater, M. Virtual reality in the assessment, understanding and treatment of mental health disorders. *Psychol. Med.* **2017**, *47*, 2393–2400. [CrossRef] [PubMed]
17. Serino, S.; Dakanalis, A. Bodily illusions and weight-related disorders: Clinical insights from experimental research. *Ann. Phys. Rehabil. Med.* **2017**, *60*, 217–219. [CrossRef]
18. Normand, J.M.; Giannopoulos, E.; Spanlang, B.; Slater, M. Multisensory stimulation can induce an illusion of larger belly size in immersive virtual reality. *PLoS ONE* **2011**, *6*, e16128. [CrossRef] [PubMed]

19. Eshkevari, E.; Rieger, E.; Longo, M.R.; Haggard, P.; Treasure, J. Increased plasticity of the bodily self in eating disorders. *Psychol. Med.* **2012**, *42*, 819–828. [CrossRef]
20. Serino, S.; Scarpina, F.; Keizer, A.; Pedroli, E.; Dakanalis, A.; Castelnuovo, G.; Chirico, A.; Novelli, M.; Gaudio, S.; Riva, G. A Novel Technique for Improving Bodily Experience in a Non-operable Super-Super Obesity Case. *Front. Psychol.* **2016**, *7*, 837. [CrossRef]
21. Tsakiris, M.; Haggard, P. The Rubber Hand Illusion Revisited: Visuotactile Integration and Self-Attribution. *J. Exp. Psychol. Hum. Percept. Perform.* **2005**, *31*, 80–91. [CrossRef] [PubMed]
22. Scarpina, F.; Castelnuovo, G.; Molinari, E. Tactile mental body parts representation in obesity. *Psychiatry Res.* **2014**, *220*, 960–969. [CrossRef] [PubMed]
23. Scarpina, F.; Cau, N.; Cimolin, V.; Galli, M.; Castelnuovo, G.; Priano, L.; Pianta, L.; Corti, S.; Mauro, A.; Capodaglio, P. Body-scaled action in obesity during locomotion: Insights on the nature and extent of body representation disturbances. *J. Psychosom. Res.* **2017**, *102*, 34–40. [CrossRef]
24. Scarpina, F.; Migliorati, D.; Marzullo, P.; Mauro, A.; Scacchi, M.; Costantini, M. Altered multisensory temporal integration in obesity. *Sci. Rep.* **2016**, *6*, 28382. [CrossRef] [PubMed]
25. Maselli, A.; Slater, M. The building blocks of the full body ownership illusion. *Front. Hum. Neurosci.* **2013**, *7*, 83. [CrossRef] [PubMed]
26. Rohde, M.; Luca, M.; Ernst, M.O. The rubber hand illusion: Feeling of ownership and proprioceptive drift Do not go hand in hand. *PLoS ONE* **2011**, *6*, e21659. [CrossRef] [PubMed]
27. Perez-Marcos, D.; Martini, M.; Fuentes, C.T.; Rivas, A.I.B.; Haggard, P.; Sanchez-Vives, M.V. Selective distortion of body image by asynchronous visuotactile stimulation. *Body Image* **2018**, *24*, 55–61. [CrossRef] [PubMed]
28. Tamè, L.; Linkenauger, S.A.; Longo, M.R. Dissociation of feeling and belief in the rubber hand illusion. *PLoS ONE* **2018**, *13*, e0206367. [CrossRef] [PubMed]
29. Blanke, O.; Metzinger, T. Full-body illusions and minimal phenomenal selfhood. *Trends Cognit. Sci.* **2009**, *13*, 7–13. [CrossRef]
30. David, N.; Fiori, F.; Aglioti, S.M. Susceptibility to the rubber hand illusion does not tell the whole body-awareness story. *Cognit. Affect. Behav. Neurosci.* **2014**, *14*, 297–306. [CrossRef]
31. Maister, L.; Slater, M.; Sanchez-Vives, M.V.; Tsakiris, M. Changing bodies changes minds: Owning another body affects social cognition. *Trends Cognit. Sci.* **2015**, *19*, 6–12. [CrossRef] [PubMed]
32. Champe, P.C.; Richard, A. *Harvey Lippincott's Illustrated Reviews: Biochemistry*, 3rd ed.; Lippincott, Williams & Wilkins: Baltimore, ML, USA, 2003.
33. Zavorsky, G.S.; Murias, J.M.; Kim do, J.; Gow, J.; Sylvestre, J.L.; Christou, N.V. Waist-to-hip ratio is associated with pulmonary gas exchange in the morbidly obese. *Chest* **2007**, *131*, 362–367. [CrossRef] [PubMed]
34. Janjic, C. Android-type obesity and gynecoid-type obesity. *Praxis* **1996**, *85*, 1578–1583. [PubMed]
35. Puhl, R.M.; Heuer, C.A. Obesity stigma: Important considerations for public health. *Am. J. Public Health* **2010**, *100*, 1019–1028. [CrossRef] [PubMed]
36. Puhl, R.M.; Suh, Y. Health Consequences of Weight Stigma: Implications for Obesity Prevention and Treatment. *Curr. Obes. Rep.* **2015**, *4*, 182–190. [CrossRef] [PubMed]
37. Guardia, D.; Metral, M.; Pigeyre, M.; Bauwens, I.; Cottencin, O.; Luyat, M. Body distortions after massive weight loss: Lack of updating of the body schema hypothesis. *Eat. Weight Disord.* **2013**, *18*, 333–336. [CrossRef] [PubMed]
38. Dakanalis, A.; Gaudio, S.; Serino, S.; Clerici, M.; Carrá, G.; Riva, G. Body-image distortion in anorexia nervosa. *Nat. Rev. Dis. Primers* **2016**, *2*, 16026. [CrossRef]
39. Riva, G.; Gaggioli, A.; Dakanalis, A. From body dissatisfaction to obesity: How virtual reality may improve obesity prevention and treatment in adolescents. *Stud. Health Technol. Inform.* **2013**, *184*, 356–362.
40. Costantini, M.; Haggard, P. The rubber hand illusion: Sensitivity and reference frame for body ownership. *Conscious. Cognit.* **2007**, *16*, 229–240. [CrossRef]
41. Slocombe, B.G.; Carmichael, D.A.; Simner, J. Cross-modal tactile-taste interactions in food evaluations. *Neuropsychologia* **2016**, *88*, 58–64. [CrossRef]
42. Auvray, M.; Spence, C. The multisensory perception of flavor. *Conscious. Cognit.* **2008**, *17*, 1016–1031. [CrossRef] [PubMed]
43. Wallace, M.T. Multisensory Perception: The Building of Flavor Representations. *Curr. Biol.* **2015**, *25*, R986–R988. [CrossRef] [PubMed]

44. Spence, C. Multisensory flavor perception. *Cell* **2015**, *161*, 24–35. [CrossRef] [PubMed]
45. Salomon, R.; Noel, J.P.; Łukowska, M.; Faivre, N.; Metzinger, T.; Serino, A.; Blanke, O. Unconscious integration of multisensory bodily inputs in the peripersonal space shapes bodily self-consciousness. *Cognition* **2017**, *166*, 174–183. [CrossRef] [PubMed]
46. Tsakiris, M. The multisensory basis of the self: From body to identity to others. *Q. J. Exp. Psychol.* **2017**, *70*, 597–609. [CrossRef] [PubMed]
47. Pyasik, M.; Burin, D.; Pia, L. On the relation between body ownership and sense of agency: A link at the level of sensory-related signals. *Acta Psychol.* **2018**, *185*, 219–228. [CrossRef] [PubMed]
48. Maselli, A.; Kilteni, K.; López-Moliner, J.; Slater, M. The sense of body ownership relaxes temporal constraints for multisensory integration. *Sci. Rep.* **2016**, *6*, 30628. [CrossRef] [PubMed]
49. Kilteni, K.; Maselli, A.; Kording, K.P.; Slater, M. Over my fake body: Body ownership illusions for studying the multisensory basis of own-bodyperception. *Front. Hum. Neurosci.* **2015**, *9*, 141. [CrossRef] [PubMed]
50. Szalay, C.; Aradi, M.; Schwarcz, A.; Orsi, G.; Perlaki, G.; Németh, L.; Hanna, S.; Takács, G.; Szabó, I.; Bajnok, L.; et al. Gustatory perception alterations in obesity: An fMRI study. *Brain Res.* **2012**, *1473*, 131–140. [CrossRef]
51. Stafford, L.D.; Whittle, A. Obese Individuals Have Higher Preference and Sensitivity to Odor of Chocolate. *Chem. Senses* **2015**, *40*, 279–284. [CrossRef]
52. Holinski, F.; Menenakos, C.; Haber, G.; Olze, H.; Ordemann, J. Olfactory and Gustatory Function After Bariatric Surgery. *Obes. Surg.* **2015**, *25*, 2314–2320. [CrossRef] [PubMed]
53. Preston, C.; Ehrsson, H.H. Illusory changes in body size modulate body satisfaction in a way that is related to non-clinical eating disorder psychopathology. *PLoS ONE* **2014**, *9*, e85773. [CrossRef] [PubMed]
54. Holmes, N.P.; Snijders, H.J.; Spence, C. Reaching with alien limbs: Visual exposure to prosthetic hands in a mirror biases proprioception without accompanying illusions of ownership. *Percept. Psychophys.* **2006**, *68*, 685–701. [CrossRef] [PubMed]
55. Piryankova, I.V.; Wong, H.Y.; Linkenauger, S.A.; Stinson, C.; Longo, M.R.; Bülthoff, H.H.; Mohler, B.J. Owning an overweight or underweight body: Distinguishing the physical, experienced and virtual body. *PLoS ONE* **2014**, *9*, e103428. [CrossRef] [PubMed]
56. Wan, X.; Spence, C.; Mu, B.; Zhou, X.; Ho, C. Assessing the benefits of multisensory audiotactile stimulation for overweight individuals. *Exp. Brain Res.* **2014**, *232*, 1085–1093. [CrossRef] [PubMed]
57. Pavani, F.; Zampini, M. The role of hand size in the fake-hand illusion paradigm. *Perception* **2007**, *36*, 1547–1554. [CrossRef] [PubMed]
58. Kilteni, K.; Normand, J.M.; Sanchez-Vives, M.V.; Slater, M. Extending body space in immersive virtual reality: A very long arm illusion. *PLoS ONE* **2012**, *7*, e40867. [CrossRef] [PubMed]
59. Van der Hoort, B.; Guterstam, A.; Ehrsson, H.H. Being Barbie: The size of one's own body determines the perceived size of the world. *PLoS ONE* **2011**, *6*, e20195. [CrossRef]
60. Schwartz, M.B.; Brownell, K.D. Obesity and body image. *Body Image* **2004**, *1*, 43–45. [CrossRef]
61. Longo, M.R.; Azañón, E.; Haggard, P. More than skin deep: Body representation beyond primary somatosensory cortex. *Neuropsychologia* **2010**, *48*, 655–668. [CrossRef]
62. Riva, G. The Neuroscience of Body Memory: From the Self through the Space to the Others. *Cortex* **2018**, *104*, 241–260. [CrossRef] [PubMed]
63. Smeets, M.A.; Klugkist, I.G.; Rooden, S.V.; Anema, H.A.; Postma, A. Mental body distance comparison: A tool for assessing clinical disturbances in visual body image. *Acta Psychol.* **2009**, *132*, 157–165. [CrossRef] [PubMed]
64. Peuskens, H.; Vanrie, J.; Verfaille, K.; Orban, G.A. Specificity of regions processing biological motion. *Eur. J. Neurosci.* **2005**, *21*, 2864–2875. [CrossRef] [PubMed]
65. Vocks, S.; Legenbauer, T.; Rüddel, H.; Troje, N.F. Static and dynamic body image in bulimia nervosa: Mental representation of body dimensionsand biological motion patterns. *Int. J. Eat. Disord.* **2007**, *40*, 59–66. [CrossRef] [PubMed]
66. Cazzato, V.; Siega, S.; Urgesi, C. "What women like": Influence of motion and form on esthetic body perception. *Front. Psychol.* **2012**, *3*, 235. [CrossRef]
67. Corna, S.; Aspesi, V.; Cau, N.; Scarpina, F.; Gattini Valdés, N.; Brugliera, L.; Cimolin, V.; Capodaglio, P. Dizziness and Falls in Obese Inpatients Undergoing Metabolic Rehabilitation. *PLoS ONE* **2017**, *12*, e0169322. [CrossRef]

68. Jewell, G.; McCourt, M.E. Pseudoneglect: A review and meta-analysis of performance factors in line bisection tasks. *Neuropsychologia* **2000**, *38*, 93–110. [CrossRef]
69. Girardi, M.; McIntosh, R.D.; Michel, C.; Vallar, G.; Rossetti, Y. Sensorimotor effects on central space representation: Prism adaptation influences haptic and visual representations in normal subjects. *Neuropsychologia* **2004**, *42*, 1477–1487. [CrossRef]
70. Probst, M.; Vandereycken, W.; Vanderlinden, J.; Van Coppenolle, H. The significance of body size estimation in eating disorders: Its relationship with clinical and psychological variables. *Int. J. Eat. Disord.* **1998**, *24*, 167–174. [CrossRef]
71. Shafran, R.; Fairburn, C.G. A new ecologically valid method to assess body size estimation and body size dissatisfaction. *Int. J. Eat. Disord.* **2002**, *32*, 458–465. [CrossRef]
72. Longo, M.R. Implicit and Explicit Body Representations. *Eur. Psychol.* **2015**, *20*, 6–15. [CrossRef]

14

Analysis of Usage Data from a Self-Guided App-Based Virtual Reality Cognitive Behavior Therapy for Acrophobia: A Randomized Controlled Trial

Tara Donker [1,2,3,*], Chris van Klaveren [4], Ilja Cornelisz [4], Robin N. Kok [5,6] and Jean-Louis van Gelder [7,8]

1 Department of Clinical, Neuro and Developmental Psychology, Section Clinical Psychology, Vrije Universiteit Amsterdam, Van der Boechorststraat 1, 1081 BT Amsterdam, The Netherlands
2 Amsterdam Public Health Research Institute Amsterdam, Van der Boechorststraat 7, 1081 BT Amsterdam, The Netherlands
3 Department of Psychology, Laboratory of Biological and Personality Psychology, Albert Ludwigs-University of Freiburg, Peter-Kaplan Meierstrasse 8, 79104 Freiburg im Breisgau, Germany
4 Department of Education Sciences, Section Methods and Statistics and Amsterdam Center for Learning Analytics, Vrije Universiteit Amsterdam, Van der Boechorststraat 1, 1081 BT Amsterdam, The Netherlands; c.p.b.j.van.klaveren@vu.nl (C.v.K.); i.cornelisz@vu.nl (I.C.)
5 Department of Psychology, University of Southern Denmark, Campusvej 55, 5230 Odense, Denmark; rkok@health.sdu.dk
6 Centre for Innovative Medical Technology, Odense University Hospital, Indgang 101, 5000 Odense, Denmark
7 Institute of Education and Child Studies, Leiden University, Pieter de la Court building, 4th floor, Wassenaarseweg 52, 2333 AK Leiden, The Netherlands; jlvangelder@gmail.com
8 Max Planck Institute for the Study of Crime, Security and Law, Department of Criminology, Günterstalstraße 73, 79100 Freiburg, Germany
* Correspondence: t.donker@vu.nl

Abstract: This study examined user engagement with ZeroPhobia, a self-guided app-based virtual reality (VR) Cognitive Behavior Therapy for acrophobia symptoms using cardboard VR viewers. Dutch acrophobic adults (n = 96) completed assessments at baseline and immediately following treatment. Primary outcome measures were the Acrophobia Questionnaire (AQ) and the Igroup Presence Questionnaire (IPQ). Usage data consisted of number of VR sessions practiced, practice time, and fear ratings directly after practicing. Results show that of the 66 participants who played at least one level, the majority continued to finish all levels, spending on average 24.4 min in VR. Self-reported fear consistently decreased between the start and finish of levels. Post-test AQ scores depended quadratically on time spent in VR. Higher pre-test AQ scores were significantly associated with subjective anxiety after the first level and a reduction of post-test AQ scores, but not with number of sessions, suggesting it might be more beneficial to play one level for a longer time period instead of practicing many VR levels. Results also show an optimum exposure level at which increasing practice time does not result in increased benefit. Self-guided VR acrophobia treatment is effective and leads to consistent reductions in self-reported anxiety both between levels and after treatment. Most participants progressed effectively to the highest self-exposure level, despite the absence of a therapist.

Keywords: acrophobia; cognitive behaviour therapy; mobile app; virtual reality; usage data

1. Introduction

Given the global challenge of access to evidence-based psychological treatment for common mental health disorders, there is an evident need for affordable and scalable self-help interventions [1]. Reasons for limited access include a lack of mental health professionals and high treatment costs [2]. Digital interventions may offer a solution. Several meta-analyses of randomized controlled trials (RCTs) have demonstrated effectiveness for digital interventions, mostly online, for treating common mental disorders such as anxiety disorders [3–5]. Innovations in this field comprise virtual reality (VR) and mobile applications (apps) [2]. There is empirical evidence that such interventions can be similar in effectiveness compared to face-to-face treatment [1,6–10]. For example, Morina et al. [9] demonstrated in their meta-analysis that results of behavioral assessment at post-treatment and at follow-up revealed no significant differences between VRET and exposure in vivo. Furthermore, in our study [1] we showed that results of an VR-CBT-based app were comparable to results found in studies investigating the effectiveness of traditional CBT. However, less is known about how user adherence and engagement relates to effectiveness of these interventions, especially with regard to VR and mobile app-based interventions. One exception is the study of Hong et al. [11] in which the effectiveness and usage of a mobile-based self-training VR program for acrophobia was investigated. Interestingly, heart rate (HR) and gaze down percentage were also included in this study. Using a pre-post study design with two arms (high and low acrophobic symptoms), Hong et al. demonstrated that participants with higher acrophobia symptoms derived more benefit from the VR program compared to those with lower acrophobia symptoms. Furthermore, they found a negative correlation with gaze-down percentage in the high acrophobia symptom group compared to the low acrophobia symptom group. In this study, subjects attended a VR-center and had contact with research staff. Treatment efficiency and effectiveness could be enhanced by a better understanding of how intervention usage affects outcome [12–14]. For example, treatment efficiency can be improved through the identification of redundant elements that do not contribute to symptom reduction. Treatment effectiveness can be increased by identifying where participants drop-out and improving that element to reduce drop-out. Exploring usage data of fully self-guided interventions is of particular importance due to the lack of human oversight and the resulting inability to adjust the course of such interventions [12]. An analysis of usage data can be beneficial in optimizing the uptake and continued use of these self-guided interventions.

Recent studies examining usage data of digital interventions have demonstrated that highly active users completing more modules predict better outcomes for eating disorders, smoking cessation and depression [15–19]. Previous studies also demonstrated that higher activity during the first week of treatment is a predictor of better adherence for web-based interventions [20,21]. Moreover, more concise and shorter interventions achieve better usage rates compared to extensive interventions [22]. However, in a recent review, Donkin et al. [15] concluded that several potential usage metrics (number of log-ins, time spent online) were inconsistently associated with outcomes for online interventions for psychological disorders. Only the relation between proportion of completed modules and outcome emerged as a consistent association [15,16]. Previous research into VR treatment indicated that presence plays an important role in the effectiveness of a program [23]). For example, in our study reporting the main results of this trial we found that a larger reduction in acrophobia symptoms was associated when the feeling of being present in the virtual environment was higher [1].

The efficacy of VR interventions for acrophobia has been well-documented (for an overview, see [24]. However, with few exceptions (e.g., [25]) usage data of virtual reality (mobile app) interventions for common mental disorders has remained largely unexplored. For self-guided VR interventions, participant retention is important as there is no therapist oversight into the process. The aim of the present study was to examine usage of, and engagement, with, ZeroPhobia, a fully self-guided app-based virtual reality Cognitive Behavior Therapy (VR-CBT) for acrophobia, using mobile phones and a low-cost (cardboard) virtual reality viewer, and to determine user metrics contributing to effectiveness. The most important element of CBT for anxiety disorders is exposure, in which the participant is repeatedly confronted with the feared object or situation, thus learning that the expected disaster is not happening. This, in turn, leads to decreases in anxiety symptoms [26]. We specified the following exploratory hypotheses: (1) higher VR activity (number of completed VR sessions, practice time in VR) is associated with reduced post-test acrophobia symptoms; (2) higher presence scores on the IPQ are correlated with stronger decreases in anxiety ratings directly after practicing with exposure in the VR environment; (3) higher acrophobia symptoms at pre-test correlate positively with VR anxiety ratings and VR activity, and negatively with a reduction in acrophobia symptoms at post-test; and (4) post-session anxiety levels consistently decrease compared to pre-session anxiety levels after repeated practice in the VR environment.

2. Materials and Methods

2.1. Study Design and Procedure

In the current study, we carried out a secondary analysis of a previously published outcome study [1]. Details of the materials and methods are described elsewhere and will therefore not be dealt with in detail here [1,27]. In short, in this single-blind RCT, participants were recruited from the Dutch general population through websites, magazines and local media. Ethical approval was received from the Medical Ethics Committee of the VU University Medical Center (registration number 2016-563, Trial registration: NTR6442) [1]. Participants were randomized into two groups: intervention or waitlist. The research team was blind to treatment allocation. All materials were completed online without researcher intervention. Trial Registration: Nederlands Trial Register http://www.trialregister.nl identifier: NTR6442 (prospectively registered).

2.2. Participants

Participants (18–65 years) who provided written informed consent by email or mail, who scored at least 45.45 on the Acrophobia Questionnaire (AQ)-Anxiety [28,29], had access to an Android smartphone (Android v.5.1 Lollipop or higher, 4.7–5.5 inch screen and gyroscope) were included in the study. Participants with insufficient Dutch language skills, or participants receiving current phobia treatment or psychotropic medication < 3 months were excluded from the study, as well as participants having severe depression (Patient Health Questionnaire [PHQ-9], [30]; total score > 19) or suicidality (Web Screening Questionnaire; WSQ, score ≥ 3; [31]). Enrollment commenced 24 March and ceased 28 September 2017.

2.3. Intervention: ZeroPhobia

ZeroPhobia-Acrophobia consists of six animated and engaging modules using 2D animations which provide background information and explain key concepts (e.g., the fear curve). The annimations are accompanied by an explanatory voice-over and an animated virtual therapist (modelled after the first author) about the nature and origins of the phobia, how to deal with it, setting goals, exercises, getting through difficult moments, cognitive behavioral therapy to deal with negative thoughts and practicing with challenging situations. The modules take between 5 and 40 min to complete. Exposure, the core of the treatment, is realized through gamified mobile VR and four 360° videos covering the entire acrophobia exposure spectrum. Participants started using the VR and the 360° videos from Module 3 onwards and navigated through the virtual environment using gaze control. Gaze control is a method for the hands-free selection of objects and the activation of functions within a virtual environment. By looking at an object or button in the center of the field of view for a specified period of time, e.g., 2 s, the object or button is selected or activated. In ZeroPhobia, large arrows served as interactive buttons used for navigating the virtual environment. By gazing at an arrow, a user moved to the location of the arrow. Similarly, items that needed to be collected, as part of the assignments in the various levels, could be selected by looking at them. The cardboard viewer could be strapped to the head. The VR involved a gamified virtual theater. In the game participants had to complete a series of increasingly challenging tasks (e.g., changing a light bulb on a small ladder, connecting speakers at the edge of the stage, going up a high ladder to repair a small damaged platform, fixing a spotlight on the highest balcony, saving a cat while being on a gangway high above the stage). In each level, participants had to look at assets located on the theatre floor that needed to be collected, hence encouraging them to look down and face their fears [27]. For more details on the VR environments used, see [1,27].

Because any VR setup that generates frame rates below 90 frames per seconds is likely to induce disorientation, nausea and other negative user effects, the frame rate was increased to an optimal level to minimize the risk of cybersickness. Furthermore, there were no quickly moving objects and it was not possible for the user to move quickly through the VR environment. Battery drainage was reduced by keeping the VR levels at an optimum duration meaning that playing a VR level did not exceed 10 min, although participants were at liberty to practice in VR as long as they felt like they needed. Battery drainage was further for small degree lessened indirectly by removing the back cover off the phone, which reduced overheating. The app provides safety instructions to participants before entering the VR environment. For example, participants were instructed to remove all sharp objects in their environment prior to commencing with VR-exposure, to avoid possible injuries. Also, they were instructed to start practicing in VR while seated. Only once anxiety decreased, participants were encouraged to practice standing up. They were also instructed to take off their VR viewer immediately if they felt they might fall.

For the current usage analyses, only information from the interactive VR environment was used, not the 360° videos. This is because the majority of participants were unable to view the 360° videos due to technical limitations of their smartphone (they encountered a black screen). They could, however, view the 360° videos on YouTube. The trial was delivered over a 3-week period during which participants were at liberty to practice with ZeroPhobia as often and as long as they wanted [1]. Weekly standardized motivational e-mails with reminders to start or continue with ZeroPhobia were sent to participants during the intervention period. For details, see [27] and for ZeroPhobia screenshots Figure S1. The VR environment was created with the Unity game engine (version 2017.3.0f3; Unity Technologies, San Francisco, CA, USA).

2.4. Outcomes

All questionnaires were completed online. Measures were taken at baseline (pre-test), immediately after the intervention (posttest), and 3 months after the intervention (follow-up). Participant characteristics measures were collected at baseline, while symptom measures were administered at each time point. All assessments were programmed with Survalyzer software [32]. See [27] for details on outcome measures. The primary outcome was the 20-item Acrophobia Questionnaire (AQ) [28]. The AQ is a widely-used validated instrument [29]. The anxiety subscale is measured using a 7-point Likert scale (0 = not anxious to 6 = extremely anxious). Total score ranges is 0–120. The avoidance subscale uses a 3-point Likert scale ("I would not avoid it" to "I would not do it under any circumstances"). Secondary outcomes included in this study were the Igroup Presence Questionnaire (IPQ); [33] to assess presence in VR, and usage. Because the IPQ is widely used in VR research and to be able to compare results on presence with previous studies, we chose the IPQ instead of other measures targeting presence. Usage data consisted of practice time in VR (for each level [time between entering and exiting the VR level] and in total [the sum of all practice time in VR per patient in minutes]), number of sessions (were one session is defined as repeatedly practicing with the same level) and anxiety ratings directly after practicing a session in the VR environment. As described in [27], participants were encouraged to progress to a more difficult level as soon as self-reported fear dropped below 4 on a 10-point scale. For self-reported fear between 4–7, participants were advised to try the same level again, and for self-reported fear levels 8–10 they were strongly advised to keep practicing the current level. Participants could not continue to the next level without self-reporting fear under 4.

2.5. Usage Data Retrieval

Usage data was retrieved from the ZeroPhobia app to a server which then stored the data on a database, on a secure (SSL) website. All communication between the app and the database was encrypted by means of a certificate. To prevent others (non-participants) from contaminating the database with data, adding new data was only possible by sending the correct key from one of the participants in the study. The data was pseudo-anonymized, meaning that data was anonymized but linked with the trial identifier consisting of four numbers. Examples of database reads are time spent in a VR level, time stamps (start and end time of a participant in the VR environment) that enabled us to exactly determine duration of practice time for each VR level, and experienced anxiety levels after each VR level played.

2.6. Statistical Analyses

Demographic and clinical characteristics are presented in terms of means and SDs. Usage data are presented in terms of means, SDs, and minimum and maximum observations for two groups: (1) all participants and (2) participants who have at least experienced one VR session. The primary outcome (AQ) was replicated using the same imputation methods and covariates as performed in Donker et al. [1], with the exception that the model was not estimated with OLS but instead with Maximum Likelihood Estimation. This estimation method is convenient as it allows parameterization of the treatment effect such that associations with the usage covariates can be directly estimated. Two-sided p-value < 0.05 indicated statistical significance. STATA version 14.2 (StataCorp LP., Texas, TX, USA) were used for the analyses. A data monitoring committee was not required by the Ethics Committee because of the expected low safety risk of the participants.

3. Results

3.1. Sample, Baseline Characteristics and Cybersickness

Details of the participant flow and drop-out are described elsewhere [1,27]. In short, of 663 individuals who signed up for participation, 291 were ineligible (e.g., due to phone ineligibility) and therefore excluded from participation. In total, 193 participants filled in the baseline assessment and were randomly assigned to the VR-CBT app condition (n = 96) or to the wait-list control condition. The pre-treatment attrition rate was 23% in the app condition because of illness (1 [1%]) or an incompatible smartphone (21 [22%]) [1]. Of the total sample (N = 96), the mean age was 41 years (SD = 13.73) and 66 (68.75%) of them were female. Most participants completed postsecondary education (n = 84; 87.5%). The mean AQ baseline score was 85.16 (SD: 18.42). Of the 96 randomized participants, 21 (23%) could not download ZeroPhobia on their smartphone because the smartphones were lacking a gyroscope (required for experiencing VR) and one (1%) did not start ZeroPhobia because of illness, leaving the sample with n = 74 participants.

3.2. General VR Usage Data

Of the 74 participants, 66 participants (68.8%) experienced at least one VR session. Usage data for these 66 participants are shown in Table 1, where the total VR duration time of active users is 24.4 min, with a minimum of 0.6 min (36 s) and a maximum of 71.05 min. On average, active participants practiced with around nine VR sessions. As can be seen, the anxiety ratings of participants are substantially different for practicing with level 1 compared to the highest level they attained (for most participants, this was level 5). The anxiety rating after playing a more difficult level, was on average lower than the anxiety rating after playing level one for the first time. When the anxiety ratings after playing a certain level for the first time were compared with anxiety ratings after playing a certain level for the last time (e.g., the anxiety rating after having played level 4 for the last time as compared to playing level 4 for the first time), we noted that anxiety was reduced by around 1.3 points on average (range: 1–10).

Table 1. Overall descriptive Statistics of Usage Data for Users who Experienced at least one VR session.

Variable	N	Mean	SD	Min	Max
Total					
Duration (total VR time in minutes)	66	24.384	16.127	0.600	71.050
Anxiety rating after playing level 1 [1]	66	3.545	2.288	1.000	10.000
Anxiety rating of highest attained level [2]	66	3.227	1.830	1.000	9.000
Anxiety rating after playing level first time [3]	66	4.576	2.308	1.000	10.000
Anxiety rating after playing level last time [4]	66	3.227	1.830	1.000	9.000
Number of VR sessions	66	9.167	5.365	2.000	25.000
Women					
Duration (total VR time in minutes) [1]	47	23.516	15.744	0.600	58.967
Anxiety rating after playing level 1 [2]	47	3.894	2.343	1.000	10.000
Anxiety rating of highest attained level [3]	47	3.149	1.818	1.000	9.000
Anxiety rating after playing level first time [4]	47	4.596	2.242	1.000	10.000
Anxiety rating after playing level last time [5]	47	3.149	1.818	1.000	9.000
Number of VR sessions	47	9.085	5.344	2.000	24.000
Men					
Duration (total VR time in minutes)	19	26.532	17.289	3.517	71.050
Anxiety rating after playing level 1 [2]	19	2.684	1.945	1.000	7.000
Anxiety rating of highest attained level [3]	19	3.421	1.895	1.000	9.000
Anxiety rating after playing level first time [4]	19	4.526	2.525	2.000	10.000
Anxiety rating after playing level last time [5]	19	3.421	1.895	1.000	9.000
Number of VR sessions	19	9.368	5.560	3.000	25.000

[1] Grubbs test was conducted to test for outliers and confirmed the apparent absence of outliers. Please see Figure S2 for details on the variation in practicing duration. [2] anxiety rating after playing level 1 (the easiest level: changing a light bulb on a small ladder) for the first time. [3] anxiety rating after playing the highest level (for that person) for the last time, which is level 5 for most participants (range: 1–10). [4] anxiety rating after playing a level for the first time [5] anxiety rating after playing a level for the last time (range: 1–10).

A paired *t*-test indicated that this difference was statistically significant (t (280) = 12.28, $p < 0.0001$) (see Table 2).

Table 2. Level-specific Statistics of Usage Data for Users who Experienced at least one VR session.

Variable	N	Mean	SD	Min	Max
LEVEL 1					
Time spent in level (minutes) [1]	65	2.289	2.109	0.317	11.483
Initial anxiety [2]	65	3.554	2.305	1	10
Final anxiety [3]	65	2.092	0.861	1	5
Number of sessions in level [4]	65	2.046	1.556	1	8
LEVEL2					
Time spent in level (minutes)	62	5.322	5.334	0.283	36.350
Initial anxiety	62	4.129	2.229	1	10
Final anxiety	62	2.645	1.527	1	10
Number of sessions in level	62	2.177	1.337	1	6
LEVEL 3					
Time spent in level (minutes)	57	7.768	5.222	0.967	23.367
Initial anxiety	57	5.070	2.638	1	10
Final anxiety	57	2.877	1.489	1	9
Number of sessions in level	57	2.281	1.278	1	7
LEVEL 4					
Time spent in level (minutes)	50	6.742	5.639	1.100	29.517
Initial anxiety	50	4.700	2.517	1	10
Final anxiety	50	2.940	1.096	1	7
Number of sessions in level	50	2.260	1.724	1	11

Table 2. *Cont.*

Variable	N	Mean	SD	Min	Max
LEVEL 5					
Time spent in level (minutes)	47	7.463	4.678	1.5	19.883
Initial anxiety	47	4.213	2.010	1	9
Final anxiety	47	2.872	1.035	1	7
Number of sessions in level	47	2.000	1.351	1	8
TOTAL					
Time spent in level (minutes)	281	5.727	5.114	0.283	36.350
Initial anxiety	281	4.302	2.397	1	10
Final anxiety	281	2.655	1.270	1	10
Number of sessions in level	281	2.153	1.450	1	11

[1] Total time spent in this level, in minutes. [2] Self-reported anxiety after playing this level for the first time (range: 1–10). Self-reported anxiety after playing this level for the last time (range: 1–10).[4] Number of sessions spent in this level.

3.3. Level-Specific Usage Data

As can be seen in the level-specific usage results in Table 2, the self-reported anxiety of users was, on average, relatively low (M = 4.302, SD = 2.397) when finishing levels for the first time (initial anxiety). The final anxiety numbers show that on average, users exited a level with a self-reported anxiety level of 2.665 (SD = 1.270). This shows that most users complied well with the advice to 'level up' after self-reported anxiety had dropped below 3, however some users chose to replay a level up to 11 times (level 4).

3.4. Replication of Main Results

An intent-to-treat analysis showed a significant reduction of acrophobia symptoms at post-test at 3 months for ZeroPhobia compared with the controls ($b = -26.73$ [95%CI, −32.12 to −21.34]; $p < 0.001$; $d = 1.14$ [95%CI, 0.84 to 1.44]). Using the ML-estimation procedure, similar results for ZeroPhobia effectiveness were found compared to original study (b(SE) = −26.7 (2.73), noting a slight difference in standard error due to using a ML-estimation rather than an ordinary least squares approach as in [1].

3.5. Hypothesis 1: More VR Activity Is Associated With Lower Post-Test AQ Scores

To test the hypothesis that more VR activity is associated with a greater reduction in AQ scores at post-test, we modelled the post-test scores of the AQ with the pre-test scores on the AQ, the number of sessions played and a linear and quadratic parameter of practice time in minutes. The results show that practice time and the number of sessions result in lower post-test AQ scores, although number of sessions is not statistically significant. Post-test AQ scores depends quadratically on time spent practicing (Practice Time: b(SE) = −1.07(0.391); $p < 0.05$; PT^2: b(SE) = 0.018(0.005); $p < 0.05$). The association with number of sessions was not statistically significant. To test for robustness, this analysis was performed with and without baseline covariates in the model, but results did not change significantly. With respect to the estimated association between the number of sessions and Post-test AQ scores, we note that the inclusion of background characteristics does not change the estimated coefficient, but it does make the association insignificant. The insignificant result may be the result of lack of statistical power.

In Figure 1 the association between decrease in AQ scores and practice time and number of sessions is represented graphically, where darker areas denote a greater reduction in AQ scores at post-test. These results suggest the existence of a 'sweet spot', an optimum level of exposure at which increasing practice time does not result in an increased benefit and that it does not significantly depend on the number of sessions. The optimum level of practice time in the VR environment was found to be 25.5 min.

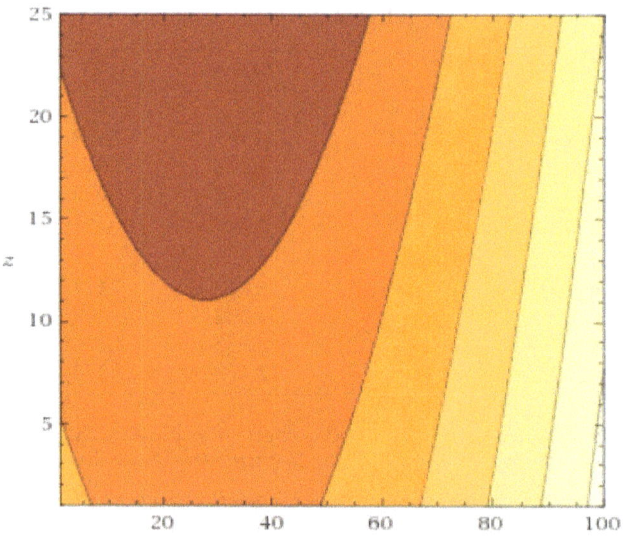

Figure 1. Practice Time (x-axis) vs. Number of Sessions (z-axis). Figure 1 visualizes the estimated function $AQ\_Total\_Post = -1.02x + 0.02x^2 - 1.17z - 12.85$ and plots a contour plot for $x = 1$ *to* 100 and $z = 1$ *to* 25. It thus represents a contour plot in which the outcome differences for the observed combinations of practice time (x-axis) and number of sessions (z-axis). The darker the color, the larger the outcome difference.

3.6. Hypothesis 2: A Higher Level of Presence Is Associated with Greater Decrease in Post-Session Anxiety

To test this hypothesis, we tested the association between the IPQ scores post-test and the treatment effect while controlling for baseline covariates. We also controlled for practice time, and pre-test AQ scores, as this would be associated with treatment effect. Because not all participants filled in the IPQ at post-test (12/66 missing, 21.2%), this variable was also modeled.

The results showed that those who filled out the IPQ, a higher level of presence was associated with a larger reduction of AQ scores post-test b(SE) = −0.914 (0.225), $p < 0.001$, confirming our hypothesis. The addition of the IPQ variable to the model did not change the parameter for the AQ pre-test scores, indicating that presence is not associated with pre-test AQ scores. The practice time coefficient did change after the introduction of presence into the model, indicating that presence and practice time covary, which is evidenced by the high correlation between presence and linear and quadratic play time ($r = 0.599$ and $r = 0.481$ respectively).

3.7. Hypothesis 3: Associations between Scores

We hypothesized that the AQ pre-test scores were significantly associated with VR anxiety ratings after the first session. Moreover, we hypothesized that the AQ pre-test scores would be significantly associated with a reduction in acrophobia symptoms, but not with VR exercise time. The results showed that the pre-test AQ scores were significantly associated with the subjective fear rating after the first session (r = 0.134, p <0.05) and a reduction in AQ scores at post-test (r = −0.312, $p < 0.05$). However, contrary to our hypothesis, AQ pre-test scores were not associated with either linear practice time (r = 0.006, p >0.05) or quadratic practice time (r = −0.003, $p > 0.05$).

3.8. Hypothesis 4: Repeated Activity in a VR Level Leads to a Consistent Decrease in Post-Level Anxiety

We hypothesized that, consistent with general expectations about exposure therapy, self-reported fear would show consistently lower scores after a session when compared to before a level, since repeated exposure should result in lower fear levels after a session. As can be seen in Table 3, this is the case for each level, with an average drop of 1.35 points (SD 2.24) per level. As seen in the minimum and maximum scores, some participants exit levels with higher fear ratings than they started with, indicating unsuccessful exposure exercises.

Table 3. Mean decrease in self-reported fear after completing each session.

Variable	N	Mean	SD	Min	Max
Level 1	4	−3.500	3.873	−9	0
Level 1–2	6	−0.833	2.562	−6	1
Level 1–3	6	−0.167	2.562	−4	4
Level 1–4	11	−1.545	2.911	−6	4
Level 1–5	39	−1.333	1.644	−6	0
TOTAL	66	−1.345	2.243	−9	4

4. Discussion

To our knowledge, this is the first study to look at self-guided VR exposure on a session-to-session basis. As self-guided exposure relies strongly on the participant to guide the progress through increasingly more challenging sessions, the inter-session data provides relevant information to guide future development of similar interventions. Moreover, successful exposure therapy relies on adequately modulating how challenging the different sessions are. This makes it important to verify that successful exposure took place within a session—as witnessed by a decreased anxiety level after a session as compared to before a session—in the absence of a therapist to guide this. Consistent with expectations from exposure therapy, the results indicate that overall, participants reported a decrease in fear as they progressed through the levels. It should be noted, however, that for some participants the exit scores remained relatively high, indicating unsuccessful exposure. The results further demonstrated that post-test AQ scores depended quadratically on time spent practicing, but not with the number of sessions practiced, indicating that it might be more important to play one level for a longer period of time instead of practicing many VR levels. Moreover, it was shown that, in line with previous research, a higher presence was associated with better outcomes [23].

Most participants advanced through all five of the VR exposure levels, indicating that—even in the absence of a therapist—self-guided VR therapy in the home setting is feasible and can be effective, even with rudimentary equipment such as a cardboard VR viewer and the participants' own smartphones. Importantly, the relatively high number of participants who completed all levels shows that the app was engaging and convincing enough to persuade participants to keep practicing. This motivational aspect is reflected by the number of sessions participants practiced, where on average participants tried each level at least twice, and in some cases up to 11 times. One explanation is that the threshold set for going to a subsequent level through levels (a self-reported fear of less than 4) added an element of challenge to the exposure, motivating participants to keep trying a level to unlock the next [34]. However, evidence for the success of gamification in smartphone apps is currently lacking [35].

Although existing VR interventions have been envisaged as solutions to be used in guided form under the supervision of a therapist (see e.g., [24]), ZeroPhobia was designed as a fully self-guided intervention with no therapist oversight. Therefore, it was crucial to monitor participant progression to verify whether successful in-virtuo exposure was taking place. When practicing with exposure exercises, it is important to correctly pace the increase in difficulty and challenge. Progressing too quickly through levels could result in excessive anxiety, leading to dropout, while practicing at an easy level for too long is inefficient and may lead the participant to disengage because it is not challenging enough. In ZeroPhobia it seems that these decisions were in line with the recommendations on pacing progress through the levels as shown in the app. In Table 2 it is shown that the average final anxiety scores in the levels were all below 4, since participants could not progress unless their self-reported fear had dropped under 4. This is visible in the self-reported fear levels after practicing a level for the first time. These averages also show that participants tended to 'level up', and not unhelpfully linger in levels. As most participants progressed to the highest level of the VR exposure game (level 5), it was not possible to find a reliable cut-off value for number of levels that should be completed, or to find a level that should minimally be attained for deriving clinical benefit; but the corollary is that participants chose to persist with the exposure exercises until the end, indicating successful and perhaps even enjoyable exposure experiences. However, we did find that increased activity was related to lower AQ scores at post-test. Results also demonstrated an association between decrease in AQ scores and practice time and number of sessions, suggesting the existence of a 'sweet spot', an optimum level of exposure at which increasing practice time does not result in increased benefit. In this study we found that participants derive most benefit when the practice time in the VR environment is 25.5 min irrespective of the amount of VR sessions. However, these results need to be interpreted with caution because it is unknown how many participants practiced for how long with the 360 videos.

The results showed that the pre-test AQ scores were significantly associated with the subjective fear rating after the first session and a reduction in AQ scores at post-test. This would suggest that those with higher acrophobia symptoms could derive more benefit from the VR exposure. This is also in line with previous research findings [11]. It could however also be a floor effect, where participants with already relatively low acrophobia symptoms have relatively little to gain from the intervention. Regardless, the results show that the VR environment offers a safe and engaging way to self-guided exposure, even for those with more severe complaints.

Limitations

The current study had several limitations. Firstly, all the hypotheses in this study were exploratory in nature, leading to the possibility of false positive findings. Secondly, more granular data in terms of logins and time spent in app modules would have been helpful for a more detailed view of user activity within the VR sessions. Thirdly, we did not have access to usage data of the 360 videos from YouTube. This means that several participants have practiced with 360° video exposure which could also contribute to a decrease in anxiety ratings at post-test. The optimum level of exposure time is a conservative estimate therefore. Fourthly, we did not systematically conduct data on the performance of the cardboard VR viewer during the sessions, therefore we are unable to evaluate the interaction of the performance of the VR viewer on its usage and effectiveness. However, only one participant contacted the research team to request a new viewer because the one originally provided to them had broken. Fifthly, due to a small sample size, some insignificant result may be the result of lack of statistical power. The great inter-subject variability in usage is remarkable. It might be that, depending on the personal history, VR stimulation will work at one moment of exposure, without a tool to identify the triggering event, conditioning success of fear reduction. Sixthly, data quality can be a problem in an uncontrolled environment, when only relying on self-report measures and no biological measures. However, research has demonstrated that self-report measures can have good to excellent validity when compared to a diagnostic interview [36]. Furthermore, participants can be more honest with filling in the questionnaires, as the computer has no 'eyebrows' [37]. Moreover, in a meta-analysis targeting VR interventions, Morina et al. [9] concluded that the behavioural measurement effect sizes were similar to those calculated from self-report measures in the VR studies, indicating no differences between the two types of measurements. Furthermore, we have conducted robustness analysis which confirmed that the VR-CBT ZeroPhobia app had a strong impact on the anxiety for heights, even when analyzed very conservatively in a randomized controlled design, and that the general anxiety effect did not drive the results. Lastly, as yet we have no data on external validity, especially on whether the effects of the VR exposure translate to decreased acrophobia and acrophobic avoidance in real-world settings, and commensurate increases in quality of life.

Future research is needed to replicate the main results of the study, especially with regard to external validity and translational effects in real life. Furthermore, more granular data on, e.g., eye gaze could generate valuable information on which cues participants choose to engage with, as even in VR participants can choose to look away from the fear-inducing stimulus. It would also be interesting to investigate whether adding sound to the VR experience effects the feeling of presence.

5. Conclusions

In sum, our findings show that self-guided VR for acrophobia symptoms is feasible, effective, and follows the same general patterns in terms of self-reported fear reductions as one would expect from therapist-guided exposure exercise. The results indicate that participants were engaged with ZeroPhobia as can be seen by the majority of them advancing through all VR exposure levels. Overall, fear levels decreased when participants progressed through the levels. Furthermore, our results suggest that it might be more beneficial to play one level for a longer period of time instead of practicing many VR levels and the existence of a 'sweet spot', an optimum level of exposure at which increasing practice time does not result in increased benefit. In this study we found that participants derive most benefit when the practice time in the VR environment is 25.5 min irrespective of the amount of VR sessions. Finally, the importance of feeling present in the VR environment is stressed out as a higher reported presence was associated with better outcomes. Further research is needed to see if the gains from VR translate into long-term sustained results, both in virtual and in real-life situations.

Author Contributions: T.D. conceptualized the study, conceived the study, designed the study, contributed to survey design and data collection and wrote the manuscript. C.v.K. and I.C. performed the data analysis, wrote the method and result section and critically revised the manuscript. R.N.K. interpreted and drafted the results and discussion section and critically revised the manuscript. J.-L.v.G. contributed to the concept and design of the study and provided administrative, technical and material support and critically revised the manuscript. All authors contributed toward drafting and critically revising the paper, gave final approval of the version to be published, and agreed to be accountable for all aspects of the work. All authors have read and agreed to the published version of the manuscript.

Acknowledgments: The authors extend their gratitude to all the participants of the study, Bruno de Vos for designing ZeroPhobia, Doruk Eker for programming ZeroPhobia, Rufus van Baardwijk for ZeroPhobia sound, and Stefanie van Esveld and Niclas Fischer for assistance in data recruitment and data collection.

References

1. Donker, T.; Cornelisz, I.; van Klaveren, C.; van Straten, A.; Carlbring, P.; Cuijpers, P.; van Gelder, J.L. Effectiveness of self-guided app-based virtual reality cognitive behavior therapy for acrophobia: A randomized clinical trial. *JAMA Psychiatry* **2019**, *76*, 682–690. [CrossRef] [PubMed]
2. Fairburn, C.G.; Patel, V. The impact of digital technology on psychological treatments and their dissemination. *Behav. Res. Ther.* **2017**, *88*, 19–25. [CrossRef] [PubMed]
3. Andersson, G.; Carlbring, P.; Titov, N.; Lindefors, N. Internet interventions for adults with anxiety and mood disorders: A narrative umbrella review of recent meta-analyses. *Can. J. Psychiatry* **2019**. [CrossRef] [PubMed]
4. Andersson, G.; Cuijpers, P.; Carlbring, P.; Riper, H.; Hedman, E. Guided Internet-based vs. face-to-face cognitive behavior therapy for psychiatric and somatic disorders: A systematic review and meta-analysis. *World Psychiatry* **2014**, *13*, 288–295. [CrossRef] [PubMed]
5. Berger, T.; Boettcher, J.; Caspar, F. Internet-based guided self-help for several anxiety disorders: A randomized controlled trial comparing a tailored with a standardized disorder-specific approach. *Psychother. Chic.* **2014**, *51*, 207–219. [CrossRef] [PubMed]
6. Fodor, L.A.; Coteț, C.D.; Cuijpers, P.; Szamoskozi, S.; David, D.; Cristea, I.A. The effectiveness of virtual reality based interventions for symptoms of anxiety and depression: A meta-analysis. *Sci. Rep.* **2018**, *8*, 10323. [CrossRef] [PubMed]
7. Carl, E.; Stein, A.T.; Levihn-Coon, A.; Pogue, J.R.; Rothbaum, B.; Emmelkamp, P.; Asmundson, G.J.G.; Carlbring, P.; Powers, M.B. Virtual reality exposure therapy for anxiety and related disorders: A meta-analysis of randomized controlled trials. *J. Anxiety Disord.* **2019**, *61*, 27–36. [CrossRef]
8. Opris, D.; Pintea, S.; Garcia-Palacios, A.; Botella, C.; Szamoskozi, S.; David, D. Virtual reality exposure therapy in anxiety disorders: A quantitative meta-analysis. *Depress Anxiety* **2012**, *29*, 85–93. [CrossRef]
9. Morina, N.; Ijntema, H.; Meyerbröker, K.; Emmelkamp, P.M.G. Can virtual reality exposure therapy gains be generalized to real-life? A meta-analysis of studies applying behavioral assessments. *Behav. Res. Ther.* **2015**, *74*, 18–24. [CrossRef]

10. Parsons, T.D.; Rizzo, A.A. Affective outcomes of virtual reality exposure therapy for anxiety and specific phobias: A meta-analysis. *J. Behav. Ther. Exp. Psychiatry* **2008**, *39*, 250–261. [CrossRef]
11. Hong, Y.J.; Kim, H.E.; Jung, Y.H.; Kveong, S.; Kim, J.J. Usefulness of the mobile virtual reality self-training for overcoming a fear of heights. *Cyberpsychol. Behav. Soc. Netw.* **2017**, *20*, 753–761. [CrossRef] [PubMed]
12. van den Berg, S.W.; Peters, E.J.; Kraaijeveld, J.F.; Gielissen, M.F.; Prins, J.B. Usage of a generic web-based self-management intervention for breast cancer survivors: Substudy analysis of the BREATH trial. *J. Med. Internet Res.* **2013**, *15*, e170. [CrossRef] [PubMed]
13. Ritterband, L.M.; Thorndike, F.P.; Cox, D.J.; Kovatchev, B.P.; Gonder-Frederick, L.A. A behavior change model for internet interventions. *Ann. Behav. Med.* **2009**, *38*, 18–27. [CrossRef] [PubMed]
14. Sieverink, F.; Kelders, S.; Akkersdijk, S.; Poel, M.; Siemons, L.; van Gemert-Pijnen, L. Work in Progress: A Protocol for the Collection, Analysis, and Interpretation of Log Data from eHealth Technology. In Proceedings of the Fourth International Workshop on Behavior Change Support Systems (BCSS 2016), Salzburg, Austria, 5–7 April 2016; pp. 56–60.
15. Donkin, L.; Christensen, H.; Naismith, S.L.; Neal, B.; Hickie, I.B.; Glozier, N. A systematic review of the impact of adherence on the effectiveness of e-therapies. *J. Med. Internet Res.* **2011**, *13*, e52. [CrossRef]
16. Donkin, L.; Hickie, I.B.; Christensen, H.; Naismith, S.L.; Neal, B.; Cockayne, N.L.; Glozier, N. Rethinking the dose-response relationship between usage and outcome in an online intervention for depression: Randomized controlled trial. *J. Med. Internet. Res.* **2013**, *15*, e231. [CrossRef]
17. Van Gemert-Pijnen, J.E.; Kelders, S.M.; Bohlmeijer, E.T. Understanding the usage of content in a mental health intervention for depression: An analysis of log data. *J. Med. Internet. Res.* **2014**, *16*, e27. [CrossRef]
18. Manwaring, J.L.; Bryson, S.W.; Goldschmidt, A.B.; Winzelberg, A.J.; Luce, K.H.; Cunning, D.; Wilfley, D.E.; Taylor, C.B. Do adherence variables predict outcome in an online program for the prevention of eating disorders? *J. Consult. Clin. Psychol.* **2008**, *76*, 341–346. [CrossRef]
19. Cobb, N.K.; Graham, A.L.; Bock, B.C.; Papandonatos, G.; Abrams, D.B. Initial evaluation of a real-world internet smoking cessation system. *Nicotine Tob. Res.* **2005**, *7*, 207–216. [CrossRef]
20. Welding, K.; De Leon, E.; Cha, S.; Johnson, M.; Cohen, J.E.; Graham, A.L. Weekly enrollment and usage patterns in an Internet smoking cessation intervention. *Internet Interv.* **2017**, *9*, 100–105. [CrossRef]
21. Kelders, S.M.; Bohlmeijer, E.T.; Van Gemert-Pijnen, J.E. Participants, usage, and use patterns of a web-based intervention for the prevention of depression within a randomized controlled trial. *J. Med. Internet Res.* **2013**, *15*, e172. [CrossRef]
22. Bossen, D.; Buskermolen, M.; Veenhof, C.; de Bakker, D.; Dekker, J. Adherence to a web-based physical activity intervention for patients with knee and/or hip osteoarthritis: A mixed method study. *J. Med. Internet Res.* **2013**, *15*, e223. [CrossRef] [PubMed]
23. Gromer, D.; Reinke, M.; Christner, I.; Pauli, P. Causal interactive links between presence and fear in virtual reality height exposure. *Front. Psychol.* **2019**, *10*, 141. [CrossRef] [PubMed]
24. Wiederhold, B.K.; Bouchard, S. *Advances in Virtual Reality and Anxiety Disorders*; Springer: Boston, MA, USA, 2014; ISBN 978-1-4899-8022-9.
25. Lindner, P.; Miloff, A.; Hamilton, W.; Carlbring, P. The potential of consumer-targeted virtual reality relaxation applications: Descriptive usage, uptake and application performance statistics for a first-generation application. *Front. Psychol.* **2019**, *10*, 132. [CrossRef]
26. Beck, A.T.; Rush, A.J.; Shaw, B.F.; Emery, G. *Cognitive Therapy of Depression*; Guilford Press: New York, NY, USA, 1979.
27. Donker, T.; Van Esveld, S.; Fischer, N.; Van Straten, A. 0Phobia—Towards a virtual cure for acrophobia: Study protocol for a randomized controlled trial. *Trials* **2018**, *19*, 433. [CrossRef] [PubMed]
28. Cohen, D.C. Comparison of self-report and overt-behavioral procedures for assessing acrophobia. *Behav. Ther.* **1977**, *8*, 17–23. [CrossRef]
29. Steinman, S.A.; Teachman, B.A. Cognitive processing and acrophobia: Validating the Heights Interpretation Questionnaire. *J. Anxiety Disord.* **2011**, *25*, 896–902. [CrossRef]
30. Kroenke, K.; Spitzer, R.L.; Williams, J.B.W. The PHQ-9. *J. Gen. Intern. Med.* **2001**, *16*, 606–613. [CrossRef]
31. Donker, T.; van Straten, A.; Marks, I.M.; Cuijpers, P. A Brief web-based screening questionnaire for common mental disorders: Development and validation. *J. Med. Internet Res.* **2009**, *11*, e19. [CrossRef]
32. Survalyzer Nederland, B.V. Home. Available online: https://www.survalyzer.com/ (accessed on 2 July 2019).

33. Schubert, T.; Friedmann, F.; Regenbrecht, H. The experience of presence: Factor analytic insights. *Presence Teleoper. Virtual Environ.* **2001**, *10*, 266–281. [CrossRef]
34. King, D.; Greaves, F.; Exeter, C.; Darzi, A. "Gamification": Influencing health behaviours with games. *J. R. Soc. Med.* **2013**, *106*, 76–78. [CrossRef]
35. Edwards, E.A.; Lumsden, J.; Rivas, C.; Steed, L.; Edwards, L.A.; Thiyagarajan, A.; Sohanpal, R.; Caton, H.; Griffiths, C.J.; Munafò, M.R.; et al. Gamification for health promotion: Systematic review of behaviour change techniques in smartphone apps. *BMJ Open* **2016**, *6*, e012447. [CrossRef] [PubMed]
36. Evans, M.; Kessler, D.; Lewis, G.; Peters, T.J.; Sharp, D. Assessing mental health in primary care research using standardized scales: Can it be carried out over the telephone? *Psychol. Med.* **2004**, *23*, 157–162. [CrossRef] [PubMed]
37. Marks, I.M.; Cavanagh, K.; Gega, L. Computer-aided psychotherapy: Revolution or bubble? *Br. J. Psychiatry* **2007**, *191*, 471–473. [CrossRef] [PubMed]

UnReal? Investigating the Sense of Reality and Psychotic Symptoms with Virtual Reality

Gad Drori [1,*], Paz Bar-Tal [1], Yonatan Stern [1,2], Yair Zvilichovsky [1] and Roy Salomon [1]

[1] Gonda Brain Research Center, Bar-Ilan University, Ramat Gan 5290002, Israel; bartalpaz@gmail.com (P.B.-T.); yoniastern@gmail.com (Y.S.); zvilich@gmail.com (Y.Z.); roy.salomon@biu.ac.il (R.S.)
[2] Psychology Department, University of Haifa, Haifa 3498838, Israel
[*] Correspondence: gadidrori@gmail.com

Abstract: Distortions of reality, such as hallucinations, are common symptoms of many psychiatric conditions. Accordingly, sense of reality (SoR), the ability to discriminate between true and false perceptions, is a central criterion in the assessment of neurological and psychiatric health. Despite the critical role of the SoR in daily life, little is known about how this is formed in the mind. Here, we propose a novel theoretical and methodological framework to study the SoR and its relation to psychotic symptoms. In two experiments, we employed a specialized immersive virtual reality (VR) environment allowing for well-controlled manipulations of visual reality. We first tested the impact of manipulating visual reality on objective perceptual thresholds (just noticeable differences). In a second experiment, we tested how these manipulations affected subjective judgments of reality. The results revealed that the objective perceptual thresholds were robust and replicable, demonstrating that SoR is a stable psychometric property that can be measured experimentally. Furthermore, reality alterations reduced subjective reality judgments across all manipulated visual aspects. Finally, reduced sensitivity to changes in visual reality was related to self-reported prodromal psychotic symptoms. These results provide evidence for the relevance of SoR in the assessment of psychosis and other mental disorders in which reality is distorted.

Keywords: sense of reality; virtual reality; hallucinations; psychosis; derealization

1. Introduction

1.1. Sense of Reality

We normally and intuitively trust our sensory representation of the world to closely correspond to what "is really there" [1,2]. We term this correspondence "reality", and differentiate it from other states in which our representations of the world do not match the environment, such as dreaming and hallucinations. Intriguingly, we seem to possess a capacity to judge whether our sensory experience corresponds to the world or not, i.e., a sense of reality (SoR). This capacity is a critical aspect of the human mind, allowing us to guide our actions based on meaningful sensory signals. Abnormal SoR processing may lead to a disparity between experience and reality, resulting in hallucinations (false perceptions), which is a core symptom of psychosis. However, while SoR is an important criterion in the assessment of neurological and psychiatric health [3–5], we know little regarding its underlying cognitive mechanisms.

Previous work has focused on the mechanisms allowing the separation of internally and externally generated information in memory (i.e., source monitoring) (e.g., [6,7]). Source monitoring paradigms typically evaluate the ability to remember the source of a stimuli (e.g., was this word previously seen or imagined?) (e.g., [8]). This research has been based on the proposition that hallucinations are grounded in failures to discriminate the source of the information correctly (i.e., perception vs. imagery or memory). Thus, while the discrimination of imagery, perception, and memory has been studied extensively (e.g., [5,9,10]), the ability to discriminate between real and false perceptions in real time (i.e., perceptual reality monitoring) is poorly understood. This discrimination is essential as distortions of perceptual reality in the form of hallucinations or illusions originating from neurological, psychiatric, pharmacological, medical, or psychological origins are commonplace [11,12]. Despite the importance of this issue, there is scarce knowledge regarding 'how do we decide what is real?', or in other words, 'how do we form a SoR?'

1.2. A Theoretical Framework of SoR

There is growing evidence that perception is an inferential process [13–15]. For instance, "predictive coding" frameworks suggest that perception arises through a process of inferences (*predictions*) about the likely causes of sensory information (i.e., *likelihood*). These *predictions* are based on previous experience, through which higher levels in the hierarchy attempt to predict the signals arising from the lower levels [14,16,17]. When an unusual sensory event (e.g., a pink elephant) violates predictions, a *prediction error* arises and propagates through the hierarchy until it is either "predicted away" at higher levels (e.g., I'm wearing pink glasses) or the generative model is updated (e.g., pink elephants exist) [15,18]. Perception is thus a process of inference based on our experientially acquired model of the world. Therefore, we suggest that SoR can be viewed as a probabilistic inference based on the magnitude of prediction errors expressing the fit between a given sensory signal and our model of the world [19,20]. For a given sensory event, the magnitude of the prediction error is the probability of the perception being "real" in light of one's model of the world. Thus, viewing a "pink elephant" could be taken as a veridical perception, an optical aberration, or a hallucination, based on one's model of the world.

1.3. Failures of SoR as a Conceptual Framework

Hallucinations (i.e., false perceptions) are a perplexing symptom of many psychiatric and neurological disorders. Advances in neuroscience and computational psychiatry relate hallucinations to breakdowns of predictive processes [20–22]. For example, overreliance on predictions, favoring prior expectations over sensory evidence, may lead to hallucinations [21,23,24]. On the other hand, the overweighting of sensory signals and deficient predictive processes, enabling the structuring of experience, may cause a sense of alienation from one's own actions and thoughts, causing passivity symptoms [25–27].

Intriguingly, hallucinations can be experienced with or without insight into their nature as false perceptions. For example, patients with Charles Bonnet syndrome experience complex hallucinations yet typically identify these as hallucinations [28]. Contrarily, psychotic patients often lose the ability to discern between real and hallucinatory percepts, which has been linked to poorer prognosis [29] and reduced cognitive abilities [30,31]. Thus, psychiatric hallucinations and pseudo-hallucinations include a sensory aspect (i.e., unusual or non-veridical perceptual experience) and a metacognitive aspect related to insight (i.e., assessment of the validity of the perceptual experience). Indeed, depersonalization and derealization syndromes found in several psychiatric conditions produce a sense of "unrealness" in the absence of hallucinations, suggesting a deficit in SoR without the aberrant perceptual experience [32,33]. Thus, failures of the sense of reality leading to hallucinations, depersonalization, and derealization may be driven by either abnormal prediction error signaling impacting bottom-up sensory processing, or top-down predictions affecting the subjective experience of "unrealness", or a combination of these two. Critically, psychosis typically presents both abnormal sensory experiences as well as diminished insight regarding the implausibility of these experiences. These various manifestations of psychopathology highlight the need for a better understanding of the different components of SoR.

1.4. Modeling SoR Using Virtual Reality

SoR was previously challenging to test experimentally as visual manipulations of reality were limited to specific instances, such as prism glasses or still image manipulations (e.g., [34,35]). Here, we developed and tested a novel ecological approach to the study of the SoR, using immersive virtual reality (VR). Virtual reality is now widely employed in scientific studies [36,37] and can be used to manipulate variables that could not otherwise be manipulated (e.g., [38,39]). We created a realistic immersive environment (*UnReal*, Figure 1) in which we can manipulate different visual aspects of reality, creating hallucination like visual stimuli. Importantly, the virtual reality environment allows us to parametrically manipulate such aspects, enabling us to alter reality slightly or massively. For example, we can reduce the height of the participants' first person viewpoint on the world (*shrink* condition) or increase it (*grow* condition), inducing experiences of changes of *self*, which occur in hallucinatory states (e.g., *Alice in Wonderland* syndrome [40]). Furthermore, we can also induce minute changes, which are barely noticeable by the participants, thus resembling derealization-like states.

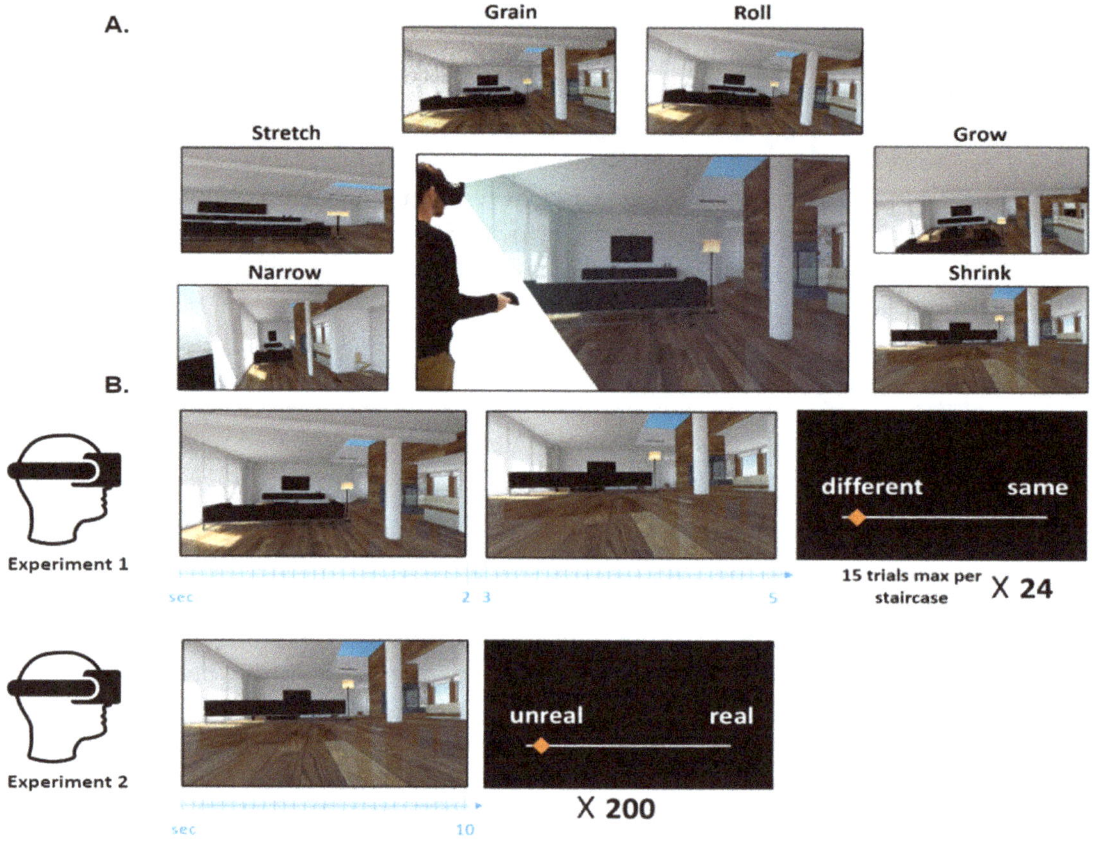

Figure 1. Experimental setup and design. (**A**) Center, illustrative image of the experimental setup and visual scenario. Participants donned a head-mounted display (HMD) and viewed the immersive virtual environment in 360° around them. The images on the sides and bottom represent the six types of alterations of the visual aspects employed, at the highest magnitude of alteration shown, for comparison, on a similar section of the virtual room. (**B**) Trial flow for the experiments. (Top) In Experiment 1, a virtual reality (VR) environment appeared for 2 s, followed by a black screen and then a second VR environment. Subsequently, participants were presented a question screen asking them to report if the two VR environments were identical or not. (Bottom). In Experiment 2, participants viewed a VR environment, which could be altered or unaltered. In each trial, they were required to judge on a continuous scale how 'real' the environment felt to them.

We selected several aspects of reality to be examined in this project, based on the phenomenology of distorted visual reality as found in psychiatric, neurological, medical, and pharmacological states [11,12,41]. These alterations of reality broadly fall into three domains: (1) *Perceptual* changes, in which the visual appearance (e.g., graininess) of the scene is manipulated; (2) laws of *nature*, in which we manipulate the visual aspects of the laws of nature (e.g., stretching of the physical world); and (3) changes of *self*, in which we manipulate the participants' sense of self through conflicts between visual signals and self-related information (e.g., changes in the first person perspective). Alterations of reality in these domains are hallmarks of the phenomenology of hallucinations in psychedelic, neurological, and psychiatric states [42–44].

1.5. The Present Study: Goals and Predictions

We report the results of two experiments investigating SoR and psychotic symptoms using immersive VR. In experiment 1, we tested the objective psychophysical sensitivity of participants to such alterations by measuring the just noticeable differences (JNDs) between altered and unaltered environments and how these are related to self-reported psychosis symptoms. In experiment 2, we tested the impact of these alterations on the subjective experience of participants, by having them make explicit reality judgments. We hypothesized that psychophysical measures of sensory processing (JNDs) would be stable within participants (low within-subject variance), demonstrating that SoR exhibits robust psychometric properties. Furthermore, we examined whether these measures of SoR are correlated to self-reported prodromal psychotic symptoms, especially for manipulations of the self that are known to be linked to schizophrenia spectrum psychosis [25,27,45]. Finally, we hypothesized that alterations of reality would consistently reduce subjective reality judgments, and this decrease will be related to the magnitude of alteration. Thus, by creating hallucination-like sensory experiences in virtual reality, we examined the impact of parametric induction of distortions on objective and subjective measures of SoR.

2. Methods

2.1. Participants

Thirty healthy participants took part in two experiments: Fifteen participated in experiment 1 (10 women, mean age 24.8 years, *SD* = 4.3 years) and 15 in experiment 2 (6 women, mean age 26.6 years, *SD* = 3.8 years). All of them were naïve to the purpose of the experiment, had normal or corrected-to-normal vision, and no self-reported psychiatric or neurological history. All participants gave written informed consent and received payment for their participation (40–50 NIS/~$15 US). The study was performed in accordance with the ethical standards of the Declaration of Helsinki, and the ethics committee of the Gonda Multidisciplinary Brain Research Center approved the experimental protocols.

2.2. Hardware

Both experiments were performed on an Intel core i7 processor and 32 GB of RAM computer running in-house software (*UnReal*, built using Unity 2018.3.2). The participants wore a head-mounted display (HMD-HTC Vive) during the experiment. Motion tracking was performed using the HTC VIVE (1.0) system. Subjects responded using the HTC VIVE touch sensitive controller (all VR hardware was manufactured by Valve Corp., Washington, DC, USA).

2.3. Experimental Design

To test the SoR experimentally, we constructed an immersive virtual environment in which we could experimentally manipulate different aspects of reality in a highly controlled fashion (*UnReal*). Here, we used an indoor variant of the *UnReal* environment modeled as an apartment with a high polygon and realistic appearance. The environment contained numerous objects and furniture as well as an animated cat (see Figure 1A for example). The participants were positioned at the center of the room, and observed the environment in 360° from a stationary point. We used a within-subject design in which all participants in each experiment underwent the same experimental protocol.

2.4. *Virtual Environment*

Unity 2018.3.2 was used to construct an environment that would reflect a normative space. The use of a Polybox's Lounge & Kitchen Pack Asset from Unity Asset Store Environment with real depth and width processing was selected, and additional furniture and accessories were added to make the room realistic. The room's width, length, and height were 13.2, 24.7, and 3.36, respectively, in the Unity unit system. The camera position was ~8.5 from the right wall when the camera was facing the TV, and 11.5 units from the TV itself.

2.5. *Alterations of Reality*

In order to test the impact of altered reality, we took advantage of the possibilities of VR to induce specific and well-controlled alterations of different aspects of visual reality. Specifically, we manipulated three domains of reality using six aspects (Figure 1A). (1) In the perceptual domain, we manipulated: (a) Graininess of the visual display (*grain*), and (b) the degree of the tilt of the virtual space (*roll*); (2) in the laws of nature domain: (c) Stretching and (d) narrowing of the width dimension of the virtual space (*stretch* and *narrow*); and (3) in the self domain: (e) Elevating and (f) lowering the participants' first person perspective (*grow* and *shrink*). As mentioned above, these specific alterations were selected based on the phenomenology of distorted visual reality as found in psychiatric, neurological, medical, and pharmacological states and their applicability within immersive virtual reality (see Supplementary Material and Figure S1 for technical details of the implementation of the alterations).

2.6. *Experiment 1: Psychophysics of Virtually Altered Reality*

2.6.1. Experimental Procedure

To assess SoR, in each trial, participants were successively immersed in two virtual environments (2-s duration each), with a black screen displayed (1-s duration) between them (Figure 1B). Critically, the two environments were identical except that one of the environments included an alteration in one of the aspects of reality mentioned above, whereas the other environment was unaltered. Participants then judged whether the environments were 'different' or 'same' in a classic psychophysics two-alternative forced choice (2AFC) paradigm. We employed a 1-up/ 2-down staircase procedure [46] to derive the JND for each of the aspects of reality. After each response, the alteration level either increased (if the participant judged environments as identical) or decreased (if the participant judged environments as different), by 40% of the current alteration. There were 6 such staircase procedures (one for each condition), which appeared four times each, thus totaling in 24 randomly intermingled staircases each containing only one type of alteration.

Preceding the experimental task, participants were instructed regarding the use of the VR system, the response controllers, as well as the course of the experiment. Then, they performed a training session in which they were acclimated to the VR environment, the experimental task, and response controllers, which lasted until they reported acclimation to the task (26 trials max). To avoid VR motion sickness effects [47], they were instructed to report any discomfort and could stop the experiment at any stage.

2.6.2. Questionnaires

Following task completion, participants completed two self-report questionnaires. The *Cardiff Anomalous Perceptions Scale* (CAPS) and the *Prodromal Questionnaire Brief Version* (PQ-B). The CAPS is a 32-item validated and reliable questionnaire of perceptual anomalies, with subscales of distress, intrusiveness, and frequency of anomalous perceptual experiences [48,49]. The PQ-B primarily serves as an initial screener questionnaire for prodromal or early psychotic symptoms. The PQ-B examines the existence of thoughts and experiences that describe cardinal symptoms of psychosis, such as suspicion, grandiosity, disorganized communication, unconventional thinking, disruptions in perception, difficulties in social functioning, and difficulties in academic or occupational functioning [50,51].

2.7. Experiment 2: Subjective Assessment of Virtually Altered Reality

Experimental Procedure

Experiment 2 examined the effects of altered reality on participants' subjective phenomenological experience of reality. In each trial, participants were placed in the center of the virtual environment and instructed to explore it in 360° degrees while standing in one spot. To ensure exploration, they were instructed to search for a target object (a teddy bear). Each trial lasted 10 s or until participants found the object, after which the room disappeared, and the response screen appeared. Participants provided a subjective rating of how 'real' or 'unreal' the environment felt on a continuous scale of 0–100 (Figure 1B). Each participant performed 200 trials. Sixty trials displayed the environment without alteration, while 140 trials included an alteration of reality in one of the aspects manipulated in experiment 1. Importantly, in each trial, only a single aspect of reality was manipulated. For each aspect of reality, there were four magnitudes of alteration (Supplementary Material Figure S1), which were identical across participants and whose values were based on a pilot study. Each magnitude for each aspect occurred five times, and the order was pseudo-randomized.

Similar to experiment 1, participants were first instructed regarding the use of the VR system, the response controller, and exposed to the environment and equipment until they felt comfortable. Then, they performed a training block of 15 trials, which were excluded from analysis, which included 3 trials with a large change in reality, 2 with mid-level magnitudes of alterations, and 10 with no alterations to practice responses.

2.8. Data Analysis

2.8.1. Experiment 1

Data was processed using in-house Matlab scripts [52]. Statistical analyses were done using JASP 0.11 [53]. To calculate JNDs, for each participant, we averaged the last five trials of each staircase to compute the mean parameter values that the staircase converged on. For each aspect of alteration, these JND values were used to calculate the variance and mean of the JNDs per condition, across the staircase procedures. Conditions with negative numerical scales (e.g., *shrink, narrow*) were converted to absolute values so that all JNDs represented the absolute distance from zero (i.e., from the unaltered condition). It should be noted that comparison across aspect ratings in both experiments was meaningful only for pairs of aspects that shared a similar scale. Therefore, *grow* and *shrink* JNDs were compared using a paired t-test and null effects were assessed using the Bayesian paired t-test, while the remaining aspects could not be directly compared. The within-subject variance of the JNDs in each aspect was calculated across the four staircases. The rate of convergence for each aspect was calculated by averaging the number of steps it took in each staircase until convergence. Pearson's r was used to test for correlations between JNDs across the different aspects. Spearman's Rho was used to test for correlations between JNDs and the CAPS and PQ-B questionnaires.

2.8.2. Experiment 2

The subjective ratings of reality in experiment 2 were averaged across participants for each magnitude of manipulation and each aspect separately. These mean values were then used for observing the change in reality ratings across ascending levels of reality manipulations in a repeated measures ANOVA (where normality was violated, a non-parametric Friedman test was performed and Greenhouse–Geisser corrections were applied when required). Pearson's r was used to test for correlations between subjective ratings of reality across aspects. Where possible, we compared subjective judgments using a paired t-test on the difference between the *real* and first level of alteration (which corresponded to the largest reduction in subjective judgements).

3. Results

3.1. Experiment 1

The average JNDs and their within-subject variance can be seen in Table 1 (see Table S3 for full descriptive statistics).

Table 1. Descriptive statistics for experiment 1.

	JND					
	Narrow	**Stretch**	**Shrink**	**Grow**	**Roll**	**Grain**
Mean	0.09	0.12	0.04	0.05	2.57	0.01
Std. Deviation	0.06	0.06	0.03	0.03	2.37	0.05
Minimum	0.04	0.07	0.01	0.01	0.31	0.03
Maximum	0.24	0.29	0.12	0.12	9.5	0.19
	Within-Subject Variability					
	Narrow	**Stretch**	**Shrink**	**Grow**	**Roll**	**Grain**
Mean	0.003	0.004	0.001	8.0e -4	0.93	0.002
Std. Deviation	0.003	0.009	0.002	0.002	1.05	0.003
Minimum	0	0	0	0	0.003	0
Maximum	0.008	0.04	0.007	0.006	3.92	0.01
	Convergence Rate					
	Narrow	**Stretch**	**Shrink**	**Grow**	**Roll**	**Grain**
Mean	5.99	8.73	7.03	6.57	5.74	6.76
Std. Deviation	1.47	0.91	1.6	1.98	2.23	1.76
Minimum	3	7	4	3	1	4
Maximum	9	10	9.5	9.75	10	10

Overall, participants showed very stable JNDs with little within-subject variability. For example, the average JND for *narrow* was ($M = 0.09$) and the average within-subject variability was ($SD^2 = 0.003$). In *stretch*, the average JND was ($M = 0.12$) and the average within-subject variance was ($SD^2 = 0.004$). The exception to this low variance was *roll*, which showed larger variance: ($M = 2.57$, $SD^2 = 0.93$). Thus, the average variability of the JNDs for all but one condition was approximately ~2.5% of the mean JND (8.2% including *roll*). This demonstrates the visual sensitivity to changes across different aspects of reality alteration and their relative consistency within participants. The *roll* condition showed greater within-subject (and between-subject) variability. We suspect this may have occurred due to some participants' compensating for the visual manipulation of *roll* by tilting their heads in the opposite direction. In addition to the consistency of the JNDs themselves, the number of trial steps needed for the staircase procedure to converge was also similar across aspects. Convergence rates ranged from 5.7 to 8.7 (trial steps) across conditions. For instance, the average *grow* and *grain* convergence rates were ($M = 6.5$, $SD = 1.98$; $M = 6.7$, $SD = 1.76$), respectively. The average convergence rate across all aspects was ($M = 6.8$, $SD = 1.05$), indicating that our staircase procedure was effective at uncovering perceptual thresholds across conditions (see Figure 2A,B. for examples of convergence rates for *grow* and *grain* and Table 1 for all conditions). Combined, the measure of within-subject variability along with the consistent convergence rate of the staircase procedures implies that perceptual thresholds of SoR exhibit stable psychometric properties that can be measured experimentally.

Examining the correlations between JNDs across the different aspects (see the correlation matrix in Figure 2D and the example correlation in Figure 2E), they exhibited high, positive, and significant correlations ranging from 0.22 to 0.95 ($M = 0.61$, $SD = 0.25$). Thus, participants with high sensitivity in one aspect were also likely to be sensitive in another aspect and vice versa. An outlier to this pattern was the *grain* aspect, which showed low levels of correlations with all other aspects ($M = 0.31$, $SD = 0.05$). Next, directly comparing JNDs for the *grow* and *shrink* aspects, which share a common parameter scale (see Figure 2C), a paired t-test revealed no significant difference between the two ($M_{Grow} = 0.05$, $SD_{Grow} = 0.03$; $M_{Shrink} = 0.04$, $SD_{Shrink} = 0.03$, $t(14) = -0.66$, $p = 0.51$, $Cohen's\ d = -0.17$). Bayesian analysis provided moderate evidence ($BF_{10} = 0.31$) for there being no difference in the perceptual sensitivity for vertical changes in both directions.

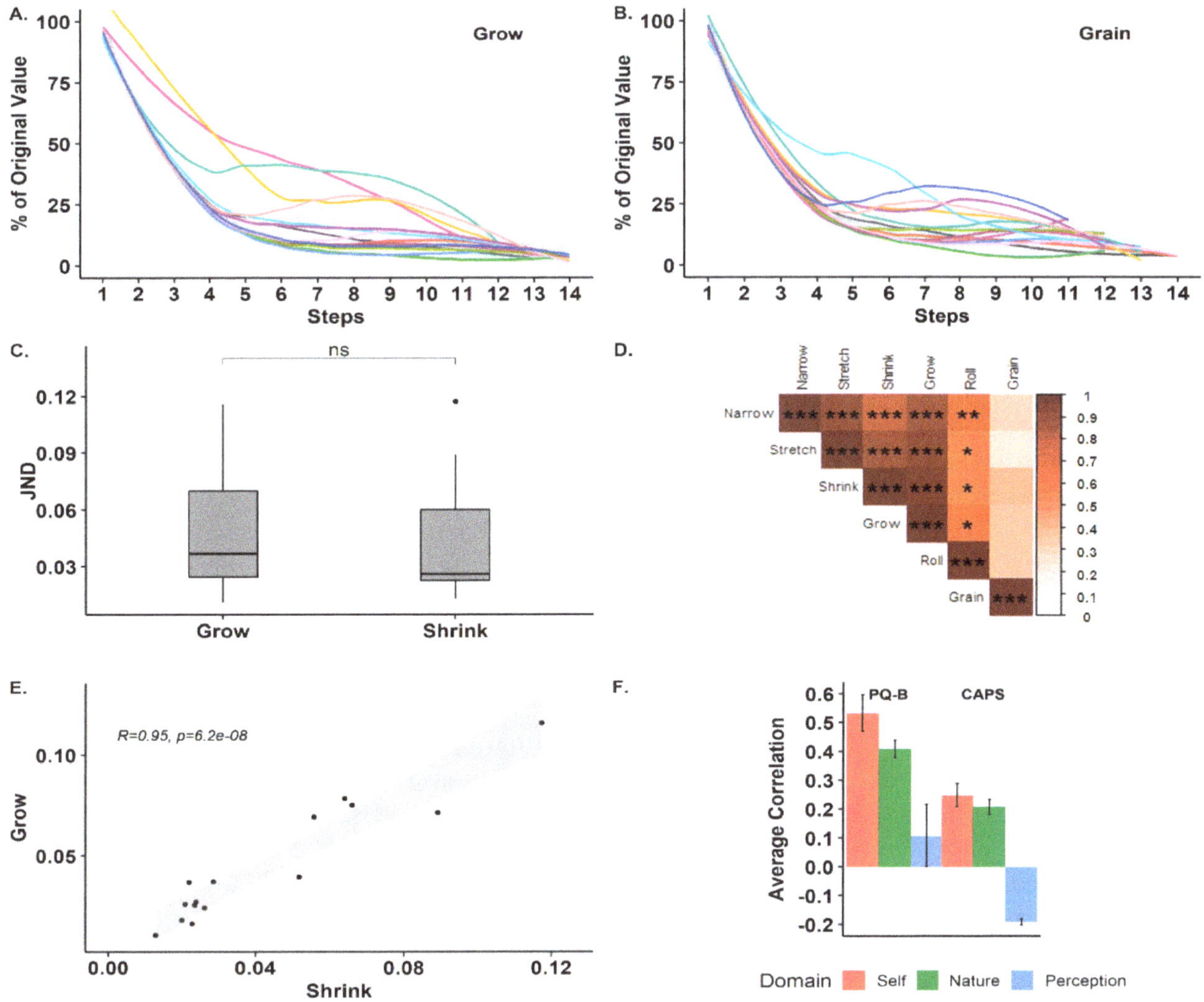

Figure 2. Perceptual thresholds for reality alterations. (**A**,**B**). Convergence rates of the staircase procedure in aspects *grow* and *grain*, respectively. *Y*-axis shows the magnitude of the reality alteration and the *x*-axis denotes the number of iterations. Note individual participants (colored lines) converged towards a stable perceptual threshold. (**C**) A comparison between JNDs of *grow* and *shrink* aspects that shared a common scale. (**D**) Pearson correlation matrix between JNDs across all aspects. Note high, positive, and significant correlations were found between all aspects' JNDs, with the exception of *grain*. (**E**) Example of correlation between participants' *grow* and *shrink* JNDs. (**F**). Averaged correlations of The *Cardiff Anomalous Perceptions Scale* (CAPS) and the *Prodromal Questionnaire Brief Version* (PQ-B) scores with JNDs shown by aspect domains (i.e., self, nature, perception).

Clinical questionnaires (CAPS and PQ-B) showed low overall scores ($M_{CAPS} = 3$, $SD_{CAPS} = 4.24$, $M_{PQ\text{-}B} = 2.8$, $SD_{PQ\text{-}B} = 3.78$) as expected in a non-clinical cohort (see Table S2 for detailed CAPS and PQ-B scores with subscales) [48,50]. Importantly, however, an analysis of the correlations between CAPS and PQ-B, with perceptual sensitivity to alterations, found that JNDs in the *grow* condition were significantly correlated with the PQ-B general score (*Spearman's Rho* $= 0.61$, $p = 0.015$), indicating that participants showing higher levels of psychotic symptoms also had reduced discrimination between 'real' and 'unreal' perceptions of *self*. Furthermore, the *grow* condition showed a high positive but non-significant (*Spearman's Rho* = 0.45, $p = 0.09$) correlation with the CAPS general score, indicating that reduced sensitivity to changes in the first person perspective (1PP) is related to abnormal perceptual experiences (see Table S1 for the full correlation matrix with subscales).

3.2. Experiment 2 (Subjective Reality Rating)

The analysis of subjective reality ratings revealed several findings. First, for the unaltered condition (*real*), the mean reality ratings were the highest ($M = 77.21$, $SD = 12.32$), demonstrating the validity of our experimental paradigm. Second, increasing magnitudes of alteration reduced the subjective reality ratings significantly for all aspects. For example, in the *grow* aspect, ratings dropped from ($M = 75$, $SD = 13.99$) in the unaltered condition to ($M = 9.57$, $SD = 8.47$) in the largest alteration magnitude, with a repeated measures ANOVA revealing a significant difference in ratings across alteration magnitudes ($F_{Grow}(2.39,14) = 79.32$, $p_{Grow} < 0.001$, $\eta^2{}_{Grow} = 0.77$). All other aspects showed similar patterns: ($\chi^2{}_{Shrink}(4) = 54.15$, $p_{Shrink} < 0.001$, $\eta^2{}_{Shrink} = 0.8$; $\chi^2{}_{Grain}(4) = 40.05$, $p_{Grain} < 0.001$, $\eta^2{}_{Grain} = 0.8$; $\chi^2{}_{Roll}(4) = 20.32$, $p_{Roll} < 0.001$, $\eta^2{}_{Roll} = 0.22$; $F_{Stretch}(4,14) = 91.91$, $p_{Stretch} < 0.001$, $\eta^2{}_{Stretch} = 0.78$; F_{Narrow} $(2.63,14) = 136.15$, $p_{Narrow} < 0.001$ $\eta^2{}_{Narrow} = 0.84$). Figure 3A–F show the average change in the ratings of subjective reality in all aspects for all levels of alteration. The *roll* condition showed a more linear reduction of reality judgments across the selected magnitudes. We note, however, that in the current design, the manipulations in different aspects are on different scales (based on a pilot experiment) and thus comparisons between different aspects are not possible, apart from the *grow* and *shrink* conditions. We thus compared the mean reduction in subjective ratings in *grow* and *shrink* between the *real* and first alteration magnitude (as this included the largest decrease in ratings across all conditions). Interestingly, in contrast with the similarity of their JNDs, a paired t-test indicated that the initial drop in reality ratings was significantly larger for the *grow* condition ($M_{Grow} = 32.12$, $SD_{Grow} = 23.19$) than for the *shrink* condition, ($M_{Shrink} = 21.18$, $SD_{Shrink} = 20.81$, $t(14) = -2.26$, $p = 0.04$, *Cohen's* $d = -0.58$, Figure 3I). Indicating that while objective perceptual sensitivity was similar, identical modulations of 1PP in the *grow* and *shrink* conditions had a differential impact on subjective reality judgments (see Table 2 and Table S4 for full descriptive statistics of the subjective ratings of reality across aspects and levels).

Third, the correlations in the reality ratings between different aspects of alteration were high, positive, and significant. Correlations between aspects ranged from 0.42 to 0.93 ($M = 0.72$, $SD = 0.17$, Figure 3G), indicating that participants' subjective judgments were similar across the different aspects. That is, participants judging the environment to be unrealistic in one aspect were also likely to do so in another aspect.

Finally, despite the fact that experiments 1 and 2 were conducted in different cohorts, we were curious regarding the relation between the objective sensitivity to alterations of reality (JNDs) and the effects of these alterations on subjective judgments. To this end, we superimposed the average JND for each aspect onto their respective average subjective ratings plot. Interestingly, for most aspects, the average JNDs (i.e., the perceptual sensitivity to a change in this aspect of reality) was found between *real* and the first magnitude of reality alteration (red diamonds in Figure 3A−F). The *roll* condition was an exception to this, with the JND found between the first and second alteration magnitudes (Figure 3C). Thus, in several aspects, the mean perceptual threshold corresponded to the point in which subjective judgments were massively reduced (e.g., *stretch*, Figure 3D). However, other aspects showed a more graded reduction of subjective reality judgments taking place at magnitudes larger than the liminal perceptual level (e.g., *narrow*, Figure 3A).

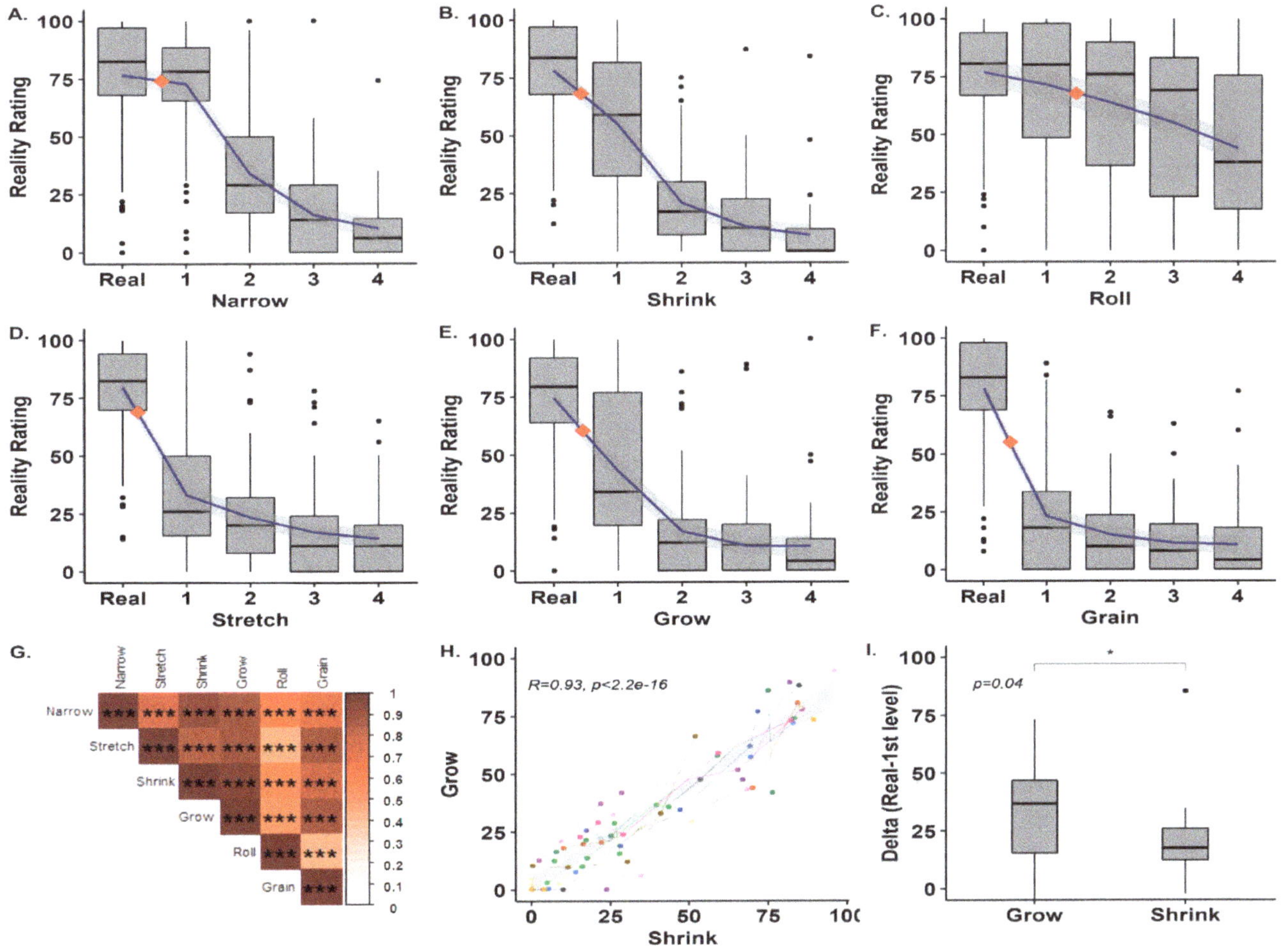

Figure 3. Subjective judgments of reality. (**A–F**) Changes in subjective reality affected the ratings of Sense of Reality (SoR) in a relatively consistent manner. Reality ratings for unaltered environments were highest while ratings for altered environments were reduced, suggesting a consistent tuning curve for SoR. (**G**) Subjective ratings for all aspects showed high, positive, and significant correlations. (**H**) Example of the correlation between participants' subjective rating of *grow* and *shrink*. (**I**) Significant difference between the drop in subjective ratings for *grow* and *shrink*, indicating an asymmetrical response for inducing changes in the first person perspective (1PP).

Table 2. Descriptive statistics for experiment 2.

	Subjective Ratings											
Alteration Magnitude	**Narrow**		**Stretch**		**Shrink**		**Grow**		**Roll**		**Grain**	
	Mean	**SD**	**Mean**	**SD**	**Mean**	**SD**	**Mean**	**SD**	**Mean**	**SD**	**Mean**	**SD**
Real	76.84	10.42	79.42	14.34	76.26	15.85	75	13.99	76.96	12.95	78.78	12.51
1	72.59	12.68	32.88	14.46	55.08	19.4	42.88	18.35	71.41	17.7	22.99	16.72
2	33.89	16.27	23.2	13.8	20.96	10.98	16.93	13.2	63.68	25.19	14.95	13.24
3	17.92	11.54	16.67	12.5	14.31	11.67	13.68	12.4	55.2	28.97	11.65	10.61
4	9.63	8.59	14.09	9.015	5.76	7.92	9.57	8.47	43.79	24.82	10.47	12.02

4. Discussion

SoR is a fundamental and ubiquitous criterion in assessing mental health, but it has been difficult to assess experimentally. This is mainly due to the lack of experimental paradigms allowing for well-controlled manipulations of reality. Employing immersive VR and a novel methodological framework, we demonstrated that both objective and subjective measures of SoR can be studied experimentally and that these show potentially meaningful correlations to clinical measures of psychosis.

4.1. The Psychophysics of SoR

In the first experiment, we examined the objective perceptual sensitivity (JNDs) to different aspects of altered reality. Our results revealed several interesting findings. First, objective perceptual thresholds for detecting alterations of reality (JND) were highly consistent within subjects, with within-subject variability in most aspects on an order of (~2.5%) of the mean JND magnitude. In addition, convergence rates were also similar across aspects. These findings suggest that JNDs for the alterations of reality are a robust and replicable psychometric measure. Furthermore, the high and significant correlations between all aspects, apart from *grain*, suggest that the perceptual thresholds across the conditions may rely on similar cognitive processes. Contrarily, JNDs in the *grain* condition were not significantly correlated with JNDs in the other conditions, suggesting that it may have been achieved in a different manner. Importantly, the PQ-B questionnaire responses, probing prodromal symptoms, were highly correlated with perceptual thresholds in the *self* domain (Figure 2F). This indicates that participants with higher ratings of psychosis-like experiences also showed lower sensitivity to changes in manipulation of the first person perspective. This finding is especially interesting given the well-established link between altered self-related processing and psychosis [25,27,45,54]. Similarly, JNDs in the *self* domain were also positively, but non-significantly, correlated with the CAPS questionnaire scores, providing converging evidence for the relationship between perceptual thresholds for reality alterations and clinical symptoms. These correlations, found in healthy participants with low levels of symptoms, are likely to be accentuated in clinical populations, and provide preliminary evidence for the viability of SoR as a diagnostic criterion.

4.2. Subjective Modulation of SoR

The second experiment measured the impact of alterations of reality on subjective judgments of reality. As predicted, we found that when the virtual environment was unaltered, most participants reported higher levels of reality judgments ($M = 77.21$, $SD = 12.32$). Furthermore, increasing magnitudes of reality alterations reduced the subjective judgments of reality (Figure 3A–F). However, as can be seen in Figure 3A–F, there were several outlier participants, which gave extremely low ratings during the *real* condition. It seems that these participants did not accept the basic premise of the task (e.g., accepting the baseline unaltered VR environment as realistic). We note that our results are robust and significant despite this; however, future experiments may benefit from prescreening for such participants.

The different aspects of reality modulated showed different rates of decrease as a function of the alteration magnitude. We note, however, that the current experiment does not allow direct comparisons between the different aspects as they use different scales (e.g., angle for the *roll* condition and percentage of height for *grow*). However, *grow* and *shrink* used the same measure and scaling factor, allowing a direct comparison between them. As predicted, when the participants' 1PP was elevated (*grow*) this reduced reality judgments significantly more than a similar magnitude of 1PP reduction (*shrink*, Figure 3I). This finding is compatible with a predictive coding framework, and specifically the notion that alterations for which we have more experience will have a smaller impact on SoR. Given that we have more experience with the reduction of our 1PP (through sitting and laying down); this had less impact on SoR compared with the *grow* condition for which we have less experience. Indeed, 1PP is considered a fundamental component of the sense of self [43]. Changes in the bodily-self have been found in both neurological (e.g., [55]) and psychiatric [27,56] conditions in which hallucinations are prevalent. Furthermore, experimentally induced changes in the sense of self impact perceptual awareness and self-consciousness [57–59].

Comparing the mean JNDs from the first experiment with the subjective judgments from experiment 2 revealed that for some aspects, the JND marked the point of the greatest reduction in subjective reality (i.e., *stretch*, *grow*, and *grain*). Thus, the perceptual threshold coincided with the subjective experience of reality, as one may expect. However, in other aspects, the largest reduction occurred at larger alteration magnitudes than the JND (i.e., *shrink*, *roll*, and *narrow*). This suggests that subjective judgments are not completely dependent on the objective threshold in certain aspects of reality. We therefore propose that JNDs can be used as standardized units to allow comparisons of SoR across the different aspects. Future experiments will capitalize upon this finding by employing participants' JNDs to normalize the levels of alterations across conditions. In turn, this will allow comparison of the impact of different alterations of reality, allowing the modeling of one's implicit model of expectations of the world. For example, this method would allow us to compute how a change in the self (e.g., 1PP modulation—*grow*) compares to an alteration in a more perceptual aspect (e.g., *grain*), as they will share a common scale.

The broader implications of this study may potentially go beyond providing a novel approach for investigating mechanisms of SoR. The current paradigm (*UnReal*) may allow both laboratory and online gathering of large data sets in diverse cohorts, enabling a starting point for a mechanistic model of SoR. The availability of a reliable mechanistic model of SoR and its clinical and behavioral correlates is bound to provide researchers and clinicians with a new set of conceptual as well as practical tools to address research questions in a large variety of neuropsychiatric and neurological disorders involving hallucinatory or dissociative symptoms. In turn, this may lead to useful measures to further support clinical diagnoses and enable clinicians to develop and employ more accurately targeted treatments, such as new neurocognitive markers for the early detection of psychosis. Finally, our paradigm may allow for the development of novel VR-based therapeutic interventions that enhance and restore SoR in clinical populations with deficits of SoR, similar to approaches in other neurological and psychiatric conditions [60–62].

4.3. Limitations

The current experiments were aimed to test our novel approach to the study of SoR and its relation to psychosis. A central limitation here is that the objective and subjective measurements of SoR were conducted in separate cohorts, thus direct within-subject comparisons were not possible. Future studies will employ both tasks within the same cohort. Furthermore, the PQ-B and CAPS questionnaires were used only in the first experiment, thus the relationship between subjective judgments and clinical symptoms of psychosis and hallucinations is yet to be assessed. Finally, both studies had low numbers of participants and thus suffered from low statistical power, which in turn limited our ability to examine individual differences, such as the effects of age and gender. Further, higher powered studies including clinical populations are needed to validate and extend these findings regarding SoR and psychosis.

4.4. Summary

The present study investigated the SoR and its relation to psychotic symptoms. By inducing hallucination-like visual experiences and testing objective and subjective measures of SoR, we found a novel psychophysical link between sensitivity to alterations of reality and prodromal psychotic symptoms. These results provide evidence for the utility of this ecological and immersive VR methodology for the scientific study of SoR and a novel tool for psychiatric clinical assessment. Future studies may employ the *UnReal* paradigm to build computational models as well as investigate the neural substrates of SoR in healthy and clinical populations. As SoR is a central benchmark in determining psychiatric and neurological wellbeing, it is critical that we acquire a fuller understanding of how SoR is constructed by the brain and mind, allowing us to provide better diagnostic and therapeutic tools.

Author Contributions: Conceptualization, R.S.; methodology, R.S., G.D. and P.B.-T.; software, Y.Z.; formal analysis, G.D. and R.S.; investigation, G.D., P.B.-T. and R.S.; resources, R.S.; data curation, G.D., P.B.-T. and R.S.; writing—original draft preparation, G.D., Y.S., P.B.-T. and R.S.; writing—review and editing, G.D., Y.S., P.B.-T. and R.S.; visualization, G.D., P.B.-T. and R.S.; project administration, G.D.; funding acquisition, R.S.; All authors have read and agreed to the published version of the manuscript.

References

1. Metzinger, T. How does the brain encode epistemic reliability? Perceptual presence, phenomenal transparency, and counterfactual richness. *Cogn. Neurosci.* **2014**, *5*, 122–124. [CrossRef] [PubMed]
2. Ratcliffe, M. *Feelings of Being: Phenomenology, Psychiatry and the Sense of Reality*; Oxford University Press: Oxford, UK, 2008; ISBN 0-19-920646-5.
3. APA. *DSM 5*; American Psychiatric Association: Arlington, VA, USA, 2013.
4. Barnes, J.; Boubert, L.; Harris, J.; Lee, A.; David, A.S. Reality monitoring and visual hallucinations in Parkinson's disease. *Neuropsychologia* **2003**, *41*, 565–574. [CrossRef]
5. Bentall, R.P.; Baker, G.A.; Havers, S. Reality monitoring and psychotic hallucinations. *Br. J. Clin. Psychol.* **1991**, *30*, 213–222. [CrossRef] [PubMed]
6. Johnson, M.K. Reality monitoring: An experimental phenomenological approach. *J. Exp. Psychol. Gen.* **1988**, *117*, 390. [CrossRef]
7. Johnson, M.K.; Hashtroudi, S.; Lindsay, D.S. Source monitoring. *Psychol. Bull.* **1993**, *114*, 3. [CrossRef]
8. Raye, C.L.; Johnson, M.K. Reality monitoring vs. discriminating between external sources of memories. *Bull. Psychon. Soc.* **1980**, *15*, 405–408. [CrossRef]
9. Garrison, J.R.; Bond, R.; Gibbard, E.; Johnson, M.K.; Simons, J.S. Monitoring what is real: The effects of modality and action on accuracy and type of reality monitoring error. *Cortex* **2017**, *87*, 108–117. [CrossRef]
10. Simons, J.S.; Garrison, J.R.; Johnson, M.K. Brain Mechanisms of Reality Monitoring. *Trends Cogn. Sci.* **2017**, *21*, 462–473. [CrossRef]
11. Ohayon, M.M. Prevalence of hallucinations and their pathological associations in the general population. *Psychiatry Res.* **2000**, *97*, 153–164. [CrossRef]
12. Blanke, O.; Pozeg, P.; Hara, M.; Heydrich, L.; Serino, A.; Yamamoto, A.; Higuchi, T.; Salomon, R.; Seeck, M.; Landis, T.; et al. Neurological and robot-controlled induction of an apparition. *Curr. Biol.* **2014**, *24*, 2681–2686. [CrossRef]
13. Rao, R.P.N.; Ballard, D.H. Predictive coding in the visual cortex: A functional interpretation of some extra-classical receptive-field effects. *Nat. Neurosci.* **1999**, *2*, 79. [CrossRef] [PubMed]
14. Clark, A. Whatever next? Predictive brains, situated agents, and the future of cognitive science. *Behav. Brain Sci.* **2013**, *36*, 181–204. [CrossRef] [PubMed]
15. Friston, K. The free-energy principle: A rough guide to the brain? *Trends Cogn. Sci. (Regul. Ed.)* **2009**, *13*, 293–301. [CrossRef] [PubMed]
16. de Lange, F.P.; Heilbron, M.; Kok, P. How do expectations shape perception? *Trends Cogn. Sci.* **2018**, *22*, 764–779. [CrossRef] [PubMed]
17. Friston, K.J.; Stephan, K.E. Free-energy and the brain. *Synthese* **2007**, *159*, 417–458. [CrossRef]
18. Wiese, W.; Metzinger, T.K. *Vanilla PP for Philosophers: A Primer on Predictive Processing*; Philosophy and Predictive Processing; MIND Group: Frankfurt am Main, Germany, 2017; ISBN 978-3-95857-302-4.
19. Lau, H. Consciousness, Metacognition, & Perceptual Reality Monitoring. *PsyArXiv* **2019**. [CrossRef]
20. Fletcher, P.C.; Frith, C.D. Perceiving is believing: A Bayesian approach to explaining the positive symptoms of schizophrenia. *Nat. Rev. Neurosci.* **2008**, *10*, 48–58. [CrossRef]
21. Corlett, P.R.; Horga, G.; Fletcher, P.C.; Alderson-Day, B.; Schmack, K.; Powers, A.R. Hallucinations and Strong Priors. *Trends Cogn. Sci.* **2019**, *23*, 114–127. [CrossRef]
22. Sterzer, P.; Adams, R.A.; Fletcher, P.; Frith, C.; Lawrie, S.M.; Muckli, L.; Petrovic, P.; Uhlhaas, P.; Voss, M.; Corlett, P.R. The Predictive Coding Account of Psychosis. *Biol. Psychiatry* **2018**, *84*, 634–643. [CrossRef]
23. Powers, A.R.; Mathys, C.; Corlett, P.R. Pavlovian conditioning–induced hallucinations result from overweighting of perceptual priors. *Science* **2017**, *357*, 596–600. [CrossRef]

24. Griffin, J.D.; Fletcher, P.C. Predictive Processing, Source Monitoring, and Psychosis. *Annu. Rev. Clin. Psychol.* **2017**, *13*, 265–289. [CrossRef]
25. Frith, C.; Done, D. Experiences of alien control in schizophrenia reflect a disorder in the central monitoring of action. *Psychol. Med.* **2009**, *19*, 359–363. [CrossRef] [PubMed]
26. Ford, J.M.; Palzes, V.A.; Roach, B.J.; Mathalon, D.H. Did I do that? Abnormal predictive processes in schizophrenia when button pressing to deliver a tone. *Schizophr. Bull.* **2014**, *40*, 804–812. [CrossRef] [PubMed]
27. Salomon, R.; Progin, P.; Griffa, A.; Rognini, G.; Do, K.Q.; Conus, P.; Marchesotti, S.; Bernasconi, F.; Hagmann, P.; Serino, A. Sensorimotor Induction of Auditory Misattribution in Early Psychosis. *Schizophr. Bull.* **2020**. [CrossRef] [PubMed]
28. Teunisse, R.J.; Zitman, F.G.; Cruysberg, J.R.M.; Hoefnagels, W.H.L.; Verbeek, A.L.M. Visual hallucinations in psychologically normal people: Charles Bonnet's syndrome. *Lancet* **1996**, *347*, 794–797. [CrossRef]
29. Perivoliotis, D.; Grant, P.M.; Peters, E.R.; Ison, R.; Kuipers, E.; Beck, A.T. Cognitive insight predicts favorable outcome in cognitive behavioral therapy for psychosis. *Psychosis* **2010**, *2*, 23–33. [CrossRef]
30. Gerretsen, P.; Menon, M.; Mamo, D.C.; Fervaha, G.; Remington, G.; Pollock, B.G.; Graff-Guerrero, A. Impaired insight into illness and cognitive insight in schizophrenia spectrum disorders: Resting state functional connectivity. *Schizophr. Res.* **2014**, *160*, 43–50. [CrossRef]
31. Nair, A.; Palmer, E.C.; Aleman, A.; David, A.S. Relationship between cognition, clinical and cognitive insight in psychotic disorders: A review and meta-analysis. *Schizophr. Res.* **2014**, *152*, 191–200. [CrossRef]
32. Baker, D.; Hunter, E.; Lawrence, E.; Medford, N.; Patel, M.; Senior, C.; Sierra, M.; Lambert, M.V.; Phillips, M.L.; David, A.S. Depersonalisation disorder: Clinical features of 204 cases. *Br. J. Psychiatry* **2003**, *182*, 428–433. [CrossRef]
33. Sass, L.; Pienkos, E.; Nelson, B.; Medford, N. Anomalous self-experience in depersonalization and schizophrenia: A comparative investigation. *Conscious. Cogn.* **2013**, *22*, 430–441. [CrossRef]
34. Harris, C.S. Adaptation to displaced vision: Visual, motor, or proprioceptive change? *Science* **1963**, *140*, 812–813. [CrossRef]
35. Mudrik, L.; Breska, A.; Lamy, D.; Deouell, L.Y. Integration without awareness. *Psychol. Sci.* **2011**, *22*, 764. [CrossRef]
36. Bohil, C.J.; Alicea, B.; Biocca, F.A. Virtual reality in neuroscience research and therapy. *Nat. Rev. Neurosci.* **2011**, *12*, 752–762. [CrossRef]
37. Sanchez-Vives, M.V.; Slater, M. From presence to consciousness through virtual reality. *Nat. Rev. Neurosci.* **2005**, *6*, 332–339. [CrossRef] [PubMed]
38. Krugwasser, A.R.; Harel, E.V.; Salomon, R. The boundaries of the self: The sense of agency across different sensorimotor aspects. *J. Vis.* **2019**, *19*, 14. [CrossRef] [PubMed]
39. Salomon, R.; Fernandez, N.; van Elk, M.; Vachicouras, N.; Sabatier, F.; Tychinskaya, A.; Llobera, J.; Blanke, O. Changing motor perception by sensorimotor conflicts and body ownership. *Sci. Rep.* **2016**, *6*, 25847. [CrossRef] [PubMed]
40. Blom, J.D. Alice in Wonderland syndrome. *Neurol. Clin. Pract.* **2016**, *6*, 259–270. [CrossRef]
41. Bentall, R. The Illusion of Reality: A Review and Integration of Psychological Research on Hallucinations. *Psychol. Bull.* **1990**, *107*, 82–95. [CrossRef]
42. Preller, K.H.; Vollenweider, F.X. Phenomenology, Structure, and Dynamic of Psychedelic States. In *Behavioral Neurobiology of Psychedelic Drugs*; Halberstadt, A.L., Vollenweider, F.X., Nichols, D.E., Eds.; Current Topics in Behavioral Neurosciences; Springer: Berlin/Heidelberg, Germany, 2018; pp. 221–256. ISBN 978-3-662-55880-5.
43. Blanke, O.; Metzinger, T. Full-body illusions and minimal phenomenal selfhood. *Trends Cogn. Sci.* **2009**, *13*, 7–13. [CrossRef] [PubMed]
44. Dudley, R.; Aynsworth, C.; Mosimann, U.; Taylor, J.-P.; Smailes, D.; Collerton, D.; McCarthy-Jones, S.; Urwyler, P. A comparison of visual hallucinations across disorders. *Psychiatry Res* **2019**, *272*, 86–92. [CrossRef]
45. Parnas, J. Self and schizophrenia: A phenomenological perspective. *Self Neurosci. Psychiatry* **2003**, *1*, 217–241.
46. Levitt, H. Transformed up-down methods in psychoacoustics. *J. Acoust. Soc. Am.* **1971**, *49*, 467–477. [CrossRef]
47. Hettinger, L.J.; Riccio, G.E. Visually induced motion sickness in virtual environments. *Presence: Teleoperators Virtual Environ.* **1992**, *1*, 306–310. [CrossRef]

48. Bell, V.; Halligan, P.W.; Ellis, H.D. The Cardiff Anomalous Perceptions Scale (CAPS): A new validated measure of anomalous perceptual experience. *Schizophr. Bull.* **2005**, *32*, 366–377. [CrossRef] [PubMed]
49. Bell, V.; Halligan, P.W.; Pugh, K.; Freeman, D. Correlates of perceptual distortions in clinical and non-clinical populations using the Cardiff Anomalous Perceptions Scale (CAPS): Associations with anxiety and depression and a re-validation using a representative population sample. *Psychiatry Res.* **2011**, *189*, 451–457. [CrossRef] [PubMed]
50. Loewy, R.L.; Pearson, R.; Vinogradov, S.; Bearden, C.E.; Cannon, T.D. Psychosis risk screening with the Prodromal Questionnaire—Brief version (PQ-B). *Schizophr. Res.* **2011**, *129*, 42–46. [CrossRef]
51. Kline, E.; Wilson, C.; Ereshefsky, S.; Tsuji, T.; Schiffman, J.; Pitts, S.; Reeves, G. Convergent and discriminant validity of attenuated psychosis screening tools. *Schizophr. Res.* **2012**, *134*, 49–53. [CrossRef]
52. MATLAB. *MATLAB 9.6.0.(R2019a)*; The MathWorks Inc.: Natick, MA, USA, 2019.
53. JASP Team. *JASP (Version 0.11.1) [Computer Software]*; Department of Psychological Methods: Amsterdam, The Netherlands, 2019.
54. Nelson, B.; Thompson, A.; Yung, A.R. Basic Self-Disturbance Predicts Psychosis Onset in the Ultra High Risk for Psychosis "Prodromal" Population. *Schizophr. Bull.* **2012**, *38*, 1277–1287. [CrossRef]
55. Blanke, O.; Mohr, C. Out-of-body experience, heautoscopy, and autoscopic hallucination of neurological origin: Implications for neurocognitive mechanisms of corporeal awareness and self-consciousness. *Brain Res. Rev.* **2005**, *50*, 184–199. [CrossRef]
56. Nelson, B.; Fornito, A.; Harrison, B.J.; Yücel, M.; Sass, L.A.; Yung, A.R.; Thompson, A.; Wood, S.J.; Pantelis, C.; McGorry, P.D. A disturbed sense of self in the psychosis prodrome: Linking phenomenology and neurobiology. *Neurosci. Biobehav. Rev.* **2009**, *33*, 807–817. [CrossRef]
57. Faivre, N.; Vuillaume, L.; Bernasconi, F.; Salomon, R.; Blanke, O.; Cleeremans, A. Sensorimotor conflicts alter metacognitive and action monitoring. *Cortex* **2020**, *124*, 224–234. [CrossRef]
58. Salomon, R.; Noel, J.-P.; Łukowska, M.; Faivre, N.; Metzinger, T.; Serino, A.; Blanke, O. Unconscious integration of multisensory bodily inputs in the peripersonal space shapes bodily self-consciousness. *Cognition* **2017**, *166*, 174–183. [CrossRef] [PubMed]
59. Park, H.-D.; Bernasconi, F.; Bello-Ruiz, J.; Pfeiffer, C.; Salomon, R.; Blanke, O. Transient modulations of neural responses to heartbeats covary with bodily self-consciousness. *J. Neurosci.* **2016**, *36*, 8453–8460. [CrossRef] [PubMed]
60. Perruchoud, D.; Pisotta, I.; Carda, S.; Murray, M.M.; Ionta, S. Biomimetic rehabilitation engineering: The importance of somatosensory feedback for brain–machine interfaces. *J. Neural Eng.* **2016**, *13*, 041001. [CrossRef] [PubMed]
61. Lubianiker, N.; Goldway, N.; Fruchtman-Steinbok, T.; Paret, C.; Keynan, J.N.; Singer, N.; Cohen, A.; Kadosh, K.C.; Linden, D.E.; Hendler, T. Process-based framework for precise neuromodulation. *Nat. Hum. Behav.* **2019**, *3*, 436–445. [CrossRef] [PubMed]
62. Freeman, D.; Reeve, S.; Robinson, A.; Ehlers, A.; Clark, D.; Spanlang, B.; Slater, M. Virtual reality in the assessment, understanding, and treatment of mental health disorders. *Psychol. Med.* **2017**, *47*, 2393–2400. [CrossRef]

Permissions

All chapters in this book were first published by MDPI; hereby published with permission under the Creative Commons Attribution License or equivalent. Every chapter published in this book has been scrutinized by our experts. Their significance has been extensively debated. The topics covered herein carry significant findings which will fuel the growth of the discipline. They may even be implemented as practical applications or may be referred to as a beginning point for another development.

The contributors of this book come from diverse backgrounds, making this book a truly international effort. This book will bring forth new frontiers with its revolutionizing research information and detailed analysis of the nascent developments around the world.

We would like to thank all the contributing authors for lending their expertise to make the book truly unique. They have played a crucial role in the development of this book. Without their invaluable contributions this book wouldn't have been possible. They have made vital efforts to compile up to date information on the varied aspects of this subject to make this book a valuable addition to the collection of many professionals and students.

This book was conceptualized with the vision of imparting up-to-date information and advanced data in this field. To ensure the same, a matchless editorial board was set up. Every individual on the board went through rigorous rounds of assessment to prove their worth. After which they invested a large part of their time researching and compiling the most relevant data for our readers.

The editorial board has been involved in producing this book since its inception. They have spent rigorous hours researching and exploring the diverse topics which have resulted in the successful publishing of this book. They have passed on their knowledge of decades through this book. To expedite this challenging task, the publisher supported the team at every step. A small team of assistant editors was also appointed to further simplify the editing procedure and attain best results for the readers.

Apart from the editorial board, the designing team has also invested a significant amount of their time in understanding the subject and creating the most relevant covers. They scrutinized every image to scout for the most suitable representation of the subject and create an appropriate cover for the book.

The publishing team has been an ardent support to the editorial, designing and production team. Their endless efforts to recruit the best for this project, has resulted in the accomplishment of this book. They are a veteran in the field of academics and their pool of knowledge is as vast as their experience in printing. Their expertise and guidance has proved useful at every step. Their uncompromising quality standards have made this book an exceptional effort. Their encouragement from time to time has been an inspiration for everyone.

The publisher and the editorial board hope that this book will prove to be a valuable piece of knowledge for researchers, students, practitioners and scholars across the globe.

List of Contributors

Carlos Suso-Ribera
Department of Basic and Clinical Psychology and Psychobiology, Universitat Jaume I, 12071 Castellón, Spain

Diana Castilla
Department of Personality, Assessment, and Psychological Treatments, Universidad de Valencia, 46010 Valencia, Spain
Ciber Fisiopatologia Obesidad y Nutricion (CB06/03 Instituto Salud Carlos III) (Ciber Physiopathology Obesity and Nutrition, CB06/03 Instituto Salud Carlos III Health Institute), 28029 Madrid, Spain

Irene Zaragozá
Ciber Fisiopatologia Obesidad y Nutricion (CB06/03 Instituto Salud Carlos III) (Ciber Physiopathology Obesity and Nutrition, CB06/03 Instituto Salud Carlos III Health Institute), 28029 Madrid, Spain

Ángela Mesas, Anna Server and Javier Medel
Pain Clinic, Vall d'Hebron Hospital, 08035 Barcelona, Spain

Azucena García-Palacios
Department of Basic and Clinical Psychology and Psychobiology, Universitat Jaume I, 12071 Castellón, Spain
Ciber Fisiopatologia Obesidad y Nutricion (CB06/03 Instituto Salud Carlos III) (Ciber Physiopathology Obesity and Nutrition, CB06/03 Instituto Salud Carlos III Health Institute), 28029 Madrid, Spain

Marta Matamala-Gomez
Institut d'Investigacions Biomèdiques August Pi i Sunyer (IDIBAPS), 08036 Barcelona, Spain
Event-Lab, Department of Clinical Psychology and Psychobiology, Universitat de Barcelona, 08035 Barcelona, Spain
Dipartamento di Scienze Umane per la Formazione 'Ricardo Massa', Università degli studi Milano-Bicocca, 20126 Milan, Italy

Birgit Nierula
Institut d'Investigacions Biomèdiques August Pi i Sunyer (IDIBAPS), 08036 Barcelona, Spain
Event-Lab, Department of Clinical Psychology and Psychobiology, Universitat de Barcelona, 08035 Barcelona, Spain
Max Planck Institute for Human Cognitive and Brain Sciences, 04103 Leipzig, Germany

Tony Donegan
Institut d'Investigacions Biomèdiques August Pi i Sunyer (IDIBAPS), 08036 Barcelona, Spain

Mel Slater
Event-Lab, Department of Clinical Psychology and Psychobiology, Universitat de Barcelona, 08035 Barcelona, Spain

Maria V. Sanchez-Vives
Institut d'Investigacions Biomèdiques August Pi i Sunyer (IDIBAPS), 08036 Barcelona, Spain
Event-Lab, Department of Clinical Psychology and Psychobiology, Universitat de Barcelona, 08035 Barcelona, Spain
Departament de Cognició, Desenvolupament i Psicologia de l'Educació, Facultat de Psicologia, Universitat de Barcelona, 08035 Barcelona, Spain
Institució Catalana de Recerca i Estudis Avançats (ICREA), 08010 Barcelona, Spain

Ngeemasara Thapa, Hye Jin Park, Ja-Gyeong Yang, Haeun Son, Minwoo Jang and Hyuntae Park
Department of Health Sciences, Graduate School, Dong-A University, Busan 49315, Korea
Laboratory of Smart Healthcare, Dong-A University, Busan 49315, Korea

Jihyeon Lee
Department of Health Sciences, Graduate School, Dong-A University, Busan 49315, Korea

Seung Wan Kang
Data Center for Korean EEG, College of Nursing, Seoul National University, Seoul 03080, Korea

Kyung Won Park
Department of Neurology, Dong-A University College of Medicine, Busan 49201, Korea

Wenceslao Peñate, Francisco Rivero, Conrado Viña, Manuel Herrero, Moisés Betancort and Ascensión Fumero
Universidad de La Laguna, 38200 La Laguna, Spain

Juan De la Fuente and Yolanda Álvarez-Pérez
Servicio Canario de la Salud, 38004 S.C. Tenerife, Spain

Cosimo Tuena
Applied Technology for Neuro-Psychology Lab, IRCCS Istituto Auxologico Italiano, 20149 Milan, Italy

Silvia Serino
MySpace Lab, Department of Clinical Neurosciences, University Hospital Lausanne (CHUV), CH-1011 Lausanne, Switzerland
Istituto Auxologico Italiano, IRCCS, Laboratorio Sperimentale di Ricerche Tecnologiche Applicate alla Psicologia, 20149 Milano, Italy

Léo Dutriaux
Institute of Neuroscience and Psychology, University of Glasgow, Glasgow G12 8QB, UK

Giuseppe Riva
Applied Technology for Neuro-Psychology Lab, IRCCS Istituto Auxologico Italiano, 20149 Milan, Italy
Department of Psychology, Catholic University of the Sacred Heart, 20123 Milan, Italy
Istituto Auxologico Italiano, IRCCS, Laboratorio Sperimentale di Ricerche Tecnologiche Applicate alla Psicologia, 20149 Milano, Italy

Pascale Piolino
Memory and Cognition Laboratory, Institute of Psychology, Paris Descartes University, Sorbonne Paris Cité, 92774 Boulogne-Billancourt, France
INSERM UMR S894, Center for Psychiatry and Neurosciences, 75014 Paris, France
Institut Universitaire de France (IUF), 75231 Paris, France

Elisa Pedroli
Applied Technology for Neuro-Psychology Lab, IRCCS Istituto Auxologico Italiano, Via Magnasco 2, 20149 Milano, Italy
Faculty of Psychology, eCampus University, Via Isimbardi, 10, 22060 Novedrate, Italy

Pietro Cipresso
Applied Technology for Neuro-Psychology Lab, IRCCS Istituto Auxologico Italiano, Via Magnasco 2, 20149 Milano, Italy
Psychology Department, Catholic University of Milan, Largo Gemelli 1, 20123 Milan, Italy

Caterina La Cascia, Filippo La Paglia and Daniele La Barbera
Department of Experimental Biomedicine and Clinical Neuroscience, University of Palermo, Piazza Marina, 61, 90133 Palermo, Italy

Annet Kleiboer
Department of Clinical, Neuro and Developmental Psychology, Vrije Universiteit, 1081-BT Amsterdam, The Netherlands

Shu Da, Yue He and Xichao Zhang
Beijing Key Laboratory of Applied Experimental Psychology, National Demonstration Center for Experimental Psychology Education (Beijing Normal University), Faculty of Psychology, Beijing Normal University, Beijing 100875, China

Rocío Herrero and Mª Dolores Vara
Polibienestar Research Institute, University of Valencia, 46022 Valencia, Spain
CIBERObn Physiopathology of Obesity and Nutrition, Instituto de Salud Carlos III, 28029 Madrid, Spain

Marta Miragall and Cristina Botella
CIBERObn Physiopathology of Obesity and Nutrition, Instituto de Salud Carlos III, 28029 Madrid, Spain
Department of Basic and Clinical Psychology and Psychobiology, Faculty of Health Sciences, Jaume I University, 12071 Castellon de la Plana, Spain

Heleen Riper
Department of Clinical, Neuro-and Developmental Psychology and the Amsterdam Public Health Research Institute, Vrije Universiteit Amsterdam, van der Boechorststraat 7, 1081 BT Amsterdam, The Netherlands
Department of Research and Innovation, GGZ inGeest Specialized Mental Health Care, Oldenaller 1, 1081 HJ Amsterdam, The Netherlands
Department of Psychiatry and the Amsterdam Public Health Research Institute, GGZ inGeest/Amsterdam UMC, Vrije Universiteit, de Boelelaan 1117, 1081 HV Amsterdam, The Netherlands

Rosa Mª Baños
Polibienestar Research Institute, University of Valencia, 46022 Valencia, Spain
CIBERObn Physiopathology of Obesity and Nutrition, Instituto de Salud Carlos III, 28029 Madrid, Spain
Department of Personality, Evaluation and Psychological Treatment, Faculty of Psychology, University of Valencia, 46010 Valencia, Spain

Patricia Otero
Department of Psychology, University of A Coruña, 15071 A Coruña, Spain

Isabel Hita and Fernando L. Vázquez
Department of Clinical Psychology and Psychobiology, University of Santiago de Compostela, 15782 Santiago de Compostela, Spain

Ángela J. Torres
Department of Psychiatry, Radiology and Public Health, University of Santiago de Compostela, 15782 Santiago de Compostela, Spain

Lisa Kooistra
Department of Clinical, Neuro-and Developmental Psychology and the Amsterdam Public Health Research Institute, Vrije Universiteit Amsterdam, van der Boechorststraat 7, 1081 BT Amsterdam, The Netherlands
Department of Research and Innovation, GGZ inGeest Specialized Mental Health Care, Oldenaller 1, 1081 HJ Amsterdam, The Netherlands

Jeroen Ruwaard and Patricia van Oppen
Department of Research and Innovation, GGZ inGeest Specialized Mental Health Care, Oldenaller 1, 1081 HJ Amsterdam, The Netherlands
Department of Psychiatry and the Amsterdam Public Health Research Institute, GGZ inGeest/Amsterdam UMC, Vrije Universiteit, de Boelelaan 1117, 1081 HV Amsterdam, The Netherlands

Alice Chirico
Psychology Department, Università Cattolica del Sacro Cuore, 20123 Milan, Italy

Claire R. van Genugten, Josien Schuurmans, Brenda W. J. H. Penninx and Johannes H. Smit
Department of Research and Innovation, GGZ inGeest, Specialized Mental Health Care, 1081 Amsterdam, The Netherlands
Department of Psychiatry, Amsterdam Public Health Research Institute, Amsterdam UMC, Vrije Universiteit, 1081 Amsterdam, The Netherlands

Femke Lamers
Department of Psychiatry, Amsterdam Public Health Research Institute, Amsterdam UMC, Vrije Universiteit, 1081 Amsterdam, The Netherlands

Harriëtte Riese and Robert A. Schoevers
Interdisciplinary Centre for Psychopathology and Emotion Regulation, Department of Psychiatry, University Medical Centre Groningen, University of Groningen, 9713 Groningen, The Netherlands

Heleen M. Riper
Department of Research and Innovation, GGZ inGeest, Specialized Mental Health Care, 1081 Amsterdam, The Netherlands
Department of Psychiatry, Amsterdam Public Health Research Institute, Amsterdam UMC, Vrije Universiteit, 1081 Amsterdam, The Netherlands
Department of Clinical, Neuro and Developmental Psychology, Clinical Psychology Section, Vrije Universiteit Amsterdam and the Amsterdam Public Health Research Institute, 1081 Amsterdam, The Netherlands
Institute of Telepsychiatry, University of Southern Denmark, 5000 Odense, Denmark

Kathleen M. Baggett, Elizabeth A. Mosley and Katy Miller
Mark Chaffin Center for Healthy Development, Georgia State University, Atlanta, GA 30303, USA

Betsy Davis, Lisa B. Sheeber and Edward G. Feil
Oregon Research Institute, Eugene, OR 97403, USA

Robert T. Ammerman
Cincinnati Children's Hospital Medical Center, University of Cincinnati College of Medicine, Cincinnati, OH 45229, USA

Federica Scarpina
Istituto Auxologico Italiano, IRCCS, U.O. di Neurologia e Neuroriabilitazione, Ospedale S. Giuseppe, 28824 Piancavallo, Italy
Istituto Auxologico Italiano, IRCCS, Laboratorio di Psicologia, Ospedale S. Giuseppe, 28824 Piancavallo, Italy

Anouk Keizer
Experimental Psychology/Helmholtz Institute, Faculty of Social and Behavioural Sciences, Utrecht University, 3584 Utrecht, The Netherlands

Jenneke Wiersma
Department of Research and Innovation, GGZ inGeest Specialized Mental Health Care, Oldenaller 1, 1081 HJ Amsterdam, The Netherlands

Massimo Scacchi
Istituto Auxologico Italiano, IRCCS, U.O. di Medicina Generale, Ospedale S. Giuseppe, 28824 Piancavallo, Italy
Department of Clinical Sciences and Community Health, University of Milan, 20122 Milan, Italy

Gianluca Castelnuovo
Istituto Auxologico Italiano, IRCCS, Laboratorio di Psicologia, Ospedale S. Giuseppe, 28824 Piancavallo, Italy
Psychology Department, Università Cattolica del Sacro Cuore, 20123 Milan, Italy

Alessandro Mauro
Istituto Auxologico Italiano, IRCCS, U.O. di Neurologia e Neuroriabilitazione, Ospedale S. Giuseppe, 28824 Piancavallo, Italy
"Rita Levi Montalcini" Department of Neuroscience, University of Turin, 10124 Turin, Italy

Tara Donker
Department of Clinical, Neuro and Developmental Psychology, Section Clinical Psychology, Vrije Universiteit Amsterdam, Van der Boechorststraat 1, 1081 BT Amsterdam, The Netherlands
Amsterdam Public Health Research Institute Amsterdam, Van der Boechorststraat 7, 1081 BT Amsterdam, The Netherlands
Department of Psychology, Laboratory of Biological and Personality Psychology, Albert Ludwigs-University of Freiburg, Peter-Kaplan Meierstrasse 8, 79104 Freiburg im Breisgau, Germany

Chris van Klaveren and Ilja Cornelisz
Department of Education Sciences, Section Methods and Statistics and Amsterdam Center for Learning Analytics, Vrije Universiteit Amsterdam, Van der Boechorststraat 1, 1081 BT Amsterdam, The Netherlands

Robin N. Kok
Department of Psychology, University of Southern Denmark, Campusvej 55, 5230 Odense, Denmark
Centre for Innovative Medical Technology, Odense University Hospital, Indgang 101, 5000 Odense, Denmark

Jean-Louis van Gelder
Institute of Education and Child Studies, Leiden University, Pieter de la Court building, 4th floor, Wassenaarseweg 52, 2333 AK Leiden, The Netherlands
Max Planck Institute for the Study of Crime, Security and Law, Department of Criminology, Günterstalstraße 73, 79100 Freiburg, Germany

Gad Drori, Paz Bar-Tal, Yair Zvilichovsky and Roy Salomon
Gonda Brain Research Center, Bar-Ilan University, Ramat Gan 5290002, Israel

Yonatan Stern
Gonda Brain Research Center, Bar-Ilan University, Ramat Gan 5290002, Israel
Psychology Department, University of Haifa, Haifa 3498838, Israel

Index

www.ingramcontent.com/pod-product-compliance
Lightning Source LLC
LaVergne TN
LVHW082144200926
848484LV00008B/2102